SYNOPSIS OF

Ophthalmology

THE OPHTHALMOSCOPY BOOK

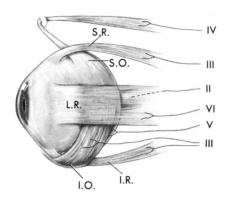

SYNOPSIS OF

Ophthalmology

THE OPHTHALMOSCOPY BOOK

William H. Havener

B.A., M.D., M.S. (Ophth.), D.Sc. (Hon.)

Professor and Chairman, Department of Ophthalmology,
The Ohio State University College of Medicine;
Member, Attending Staff, University Hospital; Member,
Attending Staff, Grant Hospital; Member,
Consulting Staff, Children's Hospital and
Mt. Carmel Hospital, Columbus, Ohio

SIXTH EDITION

with 342 illustrations and 30 color plates

The C. V. Mosby Company

ST. LOUIS   TORONTO   1984

MOSBY

A TRADITION OF PUBLISHING EXCELLENCE

Acquisition editor: Eugenia A. Klein
Assistant editor: Jean F. Carey
Manuscript editor: Judith Bange
Book design: Jeanne Bush
Production: Linda R. Stalnaker, Teresa Breckwoldt

SIXTH EDITION

The C.V. Mosby Company
11830 Westline Industrial Drive, St. Louis, Missouri 63146

Library of Congress Cataloging in Publication Data

Havener, William H.
  Synopsis of ophthalmology.

  Bibliography: p.
  Includes index.
    1. Eye—Diseases and defects. 2. Ophthalmoscope and ophthalmoscopy.   I. Title. [DNLM: 1. Eye diseases. 2. Ophthalmoscopy.   WW 140 H386s]
RE46.H32   1984   617.7   83-19522
ISBN 0-8016-2121-6

AC/MV/MV 9 8 7 6 5 4 3 2 1   01/C/060

Preface

The intent of *Synopsis of Ophthalmology* is to offer, in usable detail, information about the skills and knowledge that could reasonably be expected of a practicing physician—a person entrusted with the care of patients' sight. For proper perspective, know that 1 in 25 of your patients will lose useful sight in one eye during his or her lifetime. Half of such blindness is preventable by today's medical knowledge—if applied. Seemingly trivial details may make the difference between a well-treated seeing eye and visual tragedy. I sincerely hope that such details, as presented concisely within this book, will help prevent unnecessary blindness and disability.

The text presents functional categories rather than the usual anatomic classification. The reader is advised to use the index in addition to the table of contents when seeking specific information.

Appreciation is expressed to Miss Sallie Gloeckner, the artist whose skill has made possible many of the illustrations. The invaluable secretarial assistance of Mrs. Ruth Davis is also gratefully acknowledged.

William H. Havener

The Ophthalmoscopy Book

Skillful and intelligent use of the ophthalmoscope is the most important contribution ophthalmology can make to other physicians. No other examining instrument or technique approaches the ophthalmoscope in its capability for diagnosing such a wide variety of diseases and for assessing their severity. This sixth edition of the Synopsis is designed to help the student use the ophthalmoscope capably.

Paradoxically, the great majority of physicians freely admit to lack of skill in use of this valuable instrument and to inability to find or interpret any but the most rudimentary fundus details. How can this be? Perhaps the reason is failure of the literature to describe ophthalmoscopy adequately. After all, does an intellectual physician need to be told how to use an instrument that is just a fancy little flashlight with a few lenses? The answer is, "Yes, indeed!"

This sixth edition of the Synopsis is subtitled "The Ophthalmoscopy Book" because a major portion of it is devoted to the technique of ophthalmoscopy and the associated cerebration. You, the student and the nonophthalmologist physician, need this information, which will permit you to care for your patients more effectively.

Contents

1   The most important square inch, 1

2   Your objectives in ophthalmology, 4

3   Anatomy and physiology, 7

4   History, 16

5   Eye examination, 35

6   Laboratory testing, 70

7   Interpretation of ophthalmoscopic findings, 72

8   Applied ophthalmoscopic technique, 85

9   Macular disease, 167

10   A method of learning ophthalmoscopy, 188

11   Medical ophthalmology, 194

12   Neuroophthalmology, 210

13   Diagnosis and management of eye injury, 229

14   Diagnosis and management of the red eye, 255

15   Glaucoma, 276

16   Strabismus, 294

17   Cataract, 319

18   Retinal detachment, 326

19   Uveitis, 330

20   Disorders of the eyelids, 336

21   Errors of refraction, 351

22   Evaluation and management of reduced vision, 361

23   Ocular therapy, 371

24   Metaphysical therapy (reassurance therapy), 413

25   Evaluation of therapeutic response, 418

26   Surgery of the eye, 421

27   Ophthalmic terminology, 426

Glossary, 430

Color Plates

FOLLOWING PAGE 82

1   Red reflex

2   Albinotic fundus

3   Circumpapillary and macular chorioretinitis

4   Myopic atrophy

5   Coloboma

6   Congenital tortuosity

7   Branch retinal vein occlusion

8   Normal blond periphery

9   Preretinal hemorrhage

10   Diabetic retinopathy

11   Drusen of macula

12   Acute hemorrhagic chorioretinitis

13   Acute macular chorioretinitis

14   Myelinated nerve fibers; diabetes

15   Old chorioretinitis

16   Retinitis pigmentosa

17   Choroidal nevus

18   Amelanotic melanoma; retinal detachment

19   Senile macular degeneration

20   Disciform degeneration; angioid streaks

21   Diabetic vasculopathy

22   Diabetic retinitis proliferans

23   Hypertensive retinopathy

24   Papilledema

25   Intraocular foreign body

26   Glaucomatous cup; fundus in a black patient

27   Acute and old chorioretinitis

28   Degenerative myopia

29   Cup/disc ratios

30   Retinal detachment

SYNOPSIS OF
Ophthalmology
THE OPHTHALMOSCOPY BOOK

chapter 1 The Most Important Square Inch

Why should you be interested in the eye? Because, diagnostically and functionally, it is the most important square inch of the body surface.

To emphasize the differences in importance of various parts of the body surface from the point of view of the examining physician, let me issue a dramatic challenge. The handicap will be a barrier between examiner and patient—a barrier with an opening of 1 square inch through which the examination can be performed. My choice will be to examine the eye through this square-inch portal.

The challenge to you is that you may select any other square inch of the body surface (except the other eye) for examination. To help you, you may enlist the aid of every other physician in an entire hospital. In addition, you may have free reference to the combined library facilities of a university and may consult with any professor of the entire university staff. If you wish, you may choose anyone else to help you, with no restriction whatsoever.

We will now proceed to examine patients—I, alone, with my square inch of the eye, and you with your total team of experts, studying any other square inch of the body surface. Who do you think will be able to detect more physical diagnostic information of clinical value?

Your team does not have a chance. Let me show you why.

The eye is so intimately connected with the rest of the body that it reveals enormous amounts of general information. For example, the 12 cranial nerves provide us with a large part of our information about the brain. Of these 12, the eye examination evaluates cranial nerves II, III, IV, V, VI, VII, and VIII; in addition, it provides information about the autonomic pathways—sympathetic and parasympathetic.

The best-known connection of the eye to the brain is, of course, the optic nerve. The visual pathways, which may be studied easily, painlessly, and safely by perimetry, extend from front to back across the brain. Perimetry differentiates accurately lesions of the temporal, parietal, and occipital lobes. In addition, the optic nerve has important clinical relationships to the pituitary, the middle ventricle, the meningeal and bony structures of the base of the brain, and the sinuses.

1

The optic disc has the diagnostically useful capability of swelling (papilledema) when the intracranial pressure is elevated, from whatever cause. Also, it becomes visibly pale (optic atrophy) when its nerve fibers are damaged at any point in their course from the retina to the lateral geniculate body.

Almost the entire length of the midbrain and brainstem contributes cranial nerves that may be evaluated by eye examination. Not only the integrity of the brain but also the status of the cavernous sinus and the apex of the orbit are revealed by ocular study of the functions of cranial nerves III, IV, V, and VI.

The diagnostic value of unilateral dilatation of the pupil after head injury exists because of the sensitivity of the pupil constrictor fibers of cranial nerve III to pressure. The relationships of cranial nerve VI to the petrous ridge account for its involvement by mastoid infection. Parotid or inner ear disease may affect cranial nerve VII. Nystagmus is characteristic of involvement of cranial nerve VIII. A legion of syndromes involving these cranial nerves are described in the neurology texts.

Not only the focal lesions of trauma, vascular occlusion or hemorrhage, and neoplasm but also the diffuse diseases such as infection (meningitis, syphilis) and demyelinating disorders cause typical nerve damage. For example, retrobulbar neuritis and internuclear ophthalmoplegia are almost pathognomonic of multiple sclerosis.

Another obvious connection between the eye and the rest of the body is the vascular system. Venous flow disorders such as cavernous sinus thrombosis and carotid-cavernous fistula result in characteristic congestion of the entire orbit. The most common source of emboli to the retinal vessels is an atherosclerotic carotid artery, although emboli may also originate from diseased heart valves, as in subacute bacterial endocarditis.

Specific diseases of the vessels such as periarteritis nodosa and temporal arteritis cause ophthalmoscopically visible changes of the vessels of the retina and optic nerve. Hypertensive vascular disease, one of the most common serious human disorders, results in easily recognizable structural and nutritional retinal damage. Queer, rare conditions such as Takayashu's pulseless disease slow the retinal blood flow so greatly that actual segmentation of the blood occurs within the retinal vessels.

Hematologic disorders of all types are manifested in the fundus of the eye by their characteristic flat-topped preretinal hemorrhages and large white-centered hemorrhages. The sea-fan pattern of retinal neovascularization characteristic of sickle cell disease is unique.

Virtually all metabolic disorders affect the eye. The most common one, diabetes mellitus, causes characteristic diabetic retinopathy, ophthalmoplegia, cataract, and refractive errors. The cataract of hypoparathyroid tetany is its most serious irreversible change. Cystinosis, Hurler's gargoylism, Tay-Sachs disease, Wilson's hepatolenticular degeneration, and dozens of other rare metabolic syndromes have characteristic depositions of corneal crystals, copper rings, or other selective intraocular cellular degenerations. Exophthalmos and lid retraction mean thyroid disease, even to the layman.

Infections such as syphilis, toxoplasmosis, and histoplasmosis affect the eye with diagnostically characteristic destruction. Gonorrheal ophthalmia neonatorum was the most common cause of childhood blindness before the development of effective prophylactic and therapeutic medications and would reappear immediately if these measures were discontinued. Maternal rubella destroys eyes as well as hearts and brains.

Mucocutaneous disorders affect the delicate lid skin and conjunctiva just as they do other body surfaces. The permanent eye changes of Stevens-Johnson syndrome are the most disabling feature of this condition. The elastic tissue abnormality of pseudoxanthoma elasticum causes classic ruptures of the lamina vitrea of the fundus. Allergic and infectious blepharoconjunctivitis are extremely common skin disorders.

Many chromosomal abnormalities affect the eye. The cataractous slanted eye found in mongolism and the grossly abnormal eye of trisomy 13 and 15 are examples.

The eye is a delicate indicator of poisoning. The miotic pupil of the morphine addict and the reddened conjunctiva of the alcoholic are traditional emergency room signs. The papilledema of lead poisoning and vitamin A intoxication; the cataracts from paradichlorobenzene (and radiation), corticosteroids, and strong parasympathomimetic drugs; the yellow vision of digitalis intoxication; and the selective retinal damage from chloroquine are but a few examples of ocular poisoning.

I could go on and on about the discoveries possible in our most important square inch—the eye: metastatic cancer, intraocular parasites, hypercholesterolemia, Marfan's syndrome, tuberous sclerosis and the other phakomatoses, hysteria, and malingering. Unfortunately, all these details will not fit into an introductory synopsis.

The information described up to this point is not in any way the province of the ophthalmologist but should be the interest of the general physician, the internist, the pediatrician, the neurologist—even the surgeon! In addition to providing this information of general value, the eye is inherently valuable and deserving of medical attention in its own right. No one disputes that 90% of our information reaches our brain via sight. Not one of us could perform our medical tasks without vision. Already in grade school 10% of us need glasses, and by middle age the figure approximates 100%. Eye surgery accounts for 15% of the operations performed on patients over 65 years of age in this country. Glaucoma, our most common preventable cause of blindness, affects 2% of the population over 50 years of age. Of all the parts of the body, the eye is the most vulnerable to minor injury.

So what? Just this. If you know how, you can determine the health or disease of a large portion of the body simply by looking at the eye, the most important square inch of the body surface. No one is going to make you learn how to do this—or do it. It is your decision—if, when, and how. All I can do is hope to motivate you to start—today!

chapter 2   Your
            Objectives in
            Ophthalmology

What should you know about the eye? You seek a level of competence in ophthalmology that will be adequate for an internist, a pediatrician, a neurosurgeon, or a general physician. Reaching this goal may be simplified by defining your objectives as clearly as possible.

The following outline presents your objectives. The questions under each objective represent important examples of the type of performance expected, but they are *not* comprehensive goals.

Essential basic skills

1. Recording of an *eye history* that will identify the presence and specific location of disorders affecting the eye
    a. Can you write a concise, adequate, and accurate description of the patient's eye complaint?
    b. From your description can you suspect one or more possible diagnoses?
    c. Can you formulate questions that will help confirm or exclude your tentative diagnoses?
    d. Can you specify the physical and laboratory findings associated with your diagnoses?
2. Performing an external *ocular examination* that will identify or exclude abnormalities
    a. Can you state the precise anatomic location of an externally visible abnormality and describe its appearance?
    b. Can you measure and record distant and near visual acuity?
    c. Did your history explain each abnormal finding? If not, what additional questions should you ask?
3. Using the *ophthalmoscope* in an orderly sequence of fundus examination
    a. Can you instantly determine the transparency of the eye by observing the red reflex?
    b. Can you evaluate size, shape, color, and margins sufficiently well to determine whether a disc is normal or not?
    c. Can you follow the course of the major blood vessels and recognize abnormal constrictions, dilations, and color changes?
    d. Do you know how to use proximal illumination in the recognition and evaluation of fundus abnormality?

Required knowledge
 1. Ocular anatomy and physiology, including the visual pathways and the related cranial nerves
 2. Meaning of eye symptoms
    a. From the history, can you determine the part of the eye that is affected? Conversely, can you specify the symptoms arising from faults of various anatomic parts of the eye?
 3. Evaluation and management of reduced vision
    a. Assuming the patient can read only 20/100, are you able to differentiate between refractive error, cataract, neurologic defect, or other causes of reduced acuity?
 4. Ocular manifestations of systemic disease
    a. What are the eye findings in diabetes, hypertension, and thyroid disease?
    b. What types of eye findings suggest general, rather than local, ocular disease?
 5. Ocular manifestations of neurologic diseases
    a. Can you identify the presence of the cranial nerve paralyses affecting the eye?
    b. Can you specify the classic visual field defects associated with the various parts of the visual pathway?
    c. Can you detect these field defects by confrontation? By perimetry?
 6. Diagnosis and management of eye injury
    a. Can you evaluate the severity of an injury without further damaging the eye?
    b. Can you categorize the common types of eye injury and prescribe proper management?
 7. Diagnosis and management of the red eye
    a. Are you able to make the differential diagnosis between the common causes of a red eye?
    b. Do you know the seven red eye danger signals?
    c. How do you manage the various causes of a red eye?
 8. Glaucoma
    a. Can you estimate the C/D ratio? Do you know its significance?
    b. Do you know the symptoms of chronic glaucoma, one of our leading causes of blindness?
 9. Strabismus
    a. Can you recognize the presence, type, and amount of ocular deviation?
    b. Can you differentiate between paralytic and nonparalytic strabismus?
    c. How do you detect suppression amblyopia in a cooperative 2-year-old child? In an older child?
10. Errors of refraction
    a. When should you refer a patient for refraction?
    b. What precautions must a contact lens wearer observe? Why?
11. Degenerative diseases of the eye
    a. What are the symptoms and signs of cataract?
    b. What is the ophthalmoscopic appearance of senile macular degeneration?
12. Inflammatory diseases of the eye
    a. What are the symptoms and signs of acute iridocyclitis? Of corneal infection?
    b. What symptoms lead you to suspect acute macular chorioretinitis and how do you confirm this diagnosis?
13. Developmental abnormalities of the eye
    a. When you give supplemental oxygen to a premature infant, what should you know about its toxic effects on the eye?

14. Disorders of the eyelids
    a. Do you know how to prevent exposure keratopathy?
    b. If ptosis is present, what other ocular abnormalities should you seek?
    c. Can you evert the upper lid?
15. Orbital abnormalities
    a. What local disorders are suggested by exophthalmos? What systemic disorder?
    b. Can you estimate orbital compressibility?
16. Ocular pharmacology and medical therapy
    a. When would you use dilating drops? When not? Differentiate between cycloplegic and mydriatic effects.
    b. What ocular disasters may result from corticosteroid therapy?
    c. When do you use topical antibiotics? Anesthetics?
17. Surgery of the eye
    a. How do you repair an eyelid laceration?
    b. When should you refer a patient with suspected cataract for ophthalmologic evaluation?
18. Prevention of blindness
    a. What simple precaution is important in the school laboratory, home workshop, or industry?

Seriously, if you intend to practice medicine, you should master these few pages of objectives. Your patient's welfare requires it.

chapter 3 Anatomy and Physiology

The human eye is an incredibly complex and intricate mechanism. I could elaborate on the 120,000,000 rods and 5,000,000 cones and the other marvelous cells contained within each eye, but a detailed eye anatomy test is larger than this entire Synopsis, and all this interesting information is unnecessary in the delivery of primary-level eye care. Therefore, the purpose of this chapter is to scan only those structural and functional details directly relevant to clinical practice.

The eye (Fig. 3-1) somewhat resembles a 3-ply basketball. The three layers are the sclera and cornea (structural strength), uveal tract (nutrition), and retina (visual function).

SCLERA

The sclera (Fig. 3-2; see also Fig. 3-6) is the tough, flexible, white outer covering of the posterior portion of the eye. Anteriorly, the sclera is continuous with the transparent cornea. The circular junction between the sclera and the cornea is the limbus. Posteriorly, at the exit of the optic nerve, the sclera thins to a fenestrated membrane (lamina cribrosa) through which the axons of the optic nerve leave the eye. The front portion of the sclera, visible through the almost transparent bulbar conjunctiva, is commonly recognized as the "white of the eye."

Although the sclera is less than 1 mm thick, it is remarkably tough and is capable of withstanding intense contusions. Because of this toughness and because of the bony shield of the orbital rim and the cushioning effect of the orbital fat, rupture of the globe occurs only rarely, from the most severe blows. However, the sclera is not hard and can easily be penetrated by sharp objects (thorns, knives, small and sharp or pointed metallic foreign bodies). The shock of an ocular contusion is transmitted across the sclera and readily damages the delicate inner tissues of the eye.

The sclera is freely permeable to water and electrolytes and is not part of the blood-eye barrier.

CORNEA

The cornea (Figs. 3-3 to 3-5) is just as tough as the sclera and provides the structural strength of the front part of the eye. Its strength derives from the stroma, which constitutes

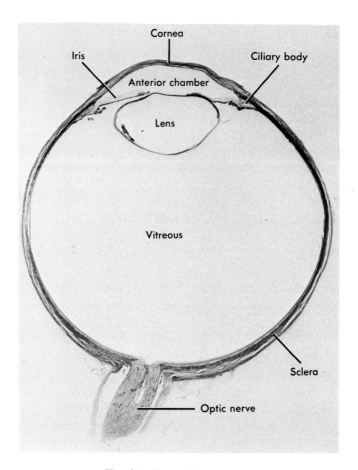

Fig. 3-1. Normal human eye.

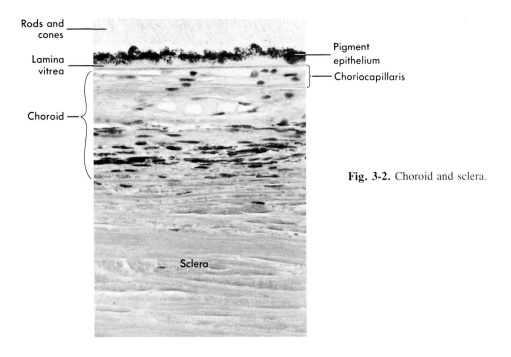

Fig. 3-2. Choroid and sclera.

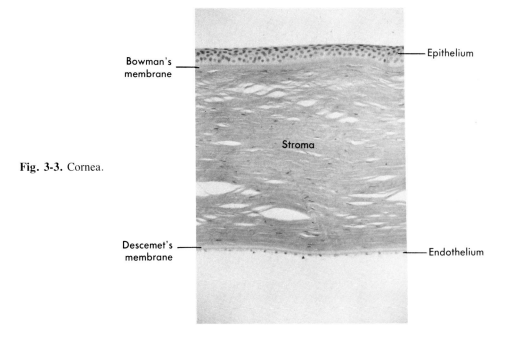

Fig. 3-3. Cornea.

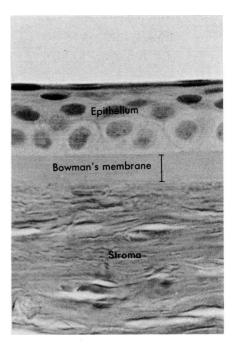

Fig. 3-4. Anterior cornea.

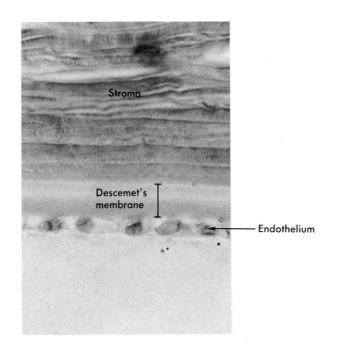

Fig. 3-5. Posterior cornea.

most of the bulk of the cornea. The stroma is freely permeable to the passage of electrolytes and water.

Most of the dioptric strength of the eye results from the corneal curvature, which provides 40 diopters of the total 60-diopter strength of the eye. (The lens provides only 20 diopters.) To serve an optical function, the cornea must be transparent. The transparency results from the regular lamellar structure and the relative dehydration of the cornea.

Corneal dehydration, maintenance of the intraocular pressure, and the resistance of the eye to entry of certain molecules (for example, antibiotics) are properties resulting from the blood-eye barrier—an electrolyte impermeable barrier within the eye. The anterior portion of the blood-eye barrier is the corneal endothelium, a single-cell-thick layer that covers the back of the cornea. Having a lipoid content 100 times greater than that of the corneal stroma, the endothelium is highly resistant to the passage of electrolytes, such as the chloride ion, which is in relative excess in the aqueous humor. Also, electron microscopy shows the endothelial cells to be connected with tight junctions, which resist leakage between the cells. Hence, the corneal endothelium is a semipermeable membrane, resistant to the passage of chloride ions, and enables osmotic force to withdraw water from the corneal stroma. Stated differently, the corneal endothelium is the "pump" that draws water out of the stroma, enabling it to be transparent.

Injury or disease of the endothelium damages the corneal pump mechanism, resulting in corneal decompensation. A decompensated cornea is edematous, thickened, and less transparent. Damaged endothelium heals only very slowly, perhaps not at all, in contrast to the rapidly regenerating epithelium.

The bulbar conjunctiva terminates at the limbus and does not cover the cornea. The corneal epithelium is a delicate layer, only 5 cells thick, and is readily abraded; yet it constitutes the main defense of the cornea against infection. The corneal stroma is relatively much more vulnerable to infection and is exposed to danger whenever epithelial loss occurs. This is the reason for prescribing prophylactic antibiotics whenever a significant break in the epithelium exists (as from contusion, abrasion, foreign body, exposure keratopathy, contact lens accident, ultraviolet burns or chemical damage).

The corneal epithelium grows with extraordinary rapidity, completely replacing itself every week. Small epithelial breaks heal overnight. Topical anesthesia paralyzes the epithelial regenerative capacity; hence, topical anesthetic drops are contraindicated for home use in the control of pain from corneal abrasion. (While anesthetized, the corneal epithelial defect will never heal.) In contrast to the permanent scarring resulting from injury to Bowman's membrane or stroma, epithelial injuries heal with no trace of scarring.

The epithelium is also lipid rich and electrolyte impermeable, like the endothelium, and maintains an osmotic pull, drawing water from the corneal stroma into the hypertonic tear film. Epithelial damage also results in corneal edema, although it is less severe than that from endothelial damage.

LACRIMAL APPARATUS

The tear film is absolutely essential to corneal health and function. Faulty lid closure or tear formation results in drying and scarring of the cornea, termed exposure keratopathy. This may result whenever the eyelids are not closed during unconsciousness; therefore, it is your duty to be sure that your patient's eyelids are closed, whether the cause of unconsciousness is anesthesia, accident, or disease.

The tear film has three constituents: a watery component from the lacrimal gland (situated in the upper, outer orbit), a mucous component from goblet cells within the conjunctiva, and an oily component from the lid margin glands. The tears are rich in immunoglobulins and constitute a major defense against infection of the eye. Tear deficiencies are common in older persons, especially in association with arthritis. Such patients often benefit from using artificial tear substitutes.

A lacrimal "pump," activated by the lid-blinking movements, propels tears into the lacrimal drainage system (puncta, canaliculi, lacrimal sac, nasolacrimal duct) to empty beneath the inferior turbinate of the nose. Epiphora (abnormal tearing) results from failure of any portion of the drainage system, including ectropion, which is a turning-out of the lower eyelid so that the lacrimal punctum does not contact the tear pool.

UVEAL TRACT

Uvea means "grape" and refers to the appearance of the internal portion of the eye remaining after the sclera and cornea have been peeled off. The dark content is now covered by the iris, ciliary body, and choroid. The primary function of these structures is nutritive. Their dark color is due to a dense melanin content.

Iris. The iris is a muscular, circular shutter, capable of spontaneously adapting the pupil aperture in response to light intensity. From the standpoint of the physician, the iris is a highly sensitive indicator of the status of sympathetic (mydriasis) and parasympathetic (miosis) innervation and cranial nerves II and III (the afferent and efferent limbs of the pupillary light reflex pathways). Relative forward displacement of the iris occurs in an eye predisposed to angle-closure glaucoma and identifies an eye that should be dilated only with caution, if at all. A perforating wound with aqueous loss may also cause shallowness of the anterior chamber. Pupil irregularity and inequality are both readily observed signs of serious intraocular disease.

Ciliary body. The ciliary body (Figs. 3-6 and 3-7) is a circular muscular and secretory structure just internal and posterior to the limbus. Inflammation of the ciliary body causes dilatation of the overlying limbal blood vessels, resulting in the circular halo of redness (limbal flush) that is so characteristic of serious intraocular inflammation.

The longitudinal muscle of the ciliary body inserts on the scleral spur. Its contraction opens the trabecular meshwork, enhancing aqueous outflow and thereby reducing intraocular pressure. Contraction of the circular muscle of the ciliary body relaxes the elastic traction of the zonular fibers on the lens (Fig. 3-8) and causes accommodation for near vision. Both these ciliary muscles receive parasympathetic innervation and respond to parasympathomimetic drugs.

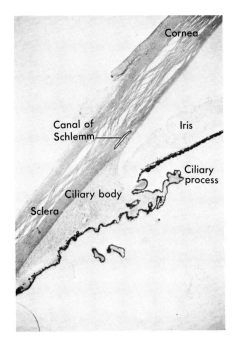

Fig. 3-6. Peripheral anterior chamber structures.

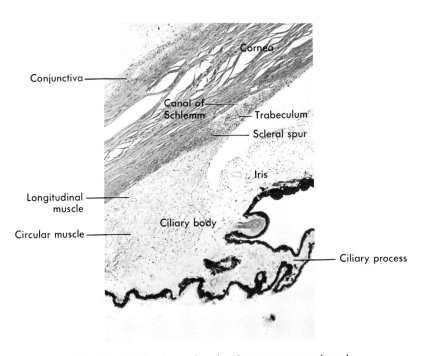

Fig. 3-7. Peripheral anterior chamber structures, enlarged.

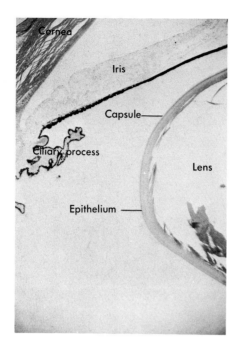

Fig. 3-8. Peripheral lens.

Cornea

Iris

Capsule

Ciliary process

Lens

Epithelium

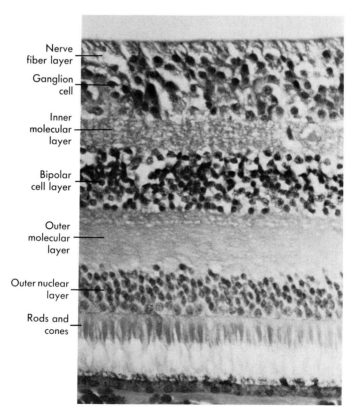

Fig. 3-9. Retina.

Nerve fiber layer

Ganglion cell

Inner molecular layer

Bipolar cell layer

Outer molecular layer

Outer nuclear layer

Rods and cones

The epithelium of the ciliary processes is capable of secreting an excess of chloride ion into the posterior chamber (the space between the lens and the iris). This chloride excess, confined within the semipermeable membranes that constitute the blood-eye barrier, develops the osmotic pull responsible for generating the normal intraocular pressure. The level of intraocular pressure is determined by the resistance to outflow of the trabecular meshwork in the anterior chamber angle (regulated by the longitudinal muscle of the ciliary body).

Choroid. The posterior portion of the uveal tract, the choroid, is a highly vascular layer that nourishes the outer half of the retina (see Figs. 3-2 and 8-2). The large choroidal vessels are external, feeding blood to the choriocapillaris, a capillary layer just beneath the retina.

RETINA

The retinal anatomy (Fig. 3-9) is described in detail in the subsequent chapters on ophthalmoscopy. The retinal pigment cell layer is the posterior part of the blood-eye barrier.

SUMMARY

The intent of this chapter is to serve as a brief introductory overview, preliminary to the chapters on history and physical examination. More detailed information on structure and function is presented where relevant to clinical practice.

chapter 4 History

The taking of a medical history is not a stenographic accounting of what the patient says. It is a probing encounter guided by an educated and active mind. A good history is an essential part of the evaluation of every patient. Indeed, with the history alone, a skilled person can arrive at the proper medical diagnosis in 80% to 90% of patients. The history provides vital guidance for the subsequent physical examination, laboratory work, and therapy. I could not possibly exaggerate the importance of your learning to take a good medical history.

Unfortunately, it is not easy for you to learn how to take a good eye history, nor for me to tell you how to do so. Still, the undertaking is well worth our mutual effort, and I do urge you to struggle through this rather long chapter. I shall present a number of different explanations and approaches to the process of history taking.

TRIAGE

The easiest application of history taking is to sort out patients in terms of the severity and urgency of their problems. This might be the goal of an appointment secretary dealing with patients over the telephone. Her instructions would specify that eye symptoms requiring immediate medical attention include:

1. Rapid loss of vision (whether straight ahead or to the side)
2. Persistent severe pain or foreign body sensation (especially if the eye is red)
3. Sudden appearance of many floating spots

Less urgent are such symptoms as gradual loss of vision, double vision, photophobia, headache, and redness. However, these symptoms do require medical evaluation, which should not be unduly delayed.

Itching, burning, irritation, and fatigue of the eyes, as well as tearing and chronic redness, are annoying symptoms but are unlikely to indicate serious disease. Appropriate medications will often relieve such symptoms.

If the patient telephoning for an appointment does not volunteer his symptoms, the secretary should inquire what they are: "How do your eyes bother you?" Many patients are unable to evaluate the urgency of their symptoms and do not understand that emergency appointments are available whenever needed.

WHAT A HISTORY IS NOT

A common (but wrong) description of how to take a history lists a large number of specific questions, linked together in a sequence. The inference is made that a good historian has learned this list and achieves success by thorough evaluation of all these answers. Such an erroneous conclusion is also advanced by efforts to adapt the computer to history taking. Here again, the thesis is that the ultimate goal is a comprehensive list of artfully designed questions, perhaps arranged in branching sequences. Not so. Such a mass of questions would be beyond the capacity of any historian and would exhaust the patients. Worse, the presentation of an impersonal and routine list of questions does not permit development of the positive interpersonal attitudes that are so important in patient care.

A history is not the comprehensive withdrawal of all facts from the patient's mind, as cider is drained from a keg. Rather, it is a selectively guided and progressive elicitation and recognition of significant information. The guidance is the hard part of a history, for it requires a knowledge of the final outcome that the questioner does not yet possess. How, then, does a beginner proceed through the labyrinth of a history when each patient is different and not even the expert is clairvoyant to know the outcome in advance?

FORMAT OF A HISTORY

Organization provides the framework for a medical record. A standard format would include:

1. General information
2. Chief complaint
3. History of the present illness
4. Past history
5. Family history

Before discussing each of these in detail, let me comment that all of this information is legally privileged and cannot be disclosed without appropriate authorization by the patient. We do not talk about identifiable patients with family, friends, or even with other professionals.

General information. A medical chart must identify the name, address, telephone number, age, sex, race, and marital status of the patient. The occupation should be clearly specified (for example, "telephone company" is not very helpful—it could mean proofreading a telephone book or climbing telephone poles). Insurance data are necessary for billing purposes. The name and address of the family physician and/or the referring physician are absolutely necessary for subsequent communications.

Chief complaint. The chief complaint might be: "Cannot see with right eye." The intent of writing down the chief complaint is to identify the primary cause of the patient's concern. For what problem did she come to you? State the chief complaint in the patient's words, not yours. In the above example, you should not come to the decision that the problem is nearsightedness and write down "myopia of the right eye." If the patient complains that she cannot see with the right eye, that is her chief complaint. At this early stage of the history you have no way of knowing whether the cause of her problem is myopia, retinal detachment, or something else. A premature statement of your diagnosis will compromise your ability to reach a correct final diagnosis.

The beginner suffers the delusion that the reason for writing the chief complaint is to satisfy the requirement of someone that the ritual of chartwriting be complete. Actually, there are three good reasons for identifying a chief complaint:

1. If you are a beginner, your repeated accurate performance provides the experience necessary for your own learning.
2. The chief complaint is your first guide to the nature of this individual patient's problem.
3. Before the patient is satisfied, someone must explain the meaning of the chief complaint and its proper management. We tend to forget this, because such an explanation will not occur until the very end of the patient's evaluation. Perhaps the beginner never even perceives this reason for identifying the chief complaint because he does not yet have the responsibility of final explanation and management. Let me repeat: *The patient's needs will not be satisfied until she has received an acceptable explanation of the meaning of the chief complaint and its proper management.*

History of the present illness. The description of the patient's chief complaint should be in sufficient detail so that the reader will understand the symptoms and the course of the disorder. The history should not be written down just as the patient states it, because most patients offer a disorganized and incomplete anecdote. You should listen and question until you have elicited material that you can write down in an orderly sequence that makes sense to you. (Later in this chapter, I will provide information that is necessary to elicit an intelligent history.)

The time sequence of the history is important. When, how fast, and in what order did events occur? The patient may tell you it happened before Aunt Minnie broke her leg. That does not help. November 1977 is the way I want to know the time of onset. Time characteristics, including the rate of onset and the duration, are necessary in differential diagnosis.

Provide specific details. "Cannot see with right eye" might mean that only distance vision is blurred, a blind spot is present in the center of the visual field, the right side of the visual field of the right eye is lost, the right visual fields of both eyes are lost, a diffuse haze obscures the entire field of the right eye, or a variety of other problems in which sight is impaired. Each of these has different diagnostic implications. To the best of your ability, question the patient about her complaint until you understand her specific problem clearly. You will find that most patients have difficulty providing precise and concise descriptions. So will you, at first. But try, and do it again, and yet again.

You also must know and write down what has previously been done about the problem. Has the patient self-medicated the symptoms or obtained medical advice? What medications have been taken, and what has resulted? Repeating a treatment that has already been unsuccessful is not sensible. If our patient who cannot see with her right eye has already tried a new pair of glasses without success, it is logical to suspect that the condition may not be amenable to correction by a new refraction. Unless you know that several of the more obvious treatments have already been tried and have failed, you cannot avoid the trap of advising the same unsuccessful remedy again. Therefore, in the history of the present illness, always include what has already been done about the problem. Be very specific as to the name and dose of the medication. And ask if the patient has faithfully used the treatment as prescribed. (At least one third of patients do not take their medications properly!)

Let us be selfish about this. What good does a detailed history of the present illness do you? What do you get out of the encounter? (Totally disregard that it permits us to help the patient; we do not care about her, for the moment.) It happens that a patient suffering from a given disease is the best source of knowledge about the symptoms of that condition. She is actually experiencing the symptoms. The historian-patient interface is a barrier between your mind and her mind. Your selfish goals are:

1. To develop skill in communication, so that you can easily and accurately cross the barrier of understanding someone else describing her experiences
2. To learn about that particular disease so that you will recognize its symptoms when you again encounter them in another patient
3. To motivate your own curiosity, so that in subsequent reading or consultation you are alert to receive the scientific explanations of why the symptoms exist

There is nothing wrong with viewing the history selfishly. The beginner feels guilty about this, thinking that he is supposed to be performing a duty of helping the patient instead of himself. But do you not also help the patient most effectively when you are personally interested? Of course you do, and this is the secret of the really effective physician. He has merged his own personal goals with those of the patient. The physician's search is for scientific understanding and the satisfaction of helping another person; the patient just wants to get well. The point is that you do these things together most effectively and enthusiastically if you recognize and accept personal benefits to yourself. If you view taking a history as just a necessary evil, you will be bored silly with the task and will probably deliver a rotten performance besides. Unfortunately, this happens all too often, to the detriment of both the patient and the historian.

Past history. The most relevant part of the past history asks if similar or related problems have existed before. If you do not yet possess enough medical knowledge to know what related problems might be, it is always reasonable to ask if the patient has in the past experienced similar symptoms or other problems with the same part of the body. For example: ''Did you ever have trouble seeing with the right eye before?'' ''Have you ever had any other trouble with your eyes?'' ''Have you had eye surgery?''

A listing of the other previous serious problems suffered by the patient helps identify the nature of the individual with whom you are dealing. Specify and date, in chronologic order, the major illnesses and operations of the patient. Be more interested in recent problems than in ancient ones. Childhood measles is not usually relevant in an 80-year-old patient.

The past use of medications is especially important. ''Are you allergic to any medication?'' must be asked of all patients and recorded. Specify the medication, the adverse reaction, and the date. Many patients are vague about their responses to medication. They do not know the name of the medicine and cannot differentiate a toxic reaction to the medicine from totally unrelated symptoms of disease. Nevertheless, if the patient thinks she has had a serious reaction to medication, describe what she thinks happened. List prescribed medication the patient has taken, the disease for which the medication was prescribed, the dates, and whether the patient is now taking the medication (how much and how often).

Allergies are so important that you should write on the chart ''No allergies'' to establish that you have really asked the question and the patient has denied allergies.

The most difficult problem with taking the past history is knowing when to stop. You could go on all day with some patients, to their great enjoyment and your nonproductive frustration. The answer to this is that the history should be as detailed as is required by the present needs of the patient. Also, if you discover by means of the history a potentially serious symptom, the consequences of which the unconcerned patient does not realize, you should follow through adequately to achieve proper management of the condition.

Family history. All major eye problems suffered by family members are relevant to an ophthalmic history. Even if a problem was the result of an injury and clearly not genetic, the experience and its consequences will affect the patient's attitudes toward her own eye problem. Of course, a great many eye conditions are inherited, including refractive error, glaucoma, cataract, strabismus, retinoblastoma, tendency toward iridocyclitis, retinal degenerative changes (including retinal detachment, macular degeneration, retinitis pigmentosa, and a host of less common retinal abiotrophies), corneal dystrophies, orbital configurations, and neuroophthalmic disorders. If genetic counseling is to be attempted, a detailed family history is essential.

ELICITING A HISTORY

I have already given you much detail about the significance of the history of the present illness. That information is a good first step, but it is not enough. You should obtain additional significant information that the patient does not recognize as being important and will not spontaneously disclose. You cannot actually do this until I have explained to you the meaning of eye symptoms (later in the chapter), but I need to explain the process now. There are six steps in the process of eliciting a complete history of the present illness:

1. *Write a concise and accurate description of the complaint.* (This information comes from the patient, as outlined under History of the Present Illness.)
2. *Enumerate the diagnoses suggested by the description.* (This step occurs in your mind, without participation by the patient.) Note that a chief complaint (such as ''cannot see with right eye'') does not usually contain enough information to permit intelligent guessing as to the diagnosis. There are too many possibilities. The purpose of the detailed description of the present illness is to obtain enough

characteristics of the problem so that you can begin to guess the nature of the problem.

3. *Ask questions designed to confirm or exclude the tentative diagnoses.* (This elicitation of significant information is again an interaction between you and the patient.) To do this, you must know enough about eye diseases to formulate the critical questions. For example, if you are considering retinal detachment, you seek a history of visual field loss progressive over a period of days or weeks, often preceded by a sudden shower of floating spots, occurring in a patient predisposed by myopia, cataract extraction, previous trauma, or family history. A given detail is said to be a *significant positive* if you expected to find it on the basis of a suspected diagnosis. For example, a recheck of the family history that disclosed a previously forgotten retinal detachment in a paternal uncle would strengthen your diagnosis of possible retinal detachment. A *significant negative* is the absence of something you expected. For example, if you guess the patient has acute glaucoma and ask whether the eye hurts, the absence of pain would certainly be unusual during such an attack. *Significance is synonymous with expectedness.* Your expectations are formulated to match your tentative diagnoses.

   Differential diagnosis requires comment. Beginners think this is a listing of all the possible causes of the problem. Not so. Differential diagnosis is the process whereby you *differentiate* between one condition and another. You seek differences rather than similarities. The best questions lead to critical differences between the relatively similar conditions. These differences may be in the symptoms elicited by the history or in the physical findings and/or laboratory results to which the developing history guides you.

4. On the basis of the tentative diagnoses, *predict the physical and laboratory findings likely to be present.* (Again, this step occurs only within the examiner's mind.) Although you might suppose all physical examinations to be the same, this is far from true. If the examiner suspects a given problem, he will perform a much more detailed examination of the involved area and will recognize the significance of a subtle, easily overlooked sign, such as the slight ptosis of an early third-nerve paralysis. Similarly, a laboratory test such as the erythrocyte sedimentation rate is appropriate in consideration of the diagnosis of temporal arteritis but is a waste of money in evaluation of glaucoma.

5. If the subsequent physical examination discloses unexpected abnormalities, ask additional questions designed to explain these physical findings. For example, finding a rusty foreign body imbedded in the back of the nonseeing right eye will lead to inquiry as to the circumstances of the old penetrating injury, previously forgotten by the patient. Always go back and forth between the history and the physical examination until the two sources of information match perfectly. *Any discrepancy between the history and the physical examination requires explanation* and may indicate the presence of an undiscovered problem or an erroneous presumptive diagnosis.

6. *Continue to add to the history* as the course of the disease unfolds. The beginner thinks the history has ended when he leaves the patient. The patient knows better—he is interested in the future: "Will I get better, how long will it take, and what is necessary to accomplish this?"

This six-step sequence of eliciting additional valuable historical material should be consciously followed by the beginner. Actually, the expert performs the same six steps. The only difference is that he knows the characteristics of the various diseases in more detail and is therefore better able to formulate the significant questions and examinations that will lead to the proper diagnosis.

PROCESSING A HISTORY

A perceptive gentleman named Bloom has analyzed intellectual functioning and concluded that our brains may work on progressively more complex levels. He states that there are six such levels: knowledge, comprehension, application, analysis, synthesis, and evaluation. This listing is called Bloom's Taxonomy of Intellectual Processes. Now, you and I are not usually impressed by these pedantic classifications, but I am convinced that this taxonomy describes our thinking processes so accurately that it is helpful as a guide to our personal learning and functioning. In fact, this taxonomy may profitably be applied to the processes of history taking.

Knowledge is the unedited information volunteered by the patient. The patient and any listener may possess knowledge. At this level, facts are not yet of medical value. Knowledge is not necessarily accurate or precise.

Comprehension is the understanding of the knowledge transmitted by the patient. By discussion, you must affirm your interpretation of what you think he said. Actually, this accomplishment is not minor. Language, thought, and comprehension barriers abound. Misinterpretations and variations of the history are so commonplace that no two physicians will produce exactly the same history from a given patient.

Application is the use of the comprehended knowledge. For purposes of understanding the taxonomy of history taking, let us accept an oversimplified definition and specify application as simply a writing down of the historical facts. (Write a concise and accurate description of the complaint. Remember, this was the first step specified that you should perform in eliciting a history.)

So far, steps that any educated person could be expected to perform have been described. The product expected is a narrative account of an episode in the patient's life. If sufficiently detailed, such a narrative is useful to a physician. However, the narrative is not a medical history.

Analysis, synthesis, and evaluation are much more sophisticated intellectual processes than are knowledge, comprehension, and application.

The *analysis* of the narrative account is a sorting out of the data into related categories. For illustration, consider the assembly of a jigsaw puzzle. One might start by sorting the pieces into similar types. All the blue pieces, possibly representing sky, would be separated from the green pieces, possibly representing vegetation. Similar groups of pieces would be gathered for each color.

Analysis presupposes the ability to distinguish separate components of the narrative history. Obviously, the greater the number of abnormal components that can be obtained from the history, the more diagnostic information available to the physician. At this level of manipulation of information, the separation of wheat from meaningless chaff is difficult. The best rule is to accept everything that seems to be abnormal. The problem is deciding what is a normal variant and can be discarded, at least temporarily.

Synthesis is the reassembly of our narrative components into recognizable disease entities. Let us return to our jigsaw puzzle analogy. Synthesis is putting the pieces together to form a recognizable part of the puzzle. Synthesis is harder than analysis because it requires a concept of the finished product—a knowledge of the disease entity that will best be described by the aggregate of the components. Unfortunately, in clinical medicine we deal not with one single jigsaw puzzle but with a mixture of many separate jigsaw puzzles. Many pieces are lost, and the remaining ones are mixed together. Unraveling the mess takes the patience of a dedicated physician.

At any rate, analysis and synthesis lead to step 2 in eliciting a history: Enumerate the diagnoses suggested by the description. Such manipulation of the data is the input made possible by professional education and experience.

Evaluation, the most critical and difficult intellectual level, is the final continuing process applied to taking history and to patient management. Evaluation involves history elicitation steps 3, 4, 5, and 6: Ask questions designed to detect significant data, whereby you can confirm or exclude tentative diagnoses. Predict the physical and laboratory findings likely to be present. Explain any discrepancy between history and physical findings. As it becomes available, add future information to the history. Diagnoses become valid only when they pass the inspection of critical evaluation. Evaluation determines whether all the available information is compatible with the working diagnosis.

In summary, the taxonomy of intellectual processes describes clearly the thinking sequences involved in the taking of a medical history.

The student may also be interested in considering the explanation of his own learning as presented in the taxonomy. The lower levels (knowledge, comprehension, and application) are basic intellectual functions and describe memory by repetition, a rather transient form of memory easily subject to error. You are well advised not to rely on these levels of learning during your education (although they are often necessary).

Analysis, synthesis, and evaluation describe an attitude of learning that forces information to make sense. Personally digested information at this conceptual level is likely to be retained for a long time, is easily refreshed, is retrievable with accuracy, and is far superior to simple knowledge. ''Programmed'' learning defeats this objective by substituting the teacher's analysis and synthesis for the student's. The main value of a ''program'' is that it permits the student to observe the way in which a subject has been analyzed by an ''expert.'' Perhaps his evaluation of the teacher's logic will be a guide to his own future performance. Unfortunately, many programs disclose the teacher's pre-occupation with knowledge—the lowest intellectual level.

USING A HISTORY

Interrelationships. A description of the context in which the physician uses a history will offer insight into the interrelationships between the history, the physical examination, laboratory determinations, the response to therapy, and general knowledge. Fig. 4-1 depicts the role of each of these five sources in reaching the central goal of proper diagnosis and management.

The concentric and radial lines may be considered to represent a maze of pathways over which the physician may pass to reach his central goal. Unfortunately, many segments of these pathways are not open; hence, the physician must often detour back and forth, seeking the information that permits him to approach better understanding and diagnosis of the given patient.

Note that the concentric lines represent general knowledge. General knowledge, being nonspecific, will *never* lead to the diagnosis of any disease. However, general knowledge does permit the physician to move back and forth between the findings of the history, the physical examination, laboratory determinations, and the response to therapy.

The most usual approach is that the history provides guidance to the symptomatic part of the body and the way in which it is affected. General knowledge, then, permits prediction of the expected physical findings. Physical examination confirms or excludes the presence of these findings and may disclose some unexpected abnormalities. Using

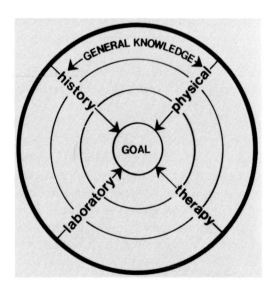

Fig. 4-1. Schematic representation of the relationship of the history, physical examination, and laboratory work to arriving at the goal of diagnosis or treatment.

general knowledge, the physician should now return to the history, to elicit historical explanation of any unexpected physical findings. By now, the physician will already have arrived at the proper diagnosis in the great majority of cases. In fact, the history alone permits the tentative diagnosis of at least 80% of patients seeking medical advice.

Laboratory studies are ordered on the basis of sufficient historical or physical data to permit prediction by general knowledge of relevant tests. Screening tests (such as blood counts or urinalysis) are routinely ordered because they will frequently disclose unexpected abnormalities. Again, the physician uses general knowledge to permit a recheck of relevant historical or physical information whenever unexpected laboratory data are encountered.

The point to be derived from Fig. 4-1 is that general knowledge permits a constant back-and-forth check between historical, physical, and laboratory findings in such a conscious search for significant positive and significant negative information. Significant positives and negatives are the criteria whereby tentative diagnoses are evaluated.

Approaching a diagnosis. Since the ultimate goal of your medical history is the making of a diagnosis, you may approach this effectively by means of the following general questions:

1. What system of the body is affected?
2. How does the system malfunction?
3. What is the most likely cause for the malfunction? (Only a limited number of general etiologies exist: congenital, degenerative, inflammatory, traumatic, neoplastic, and vascular.)

Note that these questions are not in a form that permits direct presentation to the patient. These questions are for the guidance of the physician and indicate successive goals within the history to be reached by proper utilization of both volunteered and elicited information.

Anatomic classification of eye symptoms. You are aware that the anatomic location of symptoms is helpful in guiding you to the proper diagnosis. A toothache, a bellyache, or a painful big toe obviously suggest different diagnoses. Similarly, the symptoms referable to an eye may be subdivided as they correspond to different parts of the ocular anatomy.

The anatomic drawings in Fig. 4-2 are numbered to identify structures causing characteristic symptoms. It is, in fact, possible to localize eye symptoms to these structures by use of the history alone. Start by writing down the names of the structures. (The answers follow. After you have written down as many as you can, check the accuracy of your answers.)

Now that you have written down the anatomic names, let us consider some of the characteristics of these different parts. Light enters the eye along the line *(1-2-3)*. Opacities of the transparent parts of the eye (*1*, cornea; *2*, lens; *3*, vitreous) along this axial line will blur the clarity of vision, as if you were to look through dirty glass.

The vitreous is a gel that wobbles when you move your eye. Hence, vitreous opacities

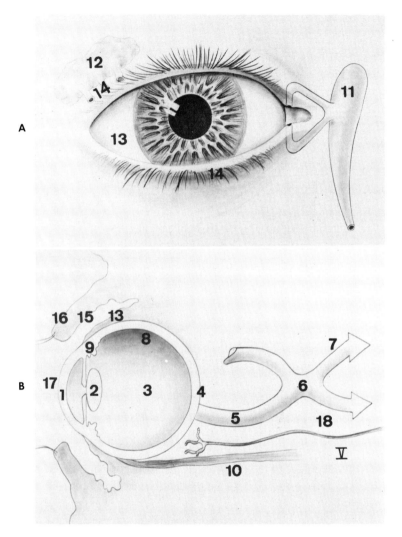

Fig. 4-2. Anatomic diagram for correlation with the history.

move or float about with eye movements and are perceived as mobile shadows called "floaters."

The retina *(8)* lines the inside of the eye as does the film within a camera. Its center *(4)*, called the macula, sees the clear detail directly straight ahead from the eye. Side vision is perceived by the more peripheral parts of the retina. Nerve fibers from the retina travel to the brain via the optic nerve *(5)*, a crossing of both optic nerves called the optic chiasm *(6)*, and more posterior pathways such as the optic tracts *(7)*. These nerve fibers from the retina to the brain are precisely arranged. Defects of these visual pathways may be exactly located by measuring the corresponding visual field defects, which do not float or move with respect to the eye.

Inflammation of the muscles within the eye (9, iris and ciliary body) is painful, especially when these muscles respond to light or accommodation.

The extraocular muscles (for example, 10, inferior rectus) align the eyes to point at the object you are observing. Faulty alignment causes double vision (diplopia). To experience this, hold your two forefingers directly in front of your nose so that one finger is about 6 inches away from your nose, the other about 18 inches. Look at either finger. How many images do you see of the finger at which are you not looking?

Tears come from the lacrimal gland (12) and escape to the nose via the lacrimal drainage system (11). The normal moisture that lubricates the eye comes from the small glands distributed throughout the conjunctiva, which lines the white surface of the eye (13, bulbar conjunctiva) and back of the eyelids (15, palpebral conjunctiva). Infection and irritation of the conjunctiva or eyelid margin (14) may cause mucoid debris to enter the precorneal tear film (17).

Cranial nerve V senses pain in the head. It is somewhat like a party telephone line—when you pick up the receiver and hear a stranger talking, you cannot tell which phone he is calling from. So also, the brain cannot always tell exactly whether pain comes from the orbit (18), the eye itself, a sinus, or a tooth. Pain from deep structures gets mixed up like this and is called "referred" pain. In contrast, the patient can usually tell fairly accurately the location from which surface pain originates.

This list of hints as to where symptoms might originate is incomplete, but let us start to guess about some symptoms. I'll name the symptom; you write down which of the labeled 18 structures might be able to cause the symptom. Guess if you want to, just so you think about it enough to have a reason for your guess.

Eye Symptom Test
Write in the anatomic structures causing the symptom.

A. _____, _____ *Glare:* unpleasant veiling sensation resulting from the scattering of light within imperfectly transparent media, like a frosty windshield.

B. _____, _____ *Photophobia:* pathologically increased, actually painful sensitivity to light.

C. *Blur:* indistinct visual detail. May be subdivided.
   1. _____, _____ *Blur:* cleared by glasses or partly closing eyelids; may vary with distance *(refractive blur).*
   2. _____ *Transient and variable blur:* cleared by blinking several times.
   3. _____, _____, _____ *Fairly constant blur:* sensation as if a fog or haze is between observer and detail.

D. _____ *Floaters:* moving opacities that change their relationship to the eye, drifting about in response to eye movements.

E. _____ *Metamorphopsia:* constant distortion or warping of central detail in one eye.

F. _____, _____, _____, _____
   Central field defects (scotomas): "straight ahead" visual loss maintaining a fixed
   relationship to the eye.
G. _____, _____ *Peripheral field defect, monocular:* loss of
   "side" vision. Patient often acutely aware of loss.
H. _____, _____, _____, _____
   Peripheral field loss, binocular: loss of "side" vision. Patient often unaware of
   loss.
I. _____ *Diplopia:* seeing double.
J. _____ *Diplopia, monocular:* persists even though the uninvolved eye is
   covered.
K. _____, _____, _____ *Pain:* foreign body
   sensation.
L. _____, _____, _____ *Pain:* deep.
M. _____, _____ *Epiphora:* tearing.
N. _____, _____ *Dryness:* burning, sandy sensation.
O. _____, _____, _____, _____
   Discharge: purulent, mucopurulent, crusting.
P. _____, _____ *Itching.*

Now check your answers.

A. Cornea, lens. *Glare,* a sensation like looking through a frosted windshield, results
   from diffuse corneal scars or from cataract. The cataract patient will characteristically
   complain that oncoming auto headlights at night scatter so much light that she cannot
   see to drive.
B. Ciliary body, iris. *Photophobia* is a severe intolerance of light associated with iridocyclitis. Corneal injury or inflammation may cause mild iridocyclitis; the resulting
   photophobia is relieved by cycloplegic therapy.
C. Blur
   1. Cornea, lens. *Blur* due to refractive error is caused by faulty combinations of the
      refractive strength of the cornea and lens and of the length of the eye. Accom-
      modative spasm of the ciliary body is an uncommon cause that may result from
      pilocarpine therapy for glaucoma. A simple test for refractive blur is to hold a
      pinhole aperture before the eye, which will improve in visual acuity if the fault is
      one of focusing (pinhole camera effect).
   2. Precorneal tear film. The presence of mucus or other surface debris on the cornea,
      or of excessive tears, will *blur* visual detail.
   3. Cornea, lens, vitreous. Opacities of the media, if situated on the axial line of
      sight, reduce vision. The ophthalmoscopic view of the fundus will be correspond-
      ingly *blurred,* confirming the accuracy of the diagnosis.
D. Vitreous. Since the semifluid vitreous humor can shift about within the eye, and
   because posterior vitreous opacities cast visible shadows on the retina, *floaters* correspond to opacities of the posterior axial vitreous. Numerous floaters of sudden onset
   may indicate serious intraocular hemorrhage or inflammation and should be considered a dangerous symptom.
E. Macula. *Distortion* of the central retina by edema, contraction of scar tissue, or other
   disorder will impart a warped or bent appearance to objects. This is characteristic of
   lesions that displace the macular retina.

F. Macula, optic nerve, chiasm, more posterior visual pathways. A *central scotoma* can result from neural damage anywhere from the retina to the brain (macula, optic nerve, tract, radiation, or cortex). If ophthalmoscopy does not show the cause, perimetry is indicated.

G. Retina, optic nerve. Loss of the *peripheral field* of view in *one eye* can be due to lesion of the retina or optic nerve. Retinal detachment, for example, causes a field loss corresponding to the portion of the retina that is detached.

H. Chiasm, tract, radiation, occipital cortex. Loss of part of the *visual field* in *both eyes* can be caused by neurologic lesions of the visual pathways at or behind the optic chiasm (or by separate lesions of each eye). Lesions of the posterior visual pathways may affect associative pathways so that the patient is entirely unaware of extensive field defects.

I. Extraocular muscles or their innervation. *Diplopia* is due to faulty alignment of the eyes. This is usually due to innervational faults, but it can be due to mechanical failure of the muscles or resistance to movement of scar tissue or orbital defects.

J. Lens. *Monocular diplopia* is characteristic of a type of nuclear cataract (double-focus lens) that breaks entering light into two images.

K. Cornea, tarsal conjunctiva, bulbar conjunctiva. A *foreign body* sensation results from irritation of the surface of the eye, especially of the exquisitely sensitive cornea. Particles imbedded on the back surface of the upper lid are particularly distressing. Corneal epithelial abrasions (or inflammatory damage) feel just like foreign bodies.

L. Ciliary body, meninges of optic nerve, orbit. *Deep pain* can originate from the ciliary body (associated evidence of iridocyclitis), the optic nerve (associated visual loss), or the orbit, or it may be referred from any structure innervated by cranial nerve V (teeth, sinuses, and so on). The retina does not experience pain. Acute glaucoma causes severe pain (also rainbow halos).

M. Lacrimal drainage apparatus, cornea. *Tearing* does not result from lacrimal gland disease. Faulty elimination of tears results from any block of the lacrimal drainage system, including ectropion of the lid, which displaces the punctum away from the tear film. Reflex hypersecretion occurs in response to ocular irritation, especially of the cornea.

N. Lacrimal gland, conjunctiva. *Dryness* of the eye results from faulty secretion by the lacrimal and conjunctival glands and may be caused by their destruction (as in chemical burns, Stevens-Johnson syndrome, or ocular pemphigus). The most common cause is Sjogren's syndrome, a generalized failure of secretory glands associated with arthritis and menopause.

O. Lid margins, conjunctiva, lacrimal drainage, cornea. *Mucopurulent discharge* is a nonspecific sign of bacterial infection and can arise from blepharitis, conjunctivitis, dacryocystitis, or keratitis.

P. Conjunctiva, lid skin. *Itching* is the classic symptom of surface allergy.

Note that multiple symptoms can originate from the same anatomic site. Obviously, this helps define the affected location. For example, corneal disease can cause loss of sight, pain, and tearing or discharge.

ETIOLOGIC DIAGNOSIS OF EYE SYMPTOMS

The history can identify not only the specific location of an eye disorder but often also the cause. To accomplish this, you must first determine the specific location, because each part of the eye suffers from its own unique diseases. For example, the lens and the optic nerve are entirely different tissues, subject to very different disorders.

Time characteristics (onset, rate of progression) provide information of great importance in etiologic diagnosis. Paradoxically, a very sudden onset is characteristic of conditions that develop very slowly, as well as of those that develop rapidly. The discovery phenomenon explains this. Many persons are unaware of slow and partial loss of vision, especially if it affects only one eye or the peripheral field of vision. Accidental covering of the good eye, or loss of sight in the good eye, results in instantaneous recognition of the problem, previously unrecognized during possibly even years of gradual development.

Embolic arteriolar occlusion affecting the retina or visual pathways should be suspected as the cause of a loss of field occurring within less than a minute. Hemorrhage obscures vision rapidly also, but not usually within a minute. Vitreous hemorrhage, for example, produces moving debris that may increase in amount for some minutes. A macular hemorrhage may develop within a few minutes.

Progressive loss of the homonymous field within minutes, recovering within a half hour, accompanied by a bright, irregular line between the seeing and the blind area, is characteristic of a migraine equivalent. Progressive loss of a monocular field over several days, preceded by a myriad of small floaters, is probably a retinal detachment. Retinal vein occlusion causes progressive diffuse blurring of one eye over several weeks.

Open-angle glaucoma and melanoma are examples of conditions that may cause visual loss so slowly as not to be noticed for many months or even years.

When the location of the fault has been identified, further relevant questioning can help in etiologic diagnosis. For example, if you have decided that the symptom of glare means the presence of a cataract, inquiry as to a family history of loss of sight due to cataract may confirm a hereditary tendency toward cataract as being at fault. If a history of central scotoma with an onset over several days and partial resolution during the subsequent month suggests retrobulbar neuritis, inquiry as to other neurologic faults may confirm the diagnosis of multiple sclerosis. Vitreous hemorrhages occur very commonly because of diabetic retinopathy. As you become acquainted with other specific disorders of the eye, you will recognize their special characteristics, concerning which proper questioning will help to identify the particular cause.

The time of onset and progression of a visual loss should be described very precisely, for this information is very helpful in differential diagnosis.

HISTORY TAKING AS THERAPY

And so are we quite done with history taking? No. There is yet more. We have obtained what we want, but has the patient received what she is seeking? After all, she is the one who initiated our relationship, and she did so because she perceived certain needs to be present. Have we met these needs, or will we do so? You may be surprised, or even skeptical, but delivery of the history is in itself one of the primary goals of every patient. Indeed, from the psychologic point of view we could redefine a history as a clear description of the objectives and goals of the patient.

Although we ordinarily think of the history as solely an information-gathering device, eliciting it is also the first of six steps required in the treatment of every patient. This dual function of the history occurs because we are actually doing two separate things for each patient. We are caring for her body and also for her mind. The concept of using a history to localize typical symptoms at the corresponding part of the visual system has been presented to you earlier in this chapter. The other aspect of history taking is as part of reassurance therapy.

Each patient should be confident that she is receiving good care. From her standpoint, this confidence is much more an emotional state than an intellectual evaluation. The deliberate use of reassurance therapy will contribute to this confidence. Note that the patient's experience includes all the personnel involved in the delivery of her care. The proportion of time spent with the nurse, the aide, or the physician can vary considerably, provided that all the essential steps of the reassurance process are covered. In other words, personnel may be interchangeable in achieving an intended outcome (reassurance of the patient). Stated differently, the nurse and secretary may contribute greatly to the reassurance process (by taking a history, for example), but the entire process includes some aspects that the nurse cannot provide. An effective physician learns to delegate part of this responsibility to his supporting personnel.

Reassurance therapy begins with the history taking, which is the patient's introduction to the medical care system. The patient's first impressions will be good or bad, depending on the skill of the historian. Note that from the patient's standpoint the history represents a large part of her verbal communication with the system and therefore assumes proportionate importance in her assessment of the system.

Step one of reassurance therapy is simply the taking of a *standard medical history,* as already described. As a student, when your role is to take the history, you may be troubled by a sense of incompleteness. You have tried to perform your task, but both you and the patient know that her needs have not been met. Her disease has not been healed by the history taking, and you both know this. You cannot reassure her as to the final outcome—only as to your quality as a historian. In fact, you should not attempt to reassure the patient during the history process; such attempts are counterproductive because they inhibit the patient from giving you further information and they betray your anxiety or impatience. Actually, permitting the patient to experience some anxiety during the history taking preconditions her to accept reassurance therapy more effectively at the appropriate later time. (Remember that reassurance therapy requires all six steps—it will not work otherwise.)

Clearly differentiate between reassurance as to the status of the patient's disease (which you should scrupulously avoid) and reassurance as to the competence of the personnel and the quality of the equipment and institution. As you leave the patient at the close of the history process, it may be reassuring to explain to her what will happen to her next as she progresses through the medical system. Avoid effusive praise that may sound suspect, but it is reassuring to volunteer something like, ''You'll like Miss Jones, the night nurse. She's nice. Call on her if you have trouble sleeping or any other problems, and she'll do her best to help you." Comparable statements are appropriate in response to any specific questions from the patient regarding the system. While you are a student, do not try to answer medical questions about this specific patient, because you do not know the answers. You can describe the process of evaluation, for example. "You'll need to have some x-rays and laboratory tests before we know those answers."

In summary, a good historian can reassure the patient that she has come to the right place for care and can impart an emotional preconditioning that will enhance the future process of reassurance with respect to the disease condition.

Step two of reassurance therapy is *evaluation of affect*. This evaluation occurs simultaneously with the taking of the history. Affect is evaluated nonverbally by interpretation of "body language." The patient's tone of voice, ease or apprehension, and mannerisms convey affect more than do her words. When you realize that you feel uneasy with a patient, she has successfully conveyed to you her concern about her problems. As a beginner, you may feel uneasy about your own inadequacies and uncertainties. This confuses your interpretation of the patient's body language. Also, you transmit your lack of confidence to the patient, which is not at all reassuring! If you sense the patient's concern about receiving part of her care from an obvious beginner, you can easily allay her fears by explaining that your role is that of preliminary evaluation, and that others will continue her evaluation very soon.

Evaluation of affect is important because it discloses the significance of the symptoms to the patient and is a guide as to how much reassurance therapy will be needed. Actually, of course, every patient you encounter is experiencing concern about her health. Without concern, she would not be there. You may also safely assume that concern increases in proportion to the severity of the disease.

A fairly accurate assessment of the degree of patient concern is helpful in guiding the quantity of future reassurance. Even more important, the specific items that require reassurance should be identified, so that they may be emphasized later. Reassurance will not be broad generalizations but must be tailored to the personal needs of the individual patient. Excessive and irrelevant attempts at reassurance are frightening, for they raise doubts where none previously existed.

Another point about body language. As you evaluate the patient, she is simultaneously probing your body language. Here she should find no evidence of anxiety or distress. With respect to betraying horror at the ravages of disease, the historian should wear an inscrutable "poker face" of concealed emotions. Poker faces are hard to maintain, however, and are not particularly reassuring. It is better, therefore, to assume a mask of helpfulness and interest. This should be easy to do if you are interested in your work and enjoy it, for these are your true emotions.

Step three of reassurance therapy is *examination of the affected part*. Examination is not only a necessity for physical diagnosis, but it also "talks" to the patient. The gentleness and assurance of your physical contact contribute greatly to her evaluation of your competence. Bear in mind that the patient cannot know the quality of information you possess or lack. She can evaluate only your voice and your touch. Roughness speaks louder than words and says clearly that you do not care very much for this patient.

Additional historical information is often derived from the physical examination. The unexpected finding of an abnormality not described in the original history will lead to additional questioning about the symptoms related to this forgotten or unknown problem.

Step four is *medical diagnosis.* The nature of the patient's problem must be properly evaluated. This step will, of course, determine the definitive medical care to be rendered to the patient.

Unlike the first three steps, which are shared experiences between the patient and the examiner, the making of the medical diagnosis belongs to the physician alone. Trained to choose, evaluate, and reject diagnoses, the orderly mind processes the most plausible possibilities, always ending in more or less uncertainty. Here is the widest divergence between the patient and the physician. The physician cannot think out loud. Invariably his probing exploration of the possibilities will come across as uncertainty—the cardinal failing of a physician, from the patient's viewpoint. The making of the diagnosis is an unshared experience, to be revealed to the patient only at her unsophisticated peril.

I do not mean to imply that medical diagnosis is necessarily an esoteric and impossibly complex mental feat that can be accomplished only by the noble physician. After all, any layman knows when he has a cold, and the diagnosis of measles is pretty obvious. But there are other times when it might be German measles and the patient might be pregnant. And will the child be blind, mentally retarded, and a cardiac cripple 7 months later? Only the experienced physician can make appropriate decisions and recommendations for the individual patient.

Step five is *explanation.* You may misunderstand this step. Although an explanation of the problem is a necessary part of reassurance therapy, is basic to the legal doctrine of informed consent, and is essential to the cooperation of your patient in treatment, the patient does *not* need to understand the medical technicalities of your explanation in order to be reassured. The explanation must, however, convey three beliefs to the patient:

1. Belief that the history and symptoms are understood
2. Belief that the proper management will be undertaken
3. Belief that the personnel are sympathetic and will be helpful

Clearly, step five describes the development of a confident attitude within the patient. A nurse, being skilled in interpersonal relationships, is ideally qualified to help in the formulation of this attitude. Also, she is skilled in reviewing medical instructions with patients, who are notoriously unable to remember the details they have first heard at a time of stress and fear.

You will recognize that explanation is designed to meet the individual questions and problems that were presented at the time of history taking. For this reason, it is ideal that the same person take the history and participate in the explanation.

The *sixth and final step is reassurance.* You cannot reassure a patient about his disease without going through the preceding five steps. It will not work.

What is reassurance? Is it saying, "Oh, don't worry"? Did you ever know anyone to worry less after such an admonition?

Reassurance may be defined as a *credible and acceptable prediction of the future.* Your statements must be believable, and their implications must be tolerable. If you have bad news, you cannot deliver it all at once, faster than is emotionally acceptable. An easy way is to predict the patient's future appropriately. Be as specific as possible with respect to the patient's particular situation. What will happen to her tomorrow? Next week? Next month? What can she do and what should she avoid? Seek out and stress all positive aspects. Do not volunteer negative and threatening facts unless she must know them (for example, informed consent to surgery requires the general knowledge that not every operation is successful).

Do not be unrealistic—serious future problems may arise if the patient's expectations exceed reality. Banish unwarranted fears—patients usually imagine worse problems than actually exist.

Your verbal communication with the patient may include history taking, explanation, and reassurance. These merge almost indistinguishably into the total emotional and factual impact you make on the patient.

SUMMARY

You should devote much time to perfecting your ability to take a history, for its importance can hardly be exaggerated. Perhaps 80% of diagnoses can be suspected on the basis of a history alone. Simultaneously, as the eliciting of a history provides you with information, it begins the formation of the patient attitudes necessary for confidence and reassurance.

PERFORMANCE

Reading about how to take a history or to play the piano is nice, but it does not result in capability to perform the given task. You must actually go forth and take histories before you learn how to do this. The following outline is suggested as a guide for you. Please use it—right away—on the next patient you can find.

1. Write a concise description of the eye complaint.
2. What diagnoses are suggested by this history?
3. What questions will help confirm or exclude these diagnoses?
4. What physical examination and laboratory findings will help confirm (significant positive) or exclude (significant negative) these diagnoses suggested by the history? (Be certain to look for these findings during the subsequent examination.)

What is your goal in taking an eye history? That you should be able to point to the part of the visual system (Fig. 4-2) that is affected, which requires especially alert physical examination. Sometimes the history will not only localize the malfunction but will be so specific as to permit an etiologic diagnosis also.

chapter 5 Eye Examination

Without the guidance of a history to pinpoint the significant physical findings, a physical examination is a mechanical routine subject to the omissions of boredom, hurry, and inattention. With respect to subtle findings (for instance, slight ptosis and minimal pupil inequality), highly important details will be overlooked unless specifically sought out. You will detect and remember only those details for which you look.

Therefore, on the basis of your history, predict the expected physical findings. From your tentative list of differential diagnoses, identify the critical physical findings that will resolve the diagnosis. Do not only look—think of your goals as you look.

Before you can perform a good eye physical examination, you require knowledge of the appearances and characteristics of the various eye disorders. During examination you are to seek out the critical features that permit identification of a specific disorder and differentiation from other conditions. As a beginner, you do not yet know such general facts, which are presented subsequently in this text. With clinical experience you will develop your knowledge and skills. No substitute equals the experience of seeing actual patients in an eye clinic under the guidance of an ophthalmologist.

MEASUREMENT OF VISUAL ACUITY

The most rewarding single test for ocular function is evaluation of visual acuity. Reduced acuity will betray the presence of a great variety of diseases as well as the need for refractive correction. Determination of visual acuity is a part of every complete physical examination.

An important reason why visual acuity should be measured before performing the rest of the eye examination is that the finding of reduced acuity will alert you to the necessity of determining the reason for visual loss and correcting this if possible.

Distance acuity is measured with a letter chart (Fig. 5-1). The chart is placed 20 feet from the patient (or a reversed chart may be mounted behind the patient's head and viewed through a mirror 10 feet away). Acuity is recorded as a fraction; the numerator represents the distance to the chart, and the denominator represents the distance at which a normal eye can read the line. Thus, 20/30 means that the patient is 20 feet away and can read the line that a normal eye can read at 30 feet; 20/200 means that he can read only the largest letter, ordinarily legible to the normal eye at 200 feet. Lesser visual acuity may be

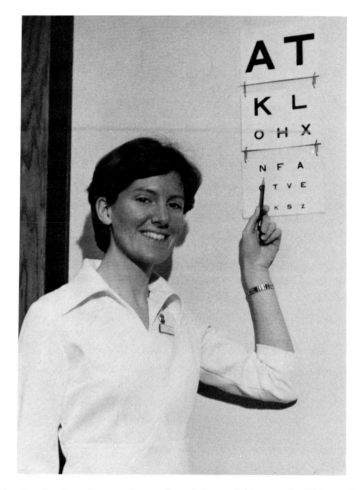

Fig. 5-1. Visual acuity chart. Inexpensive cardboard charts of this type should be available for use during a complete physical examination.

recorded by approaching the 20/200 letter until it can be identified. For example, if the patient must be within 4 feet before he can recognize the standard 20/200 letter, he has 4/200 vision.

Cruder methods of measuring reduced acuity may determine the distance at which the eye can *count fingers*. This degree of acuity is specified as CF at __ (the measured distance in feet). *Light projection accurate* indicates that the patient can tell from which direction a light source originates, in all parts of his peripheral visual field. This degree of acuity may conveniently be measured by a flashlight or ophthalmoscope light in a darkened room. If light projection is faulty, you should specify the direction in which the ability to see light is present or absent (actually, this evaluation is a very gross form of

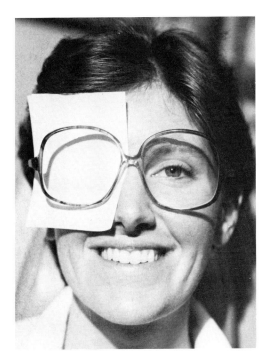

Fig. 5-2. Be sure to occlude completely the other eye during visual acuity measurement.

visual field measurement). *Light perception* is the ability to tell whether the light is on or off and is most easily determined by directing a lighted flashlight on or away from the eye in a darkened room. Stray light entering the other eye, which should be adequately covered, may confuse the results of testing a badly damaged eye. An eye is not termed ''blind'' unless it cannot even perceive light.

Acuity is examined with one eye at a time. The other eye should be occluded with an opaque card (Fig. 5-2). Always be on the alert for failure to cover the eye completely or for head turning that permits the patient to peek around the card. Such ''cheating'' may be an involuntary attempt to see with the single good eye or a deliberate fraud. *Never* allow a patient to cover his eye with his fingers, because he may see between them. Glasses should be worn if the patient customarily uses them for distance. Reading glasses will often blur distant vision.

Always coax the patient with apparently reduced visual acuity to try to read another line. Surprisingly often, he can! Illiterate patients may say they ''can't see it'' rather than admit their ignorance. Number charts answer this problem, since practically everyone can count money. Charts composed of E letters of various sizes and positions are useful for children, who simply indicate the direction in which the E is pointing. An intelligent 3½- or 4-year-old child can usually cooperate enough to permit accurate measurement of acuity (Fig. 5-3).

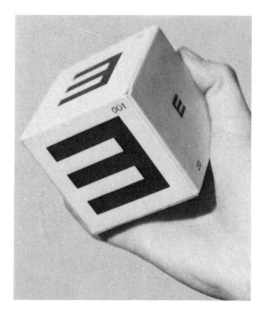

Fig. 5-3. E block for measurement of visual acuity of a child or an illiterate adult.

Measurement of near vision is particularly important in patients complaining specifically of reading difficulty or in persons over 40 years of age. With increasing age the lens of the eye becomes less flexible, resulting in loss of accommodation for near vision, which interferes with reading. This condition is referred to as *presbyopia*. Most patients who cannot read newspaper print at 1 foot while using their own reading glasses will benefit from an ophthalmologic examination and refraction. To record near vision, specify both the *size* of the smallest print legible to the patient and the *nearest distance* at which reading is possible. This distance measurement permits calculation of the amount of accommodation the patient can exert.

GENERAL INSPECTION

Watch thoughtfully as the patient walks into your examining room. Greet and welcome the patient, for this is important in developing an effective patient-doctor relationship. However, this is not a social encounter, and your purpose is to discover the patient's strengths, weaknesses, and attitudes from his actions and appearances. Facial features permit suspicion of many systemic disorders and provide clues as to pain or stress. The configuration and appearance of the eyes contribute greatly to the facial clues of importance.

From past experience we derive intuitive knowledge as to whether the face and eyes "look okay". Such intuition must be supplemented by an orderly and detailed approach whereby the physician consciously determines whether the lids, lacrimal apparatus, con-

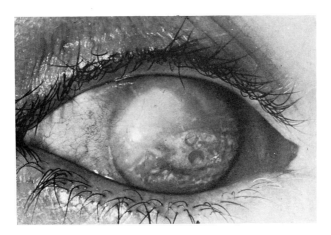

Fig. 5-4. Exposure damage to the cornea results if the lids do not close properly. Adequacy of closure of the lids should be checked during the physical examination.

junctiva, cornea, iris, extraocular muscles, and orbit are normal in appearance and function. In the beginning this approach is time consuming and unfamiliar; with experience it occurs almost automatically.

EXTERNAL EYE EXAMINATION

Lids. Lid examination has three objectives: (1) to ascertain the adequacy of protection of the eyes, (2) to seek signs that betray systemic disease, and (3) to detect local disease.

Do the lids close completely? This question should be answered in all patients and particularly in those with abnormally prominent eyes or facial paralysis. Potentially serious damage may be sustained through drying of the eye when the lids do not close properly (as in unconsciousness due to trauma, anesthesia, or serious systemic disease, or if lid defects are present) (Fig. 5-4).

Systemic disease (for example, nephrosis or myxedema) may be suspected in the presence of lid edema, provided the physician has excluded purely local inflammation and the slight bulging of lid skin commonly caused by aging. *Ptosis* (drooping of the upper lid) may be an early sign of involvement of the third nerve by any cause. Congenital defects rank high among the causes of ptosis.

Infections of glands of the lid margin (Fig. 5-5) are common. A *hordeolum* (sty) (see Fig. 20-4) is a localized infection of the small glands about the eyelashes. A *chalazion* (see Fig. 20-6) is an infection or retention cyst of the meibomian (sebaceous) glands, which lie within the tarsal plates and open on the posterior portion of the lid margins. Crusting of the lashes (see Fig. 20-2), often with very fine scales adherent at the lid margin, is an easily observed sign of surface lid infection.

Faults in position include a turning outward of the lids *(ectropion)* (see Fig. 20-21)

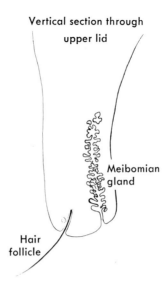

Vertical section through
upper lid

Meibomian
gland

Hair
follicle

Fig. 5-5. Cross section of the lid showing the large meibomian gland situated posteriorly and the smaller glands at the anterior edge.

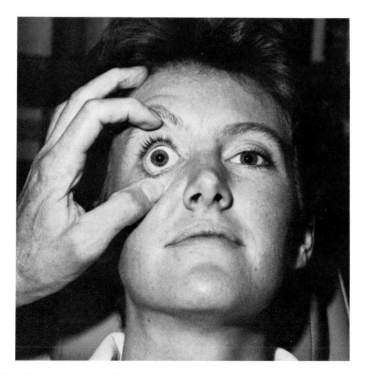

Fig. 5-6. Proper separation of the lids without any pressure against the eye.

and a turning inward *(entropion)*. The lashes normally project away from the eye. Should they be misdirected backward, as in entropion, considerable corneal irritation may be produced.

Gentle palpation of lids may be done by sliding the examining finger across the closed lid surface. In this way any masses (such as chalazion) within the lid may be felt between the finger and the eyeball and are often recognized more readily than by observation.

Great care must be taken in examining an injured eye. *Never* press over the eye when trying to separate the lids, because this may destroy the eye. Always limit manipulations to the portion of the lids overlying the bony orbital rims. The upper eyelid is elevated by pressing upward over the brow, and the lower lid is retracted by pulling down the skin overlying the cheek bone (Fig. 5-6; see also Fig. 14-2). This warning must never be forgotten when you are trying to open an injured eye for inspection. If at any time during examination of an injured eye you see that the eye has been penetrated (obvious laceration, prolapsed iris, protruding vitreous, flat anterior chamber), stop the examination immediately to avoid causing further damage by unwise manipulation.

Lacrimal apparatus. Tears are produced by the lacrimal gland, which is situated in the upper lateral orbit. A portion of this gland can often be seen beneath the retracted upper lid when the patient looks down, and must not be mistaken for a tumor. Tears are evacuated to the lacrimal sac through the lacrimal puncta, which are situated on a tiny elevation on the nasal side of both upper and lower lids. If the lower lid margin does not touch the eye (as in ectropion), tears cannot enter the punctum, and *epiphora* (pathologic tearing) will result. The lacrimal sac is a small pouch situated in the lacrimal fossa. Should passage of tears via the nasolacrimal duct to the nose be obstructed, finger pressure on the lacrimal sac (Fig. 5-7) will cause regurgitation of fluid through the punctum. The finger must be applied *inside* the lower inner orbital rim, not on the side of the nose, as is often erroneously done. This pressure will be uncomfortable. After pressing on the sac, move the finger inferiorly so as to pull down the lower lid. Any mucopurulent fluid expressed from the punctum can then be observed.

Conjunctiva. The conjunctiva is divided into two portions: palpebral and bulbar. The *palpebral conjunctiva* lines the posterior lid surface. The *bulbar conjunctiva* covers the eye up to the *limbus* (junction of the cornea and sclera). The conjunctiva is normally quite transparent, and the white color of the eye is due to the underlying white sclera. The bulbar conjunctiva is readily examined by separating the lids widely and having the patient look up, down, and to each side. Many small blood vessels are normally visible in the conjunctiva and underlying structures. Dilatation of these vessels is responsible for the various patterns of redness characteristic of many eye diseases. Both vessels and nerves penetrate the sclera at several points about 0.5 cm above the limbus. At these scleral penetrations, particularly in dark complexioned persons, uveal pigment often proliferates. These tiny black pigment dots often resemble foreign bodies, but they cannot be removed, as many an unwary beginner has learned to his sorrow. A small fleshy elevation known as the caruncle is situated in the nasal corner of the conjunctiva. Fine hairs and tiny yellowish

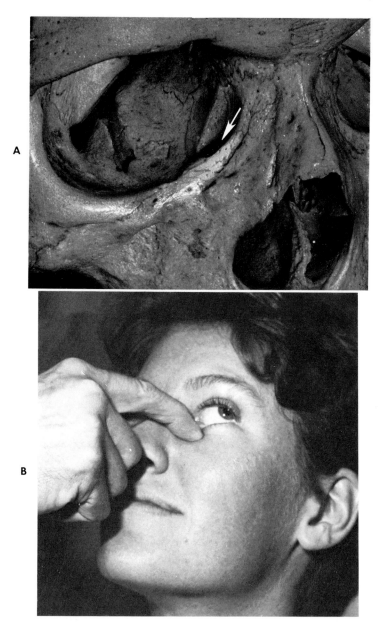

Fig. 5-7. A, The lacrimal fossa is situated *inside* the orbital rim. **B,** When examining the lacrimal sac for regurgitation of infected material, the examiner must direct pressure into the orbit, not on the nose. The patient should look upward, because this renders the punctum more readily visible.

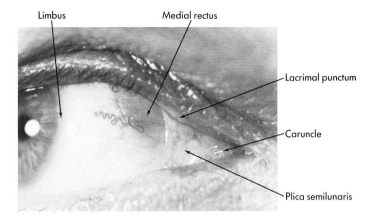

Limbus   Medial rectus

Lacrimal punctum

Caruncle

Plica semilunaris

Fig. 5-8. Inner aspect of the eye showing the caruncle and plica semilunaris.

spots (sebaceous glands) are normally seen in the caruncle and become more prominent with age. Lateral to the caruncle is a flat fold, the plica semilunaris (Fig. 5-8).

The palpebral conjunctiva overlies fleshy tissue and therefore appears more pink than the bulbar conjunctiva. Vertical yellowish striations may be conspicuous in the portion of the palpebral conjunctiva overlying the tarsal plates. These striations are the underlying meibomian glands. In response to irritation, viral infection, and particularly allergy, the lymph follicles of the palpebral conjunctiva enlarge, causing a finely nodular appearance (see Fig. 14-6), which is best seen with flashlight illumination from the side in a semi-darkened room.

The palpebral conjunctiva cannot be seen until the lids are everted. The lower lid is easily everted by sliding the skin overlying the lower orbital rim downward (Fig. 5-9). More of the conjunctiva will be exposed if the patient simultaneously looks upward.

Five simple steps are required to evert the upper lid:

1. The patient must look down. This relaxes the levator muscle, which is attached to the upper border of the tarsal plate. When the patient looks up, the tarsal plate is retracted into the orbit, a position from which eversion is impossible.

2. The patient must not squeeze the lids shut. Such contraction of the orbicularis oculi muscle effectively blocks eversion attempts. To ensure relaxation and avoid squeezing, reassure the patient, move slowly, and do not hurt him.

3. Hold the upper eyelashes. Grasping the eyelashes is facilitated by lifting the upper lid, thereby causing the lashes to protrude straight forward. Do not pull on the lashes—this only causes the patient to squeeze the lids together. Eversion is *not* accomplished by pulling the lashes upward or using them to roll the lid over a stick. In fact, pulling gently down and forward simplifies the subsequent procedure.

4. Push down on the upper tarsal border with a small stick such as an applicator or tongue blade (Fig. 5-10, *A*). The upper tarsal plate extends 12 mm above the lid

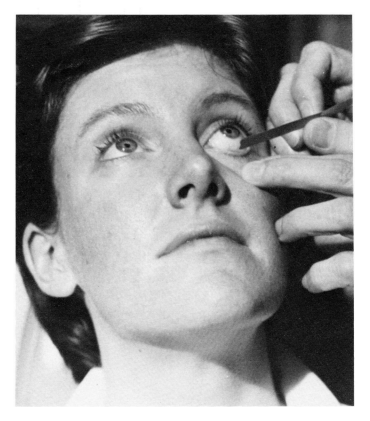

Fig. 5-9. The lower conjunctival sac is easily examined by pulling down the lower lid while the patient looks upward. A sterile fluorescein strip is being used to stain the tear film.

margin; therefore, pressure must be applied at least 1 cm above the edge of the lid margin. You will find that this simple maneuver of pushing down on the upper tarsal border is the key to easy lid eversion. Do not push in against the eye.

5. As soon as the lid is everted, appose the fingers holding the lashes to the brow, so that the lid may be held securely in eversion during inspection of the conjunctival surface (Fig. 5-10, *B*).

The examiner's left hand is used to evert the right upper lid; his right hand is used to evert the left eye. All five fingers work. The examiner's fourth and fifth fingers rest on the patient's temple and steady his hand. His middle finger pushes the patient's brow upward, raising the lid so that the lashes protrude forward and are more easily grasped. The index finger above and the thumb below hold the eyelashes firmly. The examiner lets go of the brow with his middle finger, and hereafter this middle finger is used for nothing except to help steady his hand against the patient's forehead. The lid is pulled slightly down and forward. A tongue blade in the opposite hand is used to evert the lid by pushing down on

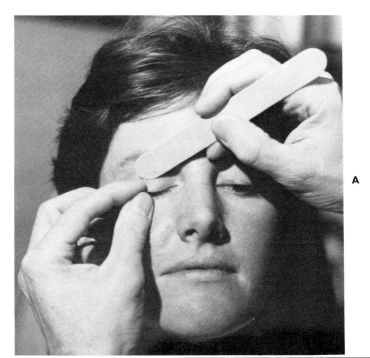

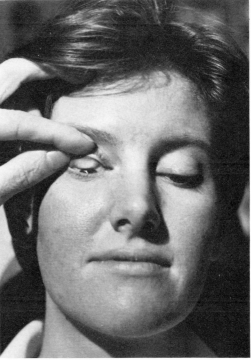

Fig. 5-10. A, The key step in everting the upper lid is downward pressure applied 1 cm above the lid margin, as the lid is pulled gently down and forward. **B,** Everted lid held in position by the thumb and forefinger.

the upper edge of the tarsal plate. The lashes are lifted by the thumb and index finger so that the lid is folded up and its margin touches the tongue blade. The index finger is slid out from behind the lid as the examiner continues to hold the lashes and lid margin against the tongue blade with his thumb. The index finger is moved nasally to hold the medial lid margin against the tongue blade just as the thumb is holding the lateral lid margin. When the index finger is in position medially, the thumb may be slid slightly lateral. Removal of the tongue blade now frees the opposite hand to hold the flashlight for inspection of the exposed palpebral conjunctiva or to use a swab to remove the foreign bodies that so often lodge here. Such equipment should be within reach, ready for use.

Because the upper lid is normally concave toward the eye, eversion causes a vertical fold to appear, usually in the nasal portion of the lid. This fold should not be misinterpreted as a mass.

To restore the everted upper lid to normal position, the examiner removes his hand completely from the patient. If the patient is still looking down, the lid remains everted. The examiner takes hold of the lashes and pulls gently forward as the patient looks up and simultaneously moves the lashes down into normal position.

Almost all medical students are much too rough during examination of the eyes. All manipulations, including eversion of the lid, must be performed far more gently than palpation of the abdomen or movement of the extremities. Move slowly, gently, and carefully, and you will retain the patient's confidence.

You communicate with each patient both verbally and nonverbally. Your nonverbal communication (via touch and attitude) is at least as important as what you say. A gentle touch will reassure the patient. Rough and painful handling of a sensitive area such as the eyelids will offend and frighten the patient. However carefully you believe you are touching the eyelids during your first physical examination, you are almost certainly pressing roughly and much too hard. Be gentle! I guarantee you that you are pressing more roughly than you think.

Cornea. Good vision requires a perfectly smooth and transparent cornea, which is normally invisible except for reflections from its surface. Two of the most common abnormalities of the cornea are *abrasions* and *opacities*. Oblique moving side illumination with a small flashlight is particularly effective in demonstrating corneal abnormalities (Fig. 5-11). Superficial irregularities are best detected by noting the defects appearing in the light reflections of the normal surface (see Fig. 13-2). Occasionally a defect casts shadows on the iris, and these shadows may be more readily visible than the corneal lesion producing them. Abrasions of the cornea are often almost invisible except when stained with fluorescein.

This staining technique simply requires instillation of a small amount of sterile fluorescein. Since dropper bottles of fluorescein are readily contaminated, fluorescein strips should be used. These individually packaged pieces of filter paper are saturated with fluorescein solution and are dried and sterilized. To use, crease the strip longitudinally before removing from the sterile envelope; then remove and place a drop or two of sterile

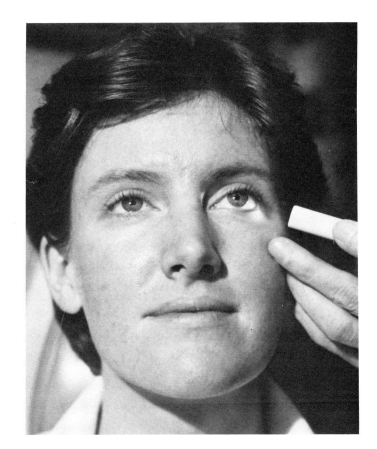

Fig. 5-11. Use of oblique moving illumination is best for examination of the cornea, anterior chamber, iris, and pupil.

water or saline solution into the crease. An alternate method is to touch the dry strip to the lower cul-de-sac, allowing the tears to dissolve the fluorescein (see Fig. 5-9). Corneal abrasions will be more clearly delineated if excess stain is washed out with saline solution.

Abrasions are stained a brilliant greenish color by fluorescein.

Oblique illumination and movement of the light also will help differentiate abrasions from corneal opacities, surface debris, deposits in the anterior chamber, and cataract. If the anterior chamber is abnormally shallow (which predisposes the eye to glaucoma and may contraindicate the use of dilating drops), oblique illumination will cast a character-istic crescent-shaped shadow on the far side of the anteriorly displaced iris (see Fig. 15-3).

An obvious opacity of the cornea may be an old scar or an active infection with leukocytic infiltration. Both are gray-white in color. Since an active corneal infection can rapidly destroy the cornea and blind the eye, it must never be mistaken as being an old scar. The appearance of a corneal scar and that of a corneal infection permit easy differentiation by an experienced observer. Other features will help a beginner. An acute corneal infection ordinarily causes severe pain and redness of the eye, with accompanying muco-purulent discharge. The history will be of recent onset, with marked loss of vision. In contrast, an old corneal scar causes no new symptoms unless degenerative changes result in a roughened and painful surface.

Corneal sensitivity (fifth nerve) is tested by touching a wisp of cotton to the center of the cornea and noting the brisk lid closure. This lid closure is a normal and important protective reflex. Approach the eye from the side so that the patient cannot see the cotton coming, because he might blink from fear. Do not touch the lashes, which also will cause blinking. Because of the great individual variation in corneal sensitivity, comparison of the corneal reflexes of the two eyes with each other is the best standard of reference (unless the patient has bilateral fifth-nerve loss). Loss of corneal sensitivity is a characteristic finding after herpes simplex keratitis.

Pupil. Normal pupils are perfectly round, are always equal in size, and constrict visibly in response to light and during accommodation. *Direct reaction to light* refers to constriction of the pupil receiving increased illumination. Constriction of the opposite pupil (even though no light increase strikes this opposite eye) is termed *consensual pupil*

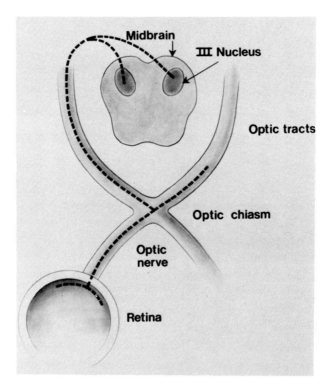

Fig. 5-12. Afferent pathway of the pupillary light reflex.

reaction. Either optic nerve may transmit the afferent part of the pupillary reflex (Fig. 5-12). Efferent pupilloconstriction stimuli are distributed evenly to both eyes via ciliary nerves (Fig. 5-13). In monocular blindness, as with a severed or diseased optic nerve, the affected eye will have no direct pupil response but will react consensually to stimulation of the opposite eye. Stimulation of the blind eye, however, will not cause consensual reaction of the opposite normal eye. If one eye is claimed to be blind, the pupillary light reflexes will provide valuable objective confirmation or refutation of this status.

The swinging flashlight test will disclose differences in afferent visual stimuli between the two eyes. Examining in a dark room, move the light rapidly from one eye to the other. You seek a dilatation of the pupil on which the light newly shines. The meaning of such a paradoxical finding is that the affected eye has a serious receptor or nerve transmission defect. Normal miosis has occurred because of the consensual pupil reaction while the opposite normal eye is illuminated. However, the direct pupil reaction of the affected eye is weaker than the consensual reaction; hence, both pupils dilate when the flashlight moves from the good eye to the affected eye. (This paradoxical dilatation is termed the

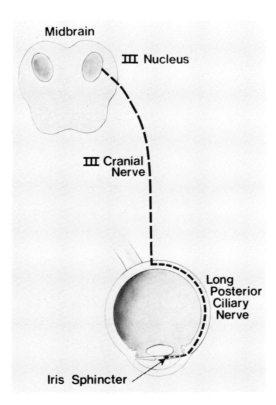

Fig. 5-13. The efferent pathway of the pupillary light reflex is distributed equally to both eyes, regardless of whether one or both eyes activate the afferent pathway.

Marcus Gunn pupil sign.) Even a dense cataract will not cause this type of abnormal pupil response.

The swinging flashlight test is a particularly important neurologic test for determination of the afferent function of the optic nerve and pupillary reflex pathways. The swinging back and forth of the flashlight is best done from below the eyes rather than from the side.

The reaction to accommodation is best tested by holding one fingertip directly in front of the eye being tested and about 4 inches away from the eye. Ask the patient to look alternately at the fingertip and at the far wall directly beyond the finger. Observation of the pupil will be greatly simplified because the eye will not move.

If the pupil reacts to light, it ordinarily may be assumed that the reaction to accommodation will be present. Do not check the light reflex with a flashlight approaching from straight ahead, because the patient will accommodate on the light source as on any other object. You should bring the light in from the side (which also is the best position during inspection of the eye). Failure to react to light with preservation of the accommodation reflex (Argyll Robertson pupil) is characteristic of central nervous system syphilis. Careful checking of the accommodation response is mandatory if light response is absent. Absence of the light reflex should not be diagnosed unless the examination has been done in a darkened room and with a bright light source.

Pupils are normally smaller in infancy and old age. Anisocoria, a readily observable difference in pupil size, occurs in 5% of apparently normal persons. Unless the patient is aware of the previous existence of such a pupil change, it should be regarded with great suspicion, because it may indicate serious neurologic or ocular disease. If normal, these pupils should react properly to light and accommodation, although the size difference may persist. Furthermore, the pupil should be perfectly round. Associated neurologic symptoms such as visual loss, redness, or pain of the eye, usually indicate that the anisocoria is a sign of disease rather than a normal variant. To aid a future physician, it is desirable to call the patient's attention to the presence of anisocoria.

Since mydriatics and miotics are frequently used medications, inquiry as to the use of drops is pertinent when examining a patient with pupil changes.

Enlargement of the pupil *(mydriasis)* may be caused by ocular injury (recent or old), acute glaucoma, systemic poisoning by parasympatholytic drugs, or local use of dilating drops. Constriction of the pupil *(miosis)* is seen in iris inflammation, in glaucoma patients treated with pilocarpine, as an effect of morphine, and physiologically in sleep.

Irregularity of pupil contour is *invariably* abnormal, occurring in iritis, syphilis of the central nervous system, trauma, and congenital defects.

Intraocular pressure. A crude estimate of intraocular pressure may be made by indentation of the eye with the examining fingers. Pressure measurement is important, because elevated intraocular pressure, known as *glaucoma*, causes slow death of nerve fibers and is responsible for 12% of blindness in the United States. The determination of intraocular pressure by finger tension is a rather crude test that will detect only gross

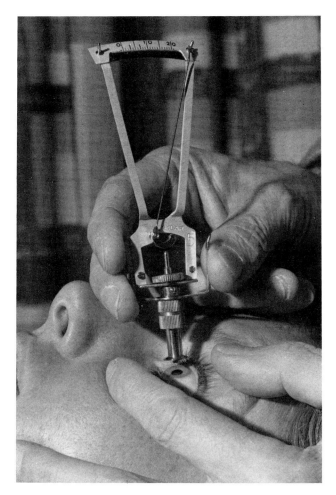

Fig. 5-14. Tonometer measurement of intraocular pressure. Pressure measurement is important in persons over 40 years of age because chronic simple glaucoma exists in 2% of patients in this age group.

pressure alterations. Greater accuracy requires use of a tonometer (Fig. 5-14). Early detection of lesser increases in pressure also requires use of a tonometer. Routine tonometry is desirable in patients over 40 years of age. This technique should be learned under the supervision of an ophthalmologist.

The technique of finger tension (Fig. 5-15) is best explained by first describing what it is *not*. You are *not* ballotting the eye in the orbit as you would a liver in an ascitic abdomen. You are *not* measuring orbital compressibility as you investigate for thyrotropic exophthalmos caused by increased orbital tissue volume. You *are* indenting the eye and feeling for the rebound of the sclera as your finger withdraws.

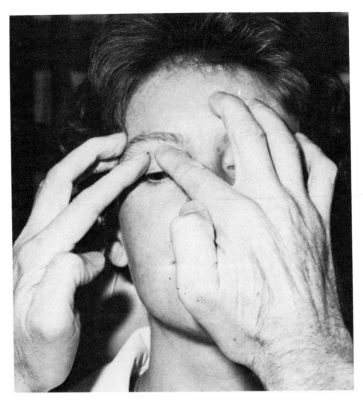

Fig. 5-15. Finger pressure technique. This gross screening procedure is effective in determining only rather large increases or decreases in pressure. This is particularly valuable in the differential diagnosis of a red eye.

The most reliable estimates of intraocular pressure are obtained by pressure on the sclera, and not on the cornea, which gives a false impression of abnormal firmness. If the patient simply closes his eyes, Bell's phenomenon will turn his cornea upward to an unpredictable degree. It is best to have him look down and then to palpate the sclera through the upper lid. One finger alone cannot distinguish between indentation of the globe and displacement of the entire eye into the orbital fat. Because of orbital compressibility, even a glass eye may seem soft to one finger. You must use two fingers, preferably both forefingers. Gentle alternating pressure is applied to the upper sclera. The advancing finger holds the whole eye in position against the orbital fat and is not used to interpret softness. The rebound of the depressed sclera against the withdrawing finger is the most reliable criterion of intraocular pressure.

To understand the technique of alternating finger pressure estimation of intraocular pressure, you need a large marble, approximately the size of an eye. Place the marble on a soft surface, such as your abdomen, which will simulate the orbital fat suspension of the eye. With one finger, press alternately firmly and lightly on the marble. Repeat with

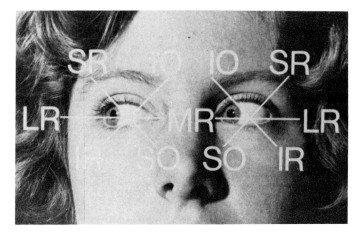

Fig. 5-16. Cardinal positions of gaze. Inability to move the eye into the positions specified indicates paralysis of the corresponding extraocular muscle.

similar pressure on your upper eyelid as you look downward. This one-finger technique cannot differentiate between indentation of the structure (eye or marble) and its displacement. You do *not* use one finger to estimate intraocular pressure; the preceding actions are requested to demonstrate to you why use of one finger will *not* produce valid results. Now alternately press with two fingers, never completely releasing pressure with either finger. You seek to maintain a constant pressure on the eye or the marble, which we will call 100% pressure. At one extreme your right forefinger should exert 90% of the pressure; the left, 10%. Conversely, at the other extreme the left forefinger should exert 90% of the pressure. Your goal is to maintain the marble pushed into your abdomen (or the eye into the orbit) at exactly the same depth at all times, using exactly the same 100% total of pressure from the combined two fingers. As you practice this, you will recognize that you can tell the eye is indented because it rebounds against the withdrawing finger, whereas the marble does not do this. The fingers should be so close together as to touch each other. Only the very gentlest pressure, barely felt by the eye, is necessary. You must use two fingers.

Extraocular muscles. Straightness of the eyes is most easily demonstrated by observing the reflection of a light on the cornea. The flashlight should be held directly in front of the examiner's eyes and the patient's gaze directed at the light (Fig. 5-16). Normally the light reflection is symmetrically situated in the two pupils. An asymmetrical light reflex will readily betray a deviating eye.

A paralyzed extraocular muscle may be one cause of ocular deviation. Muscle paralyses are best detected by moving the eyes into the six cardinal positions of gaze (Fig. 5-16). These cardinal positions are chosen because the muscle designated is paralyzed if the eye will not turn to a given position (Table 1).

Confusion often arises because of the different perspectives of the physiologist and the

Table 1. Six cardinal positions of gaze

Position to which eye will not turn	Paretic muscle
Straight nasal	Medial rectus (third nerve)
Up and nasal	Inferior oblique (third nerve)
Down and nasal	Superior oblique (fourth nerve)
Straight temporal	Lateral rectus (sixth nerve)
Up and temporal	Superior rectus (third nerve)
Down and temporal	Inferior rectus (third nerve)

clinician in the evaluation of eye movements. The physiologist is interested in the function of a muscle acting alone. The clinician wishes to detect which muscle is paralyzed. The cardinal positions are so designated because only the specified muscle can rotate the eye there. No other muscle or combination of muscles can do so.

Note that straight up and down are *not* cardinal positions of gaze. Be sure to carry the fixation point well out to the extremes of gaze in order to exaggerate a defect, thereby permitting easy recognition.

When looking far to the side, some eyes will develop a rhythmic twitching motion (end-positional nystagmus). The quick portion of end-positional nystagmus is always in the direction of gaze and is followed by a slow drift back. This differentiates end-positional nystagmus (a benign condition) from pathologic nystagmus (in which the quick component is always in the same direction, regardless of the direction of gaze).

The complaint of diplopia should initiate careful investigation of muscle function. The *cover test* is a more delicate method than simple observation to determine whether the eyes are straight, and this test is capable of recognizing deviations of less than 5 degrees. While the patient looks with both eyes at a specific fixation point (such as a flashlight), one eye is covered by a card or other type of occluder as the examiner sights over the flashlight (Fig. 5-17). Watch the uncovered eye. If this eye moved to fix on the light, it was not straight before the other eye was covered. If the uncovered eye did not move, then it was straight. Repeat the test for the other eye. Normally both eyes should be perfectly straight by this test.

The *alternate cover test* shifts occlusion back and forth from one eye to the other as the patient looks at the fixation light. Watch the eye that is just being uncovered. As shown in Fig. 5-18, an eye may turn in while covered. When occlusion is shifted to the other eye, a corrective outward movement will straighten the eye just uncovered. Simultaneously the newly covered eye will turn in by the same amount, because the angular relationship of the two eyes with each other remains unchanged. Movement of less than 5 degrees (estimated or measured by a prism) is normal in this test, since this much deviation may result from blocking binocular fusion reflexes.

A deviation recognizable by the cover test is a manifest strabismus (tropia). A deviation identifiable only by the alternate cover test is a latent strabismus, compensated for by binocular vision (phoria). See Chapter 16 for additional description.

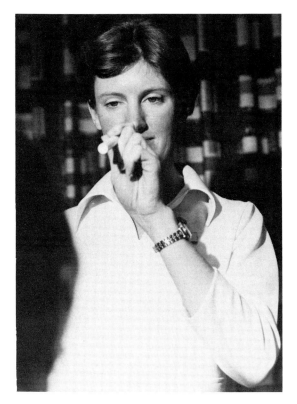

Fig. 5-17. The examiner should sight over the top of the flashlight to observe the corneal light reflexes.

Fig. 5-18. In esophoria either eye will turn in when covered, although it is perfectly straight when uncovered.

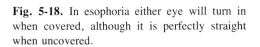

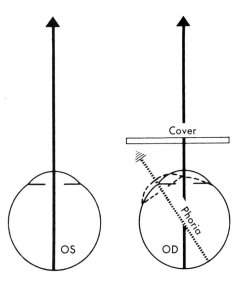

Orbit. The position of the eye in its bony socket may be altered by tumor, inflammation, trauma, thyroid disease, or developmental defect (Fig. 5-19). Forward displacement is termed *exophthalmos;* backward displacement is termed *enophthalmos.* Although abnormal prominence of the eye is recognizable by inspection, a false impression of exophthalmos may be produced by widely open lids, and enophthalmos may be simulated by a drooping upper lid.

Measurement of exophthalmos may be done by placing a millimeter ruler so that it extends straight forward from the lateral orbital rim. If the examiner sights the corneal apex over the ruler from a lateral position, he will obtain a rough measurement of the distance the cornea protrudes anteriorly from the lateral orbital rim. Normal measure-

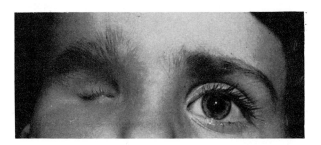

Fig. 5-19. Extreme microphthalmia has resulted in failure of the orbit and lids to develop. This cosmetic deformity could have been avoided by placing an artificial eye in the socket and making it gradually larger to force growth of the lids.

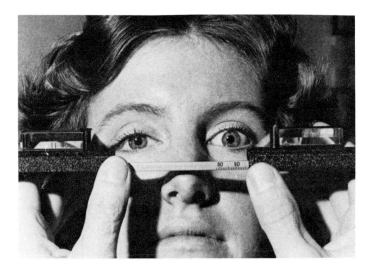

Fig. 5-20. The exophthalmometer measures the anteroposterior distance between the corneal apex and the lateral orbital rim.

ments rarely exceed 18 mm. The examiner must guard against errors of parallax in this determination. This is the principle of the exophthalmometer (Fig. 5-20).

Orbital compressibility is estimated by pressing firmly on the eye through closed lids. Normally the eye may be displaced at least 0.5 cm into the orbital fat. Increased resistance to compression results from abnormal tissue (inflammatory infiltrate or tumor) within the orbit. Sometimes a tumor mass may be palpated by introducing the little finger between the orbital rim and the eye. More effective palpation for orbital tumor is possible if the examiner stands behind the patient.

The orbital rims may be displaced by fracture. Do not mistake the occasionally palpable infraorbital and supraorbital notches for fractures. These contours are best investigated by passing a finger about the orbital edge.

Color vision. Accurate color vision testing requires use of the test charts in daylight or in illumination by special bulbs producing light of all spectral wavelengths. The incomplete spectrum of some fluorescent light invalidates color testing.

About 5% of males have inherited deficiencies in recognition and distinction of red-green wavelengths. Such color deficiencies are nonprogressive and untreatable and are not associated with other ocular or systemic defects. Severely affected individuals may have trouble in distinguishing traffic lights and in occupations requiring color discrimination.

Transmission disorders of the optic nerve (for example, retrobulbar neuritis, the demyelination of the papillomacular bundle that may occur in multiple sclerosis) impair color vision. Such acquired color defects usually persist even after the acute episode subsides and visual acuity returns to near normal; hence, color vision testing is a sensitive means of detecting conduction disease of the optic nerve.

As part of a complete neurologic examination, have the patient read the set of color plates with each eye separately. Record as a fraction: numerator (number of plates recognized) over denominator (number of plates tested). For example, OD $^3/_{14}$; OS $^{10}/_{14}$ means that a test book of 14 color plates was used for each eye, that the right eye recognized 3 plates, and that the left eye recognized 10 plates. A substantial difference such as this identifies a defect of the right optic nerve, provided that the eye itself is normal. Obviously, an eye with a dense cataract cannot read the color plates.

Visual fields. A crude estimate of the function of the visual pathways may be obtained by confrontation testing of the peripheral extent of the field of vision. With one eye covered, the patient must look steadily straight ahead at a specific fixation point, not at the test object approaching from the periphery. A small object, such as a pencil, should be used rather than a gross object, such as the hand. This object is placed behind the patient, beyond the limits of the field of vision and advanced centripetally until seen. Normally a patient should see about 50 degrees upward, 60 degrees nasalward, 70 degrees downward, and 90 degrees temporally as measured from the anteroposterior axis of the eye (Fig. 5-21). At least eight equally spaced meridians should be tested for each eye. (See the discussion on neuroophthalmology in Chapter 12 for a more detailed description of visual field measurement by use of perimetry—Fig. 5-22).

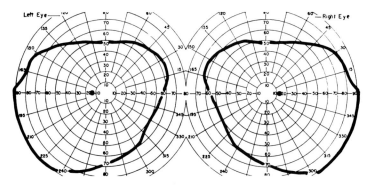

Fig. 5-21. Normal visual fields. The extent of the field in each direction is indicated in degrees.

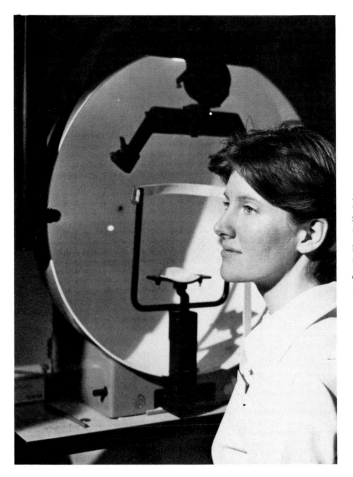

Fig. 5-22. Use of a hemispheric perimeter permits very sensitive quantitative measurements of the visual field, far superior to confrontation testing.

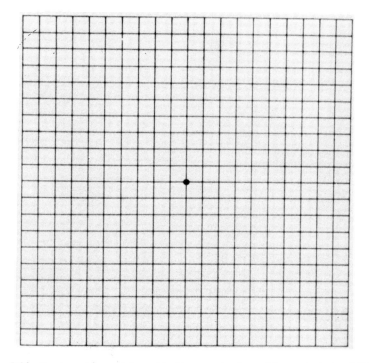

Fig. 5-23. Amsler grid, used for subjective examination of the central visual field.

Use of an Amsler grid (Fig. 5-23) is a simple and rapid way of examining the central portion of the visual field. The patient is asked to look at the central fixation dot. The eye not being examined is covered. Absence or distortion of any part of the grid pattern is described by the patient. Information derived from this measurement corresponds fairly closely to the results of perimetric examination of the central field, although the blind spot is not identifiable.

Alterations in the visual field may be the result of ocular disease (such as glaucoma or chorioretinitis) or central nervous system disease (such as syphilis or pituitary tumor).

BIOMICROSCOPY

With the aid of a slit-lamp biomicroscope, the structure of the eye may be examined under very high magnification and with finely controlled illumination (Fig. 5-24). The technique is too complex and specialized to warrant description here, but you should seek a demonstration of biomicroscopy from an ophthalmologist. The details revealed by such scrutiny are truly fascinating.

An increasing number of emergency rooms are being equipped with slit lamps, which thereby become available for use by the nonophthalmologist. Up to 10% of emergency room visits are for the evaluation of eye problems. No question about it, you can evaluate

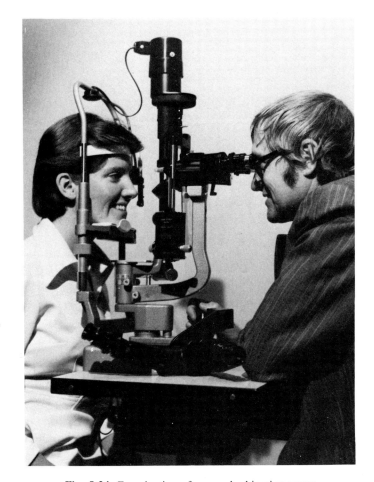

Fig. 5-24. Examination of an eye by biomicroscopy.

the status of the anterior portion of the eye much better with a slit lamp than with any other instrument.

A slit lamp is a microscope (which you already know how to use) that can be moved very precisely with a joystick. The microscope is combined with a narrow slit of light that is focused at the same point as is the microscope. All you need to do is position the slit lamp's focal point at the part of the eye to be examined. It is not all that hard to learn from demonstration by an ophthamologist.

USE OF THE OPHTHALMOSCOPE

Thorough physical examination should always include careful study of the details of the posterior eye (fundus) with an ophthalmoscope. In addition to the detection of ocular

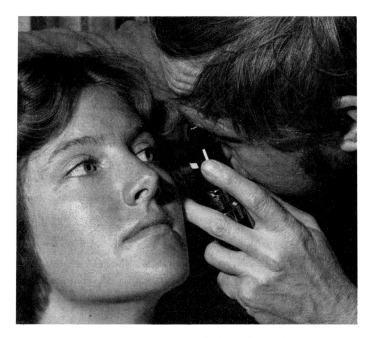

Fig. 5-25. Proper position for ophthalmoscopic examination. The ophthalmoscope is most effective if brought very close to the patient.

disease, this procedure will permit the diagnosis of many serious systemic disorders. Because a careful study of the retina, vessels, and optic disc is so often important to the diagosis of both local and systemic disease, it is often desirable to dilate the pupils, permitting a much more adequate examination of the fundus.

Successful ophthalmoscope examination requires cooperation from the patient. He must hold his eyes still. It is helpful to point out a distant object at which you want him to look (or pretent to look if your head interferes). If he is seated and you are standing, the optimal direction of gaze is about 20 degrees upward and temporally (Fig. 5-25). A darkened room is necessary for proper examination. Dilatation of the pupil with 2½% phenylephrine hydrochloride greatly simplifies the examination. Glasses need not be worn by the examiner or the patient unless a high degree of astigmatism is present. Both the examiner and the patient should keep both eyes open.

The ophthalmoscope is held in the examiner's right hand and before his right eye during examination of the patient's right eye. (The left hand and eye are used to examine the patient's left eye.) The index finger rests on the lens wheel to permit focusing during observation. The head of the ophthalmoscope should be braced firmly against the physician's brow or nose, with the viewing aperture positioned exactly in front of his eye. This position of the ophthalmoscope and physician will not be changed during any part of the examination. Because of the great importance of firm fixation of the ophthalmoscope against the examiner's head, the beginning student should place the ophthalmoscope in this position and turn his head about in various practice directions as he looks through the aperture. Failure to maintain proper position will result in misalignment of the eye and viewing aperture, with consequent loss of the fundus view.

A number of more or less useless apertures and colored filters are incorporated into most ophthalmoscopes. The small, round, white light is best for almost all purposes. The light of a modern ophthalmoscope is so bright with fresh batteries as to be uncomfortable. Adjust the light so that you can see fundus detail easily, but do not use the maximum power until the battery begins to fail. You will enjoy greater cooperation from the patient if you avoid use of excessively bright lights. It is probably easiest to start with the ophthalmoscope lens set at zero (unless the examiner has a significant spherical refractive error that can be corrected by the ophthalmoscopic lens). Red (minus) numbers focus farther away; black (plus) numbers focus nearer.

Looking through the aperture of the ophthalmoscope, which is held firmly against his head, the examiner should approach to within 1 foot of the patient and direct the light into the pupil. A uniform red glow (the red reflex) (see Plate 1) will now be seen to fill the pupil in all normal eyes. Opacities in the clear portions of the eye will appear as black defects within the red reflex. Absence of the red reflex indicates that some abnormality is blocking transmission of light through the eye or that the ophthalmoscope is not properly positioned.

Always keeping the red reflex in sight, the physician should approach the patient's eye until his forehead touches the patient's forehead. Loss of the red reflex during the approach means the light is not directed into the pupil and is best corrected by backing away until the red reflex is again located. Another possible cause for loss of the red reflex is blinking by the patient. If this interferes with the examination, the examiner's free hand may rest on the patient's head and his thumb may be gently used to elevate the upper lid. To prevent bumping the patient's nose with the ophthalmoscope, its handle should be directed down and slightly away from the patient, a position achieved by the examiner's tilting his head.

In contact with the patient's forehead, the examiner should now perceive some fundus detail, such as a vessel, pigment, or the optic disc. Whatever detail is first encountered should be brought into sharp focus by rotating the lens wheel as necessary. Because the patient's eye is only 1 inch away, the examiner will reflexly converge and accommodate. Since the amount of this accommodation may be variable, it interferes with focusing and causes the picture to blur and clear in annoying fashion. This problem is easily avoided if the examiner pretends he is looking through the patient's head at some distant landscape. Focusing should be done with the lens wheel, not by the examiner's accommodation.

In systematic examination of the fundus, the examiner should first locate the optic disc. If the ophthalmoscope light is directed into the eye from a position about 15 degrees temporal to the straight-ahead gaze of the patient, the optic disc will be the first detail seen (see Plate 2). If not located immediately, the disc may be found by following down the vessel bifurcations, just as following down the branches of a tree will lead to the trunk.

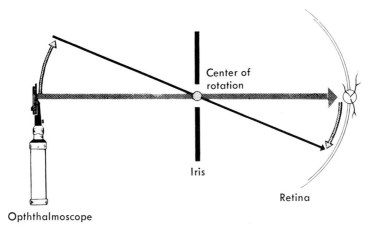

Opththalmoscope

Fig. 5-26. To look at another part of the retina requires movement of the ophthalmoscope so that the rotation of the beam of light is centered at the pupil.

When the ophthalmoscope light is moved from one part of the retina to another, the beginner will often lose the fundus view completely. This is because the light has been moved so that it no longer enters the pupil. To understand this problem and its correction, refer to Fig. 5-26, which illustrates the beam of light passing between the ophthalmoscope and the retina. Illumination of another part of the retina requires movement of the oph-thalmoscope (together with the examiner's head) in the opposite direction so that rotation of the light beam is centered at the pupil.

Dazzling light reflections from the corneal surface may be annoying, especially during examination of the posterior pole of the eye. These reflections may be avoided by moving the ophthalmoscope very slightly to one side or the other.

The beginning ophthalmoscopist is often frustrated to find that he is unable to see an area of fundus as large as that depicted in the usual photographs. This is because of the different optical system of a fundus camera. You cannot see such a large field with the direct ophthalmoscope.

Examination of the ocular fundus

A definite routine, beginning with the optic disc, should be followed in examination of the fundus, as follows.

Optic disc. The optic disc is the most conspicuous feature of the fundus, and the following details should be noted:

1. *Size*. Normal discs appear of a uniform size that is readily recognized with little experience. High myopic refractive errors magnify the disc; hyperopic errors min-ify it. For example, after cataract extraction the disc looks very small. Fundus distances are conveniently estimated in terms of disc diameters (DD). Thus, a lesion slightly larger than the disc and situated in the upper fundus may be de-scribed as being "1 × 2 DD in size and 3 DD away from the disc at the 1:30

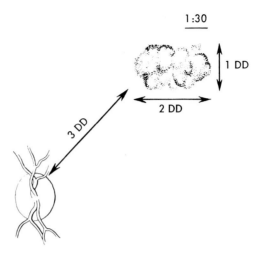

Fig. 5-27. Method of giving the position and dimensions of a lesion in terms of disc diameters.

position (Fig. 5-27). The disc is approximately 1.5 mm in diameter. All fundus details appear magnified 15 times because of the focusing effect of the cornea and lens.

2. *Shape.* The disc is normally round or vertically oval. Gross irregularities in shape and size should not be interpreted as being part of the disc but are ordinarily due to adjacent disease.

3. *Color.* The healthy disc is a creamy pink color because of the rich capillary network, the larger vessels of which are normally just visible. The center of the disc may be grayish and speckled if a deep physiologic cup exposes the lamina cribrosa. Infants have very gray discs that may easily be misconstrued as atrophic.

4. *Margins.* Ordinarily the disc outline is more or less regular, frequently with scattered pigment overlying the margins. Normally it is possible to focus clearly on these physiologic irregularities of the edges, indicating the absence of edema or inflammation. Dense pigment deposits are often situated about the disc margin, especially on its temporal side. As a normal variant, a grayish crescent of sclera is frequently visible immediately adjacent to the disc.

5. *Physiologic depression.* Most discs have a small, pale depression just temporal of the center. It may be quite large but *never* extends completely to the disc margin. It may be deep enough to permit a clear view of the fine fenestrations of the lamina cribrosa.

   The cup/disc ratio (C/D) refers to the relative size of the physiologic cup to the optic disc. This measurement is judged as the horizontal diameter and is expressed as a decimal. For example, if the horizontal diameter of the cup is approximately one third that of the disc, this measurement is recorded as (C/D 0.3. If glaucomatous excavation has destroyed the substance of the entire disc, it is recorded as C/D

1.0. In general, the C/D ratio of the two eyes should not differ by more than 0.2. A C/D larger than 0.5 should be regarded with suspicion, because it occurs in only 5% of normal eyes. The main reason for observing C/D ratios is the search for glaucoma, which causes an increasing excavation in the disc, with progressive atrophy.

Vessels. The central retinal artery and vein appear in the depths of the disk. Bifurcations are variable and may occur deep in the disc or not until the vessel reaches the retina. Each large vessel should in turn be carefully observed along its whole length from disc to periphery.

Arterioles usually are about 25% narrower than veins. Absolute size varies with the number of branches, and it is easily understood that if two veins drain an area fed by one arteriole, the arteriole will be the largest vessel. A narrow band of light, the *arteriolar light reflex,* is reflected from the center of an arteriole. Arterioles and veins may cross and entwine each other in any fashion, but *normal arterioles do not indent* or displace veins. Arteriovenous crossings should be sought out and evaluated for the presence of such abnormal indentations, which are characteristic of arteriolar sclerosis.

Veins are darker in color than arterioles and do not have a prominent light reflex. At the proximal end of the vein overlying the disc there is usually a visible slight pulsation *(spontaneous venous pulsation)* synchronous with the arteriolar pulse. It is caused by the forcing of venous blood out of the eye with each arteriolar systole. External pressure on the eye with a finger during ophthalmoscopic examination will produce venous collapse or pulsation (only at the disc end of the vein) in all normal eyes.

Size, shape, color, and margins are the features important during examination of the optic disc, the vessels, or any abnormal area found within the fundus. Indeed, description of these four aspects of almost anything is a good way to proceed. With respect to the vessels, size should be translated to vessel width, or caliber. Shape refers to the degree of tortuosity or straightness of the vessel. Color differences are most important with respect to the width of the arteriolar light reflex. The most significant margin is at an arteriovenous crossing, at which point arteriosclerotic changes may conceal the underlying vein. (see Vessels in Chapter 8.)

Macula. The macula is an area about 1 DD in size and is situated 2 DD temporal to the disc. It is avascular, not even capillaries being present in its center, and is nourished by the choroid. The minute glistening spot of reflected light seen in the center of the macula represents a pinpoint depression, the *fovea centralis.* Delicate retinal vessels run toward the fovea from all directions. Fine pigment granularity is normally seen in the macula as well as in the periphery of the retina.

If difficulty is encountered in finding the macula, instruct the patient to look directly at the ophthalmoscope light. This will place the macula in the center of the examiner's field of vision. This area deserves careful inspection, since it is the region of the retina with by far the highest visual acuity.

Periphery. Although the retina adjacent to the disc may be seen by aiming the ophthalmoscope beam in different directions, it is necessary to enlist the patient's aid to see further into the periphery. Instruct the patient to look upward as the ophthalmoscope beam is directed upward, to the left as the beam is directed to the left, to the right as the beam is directed to the right, and downward as the beam is directed downward. In this manner the entire periphery of the retina can be visualized.

Background. Various types of background exist normally:

1. Tessellated fundi are fairly darkly pigmented except for prominent, crisscrossing, linear, light orange streaks that represent choroidal vessels (see Plate 17).
2. Albinoid fundi are quite light in color, showing clearly the reddish choroidal vessels lying on the gray-white scleral background (see Plate 2).
3. Negroid fundi are uniformly quite dark.
4. Most fundi are fairly uniform in coloration and of a finely granular texture, with occasionally visible choroidal vessels. The peripheral retina is usually lighter than the central portion.

In a normal eye the pigment granularity of the retinal pigment layer and the choroidal pigment will always be easily recognizable. Linear variations of color due to the choroidal vessels are also visible. Concealment of this underlying pigmentary and vascular pattern is always abnormal and indicates the presence of an abnormal opacity between the ophthalmoscope and the retinal layer. For example, the uniform gray opacity of retina, dead from recent arteriolar occlusion, will conceal this underlying detail, as also will a layer of subretinal fluid in retinal detachment.

During routine evaluation of all areas of the fundus, be constantly aware of this normal pigmentary and vascular background mottling. Its absence denotes disease.

Light reflexes. Light reflexes are glistening movable reflections from undulations in the smooth retinal surface. They characteristically parallel the vessels and often encircle the macula. Light reflexes are more prominent in young persons than in older persons.

Media. After completion of the fundus examination, the more anterior portion of the eye may be examined by turning to higher plus (black) lenses. In sequence, the focus will be on the posterior vitreous, anterior vitreous, and lens, which appear perfectly transparent and invisible in the normal eye. Usually a +15 or +20 lens will be needed to see the iris and cornea at this close distance. About fourfold magnification of the iris results.

Any structure elevated into the vitreous cavity is abnormal. Examples include neoplasm, retinal detachment, and diabetic retinitis proliferans.

PEDIATRIC EXAMINATION

When ophthalmoscopy or external ocular examination must be performed on an uncooperative child, some type of restraint becomes necessary. Distraction with lollipops is better but will not always work. "Mummying" the child by wrapping him snugly in a sheet is the usual method of holding him still. A quicker, simpler, and more effective means of simultaneous immobilization of the head and arms is to lay the child on a cot, take hold of both his elbows, and press his arms firmly against his ears (Fig. 5-28). The parent can

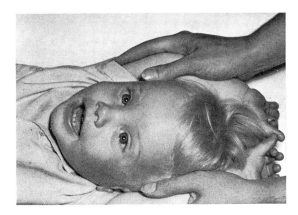

Fig. 5-28. Positioning of an uncooperative child for an eye examination by holding his arms firmly against his head.

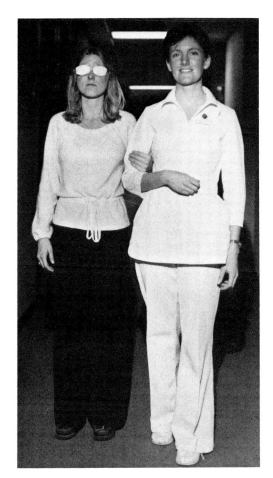

Fig. 5-29. Properly guided, a blind person can walk just as rapidly and confidently as a seeing person.

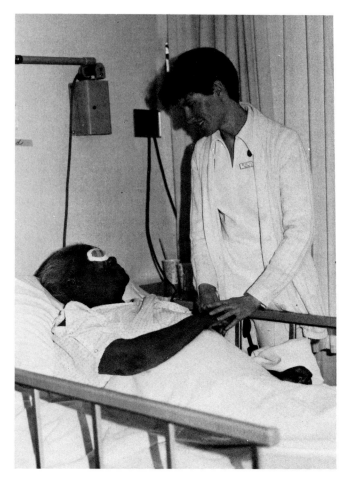

Fig. 5-30. Announce your presence, identity, and purpose when you enter a blind person's room. Under these circumstances, touch is reassuring, whereas a sudden and unexpected touch will startle and frighten a blind patient.

easily be instructed to hold the child in this way during examination. If the child moves his body and legs enough to disturb the eye examination, the parent can lean gently on the child's body by standing beside him rather than above him.

EXAMINATION OF THE BLIND ADULT

The blind adult, just as the child, also requires special consideration. If ambulatory, she needs guidance (Fig. 5-29). In trying to help, most laymen and physicians try to push the blind person where they want her to go. This is most unpleasant, as you can easily experience by closing your eyes while someone else pushes you about. Preferably, place the blind person's hand on your elbow and let her follow you. Allow proper space so that you do not lead the blind person into danger. If the blind person is slightly behind, she can sense what is ahead by your body movements as you shift direction or change pace to signal obstacles.

If confined in a strange hospital bed, the blind person is especially dependent and in need of reassurance (Fig. 5-30). Be considerate of the patient's problems, thoughtful, and gentle.

SUMMARY

Differentiation of diseased structures from the normal is the first aim of all physical diagnostic procedures. This differentiation may be relatively difficult in the presence of some of the more uncommon normal variants that superficially resemble the appearance of serious diseases. Recognition of these normal variants as such assumes considerable practical value, because it avoids unnecessarily frightening the patient and the inconvenience and expense of a consultation.

Proficiency in ophthalmoscopy is gained only through practice. Examining the eyes of every patient will soon lead to a considerable degree of skill in ophthalmoscopy and the ability to recognize normal variants.

Remember that more different types of diseases can be diagnosed with the ophthalmoscope than with any other single examining instrument except one—and that is the autopsy surgeon's scalpel!

RECOMMENDED READING

Moses, R.A.: Adler's physiology of the eye: clinical application, ed. 7, St. Louis, 1981, The C.V. Mosby Co.

Wolff, E.: The anatomy of the eye and orbit, ed. 7, New York, 1976, McGraw-Hill Book Co.

chapter 6   Laboratory Testing

The history, the physical examination, and laboratory testing are the three sources from which we derive the data base of information on which we rely to make a diagnosis and plan appropriate management. Common sense indicates that more laboratory tests will provide a bigger and better data base. Observation of the enthusiasm with which laboratory tests are ordered in teaching hospitals verifies the supposition that more testing is better. Do you really think that more is better?

Bayes theorem, published in 1763, tells us the predictive value of a finding (any finding, whether from the history, the physical examination, or laboratory testing). The value is derived from the sensitivity and specificity of the finding and the prevalence of the condition in the population under consideration. Depending on the prevalence, even the most sensitive and specific finding may vary in predictiveness from a convincing 95% to a useless 2%. Stated differently, if you order several dozen tests at random, in the hope of ''finding something,'' the predictive value of the results is so low as to be useless or even counterproductive.

The diagnostic *sensitivity* of a test or finding means the percent of positive findings in patients who have the disease. The diagnostic *specificity* means the percent of negative findings in patients who do not have the disease. *Prevalence* is the number of cases of the condition existing at a given time in a given population.

The misleading trap into which we fall is that laboratory and clinical findings may be falsely positive or falsely negative. The more highly sensitive a test, the more false-positive results it will produce. The more highly specific a test, the more false-negative results it will produce. Table 2 and Fig. 6-1 show the predictive value of an exceptionally good test: one that is 95% sensitive and 95% specific. Very clearly, prevalence is all important.

You cannot change the sensitivity or specificity of a laboratory test. Therefore, the secret of making laboratory tests work for you is to increase the prevalence of the disease. You accomplish this by means of a careful history and physical examination, whereby you come as close as possible to the diagnosis. Then, you order laboratory examinations specific for the expected disorder.

Tests performed in this way will have the highest predictive value and will produce the fewest false-positive, confusing results. Also, this approach will waste the least amount of money. (In 1975 we spent 6 billion dollars on laboratory tests.)

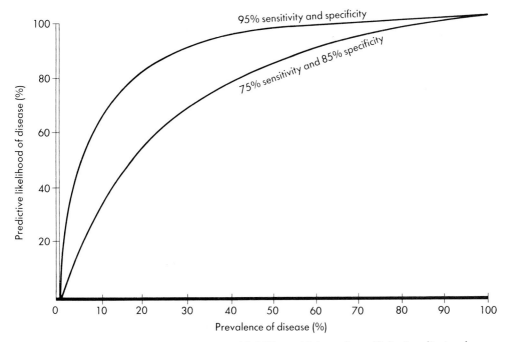

Fig. 6-1. Predictive value of a positive test with 95% sensitivity and specificity *(top line)* and one with 75% sensitivity and 85% specificity *(bottom line)*. (From Havener, W.H.: Ocular pharmacology, ed. 5, St. Louis, 1983, The C.V. Mosby Co.)

Table 2. Influence of prevalence of a disease on the likelihood of a positive test indicating the presence of the disease in a given individual

Prevalence (%)*	Predictive value of a positive test (%)
0.1	1.9
1.0	16.1
2.0	27.9
5.0	50.0
50.0	95.0

From Havener, W.H.: Ocular pharmacology, ed. 5, St. Louis, 1983, The C.V. Mosby Co.
*Effect of prevalence: sensitivity, 95%; specificity, 95%.

SUMMARY

Do not order any laboratory tests until you have asked yourself the following questions:
1. What am I looking for, and why?
2. Could this test change the diagnosis, prognosis, or management of the patient?
3. Have I concentrated the prevalence so that the test will be meaningful?

chapter 7 Interpretation of Ophthalmoscopic Findings

When the mechanical difficulties of ophthalmoscopy have been mastered through practice, the problem of interpretation of the findings arises. The resident training program has taught me that practical experience in seeing a variety of lesions is indispensable—nevertheless, description of the more common abnormal ocular appearances is helpful as a beginning.

OPACITIES OF THE CLEAR MEDIA

Observation of the red reflex is not only helpful in aligning the ophthalmoscope properly before the patient's eye but also provides immediate information as to the health of the transparent portions of the eye. A brilliant, uniform red reflex rules out almost all serious defects of the axial portion of the cornea, aqueous, lens, and vitreous (see Plate 1). Even the smallest corneal scar or cataract will produce an easily observed dark shadow. Vitreous hemorrhage or dense cataract may destroy the red reflex completely. Abnormalities of pupil shape are rendered particularly conspicuous as they outline the red reflex.

Usually the examiner can tell whether the cause of a defect of the red reflex is superficial or deep within the eye simply by ophthalmoscopic observation. Illumination with a bright flashlight is also helpful in localization. Side illumination will strike opacities of the cornea, anterior chamber, or very superficial lens. Straight-ahead flashlight illumination will show opacities within the lens or very anterior vitreous (provided the pupil is dilated). Most vitreous opacities cannot be seen with a flashlight. Hence, if an eye appears normal on external examination, a faulty red reflex will be due to vitreous opacities (provided the examiner has not overlooked a more superficial lesion). Through observation of the red reflex and oblique flashlight illumination, it is usually possible to identify the presence of even small opacities of the media and to localize them accurately in the cornea, anterior chamber, lens, or vitreous. More precise identification of the nature of many of these opacities often cannot be made by ophthalmoscopy. The bright focal illumination and high magnification of the slit-lamp microscope are required for study of diseases of the clear media.

DISC ABNORMALITIES

In the discussion on ophthalmoscopy in Chapter 5, the student is advised to observe disc size, shape, color, margins, and physiologic depression. Abnormalities are recognized by changes in these features.

Size. In most instances the appearance of an excessively large disc is due to adjacent disease (see Plate 3) that is misinterpreted as being part of the disc. This mistake is easily made and is most readily avoided by determining whether the disc itself is of normal size.

Circumpapillary chorioretinal atrophy is relatively common with age or after inflammation near the disc. It appears as a well-defined, pale doughnut or crescent completely or partially surrounding the disc. Pigment clumps are usually scattered irregularly throughout the atrophic area. This irregular pigmentation is more prominent in scars of inflammatory origin than in circumpapillary depigmentation of a spontaneous degenerative origin and thus is an important criterion in differentiation of the two conditions. Visual cells (rods and cones) are destroyed within the atrophic area; hence, the patient has an enlarged blind spot. Except for the rare instance in which the atrophy extends to involve the macula, the patient is unaware of his juxtapapillary field loss and has no symptoms. No treatment is possible or necessary. Some diagnostic interest may arise from the fact that most old circumpapillary choroiditis is associated with presumed histoplasmic choroiditis, as determined by the close correlation with positive histoplasmin skin tests in such patients.

A *myopic crescent* closely resembles circumpapillary atrophy except that the atrophy is usually limited to the temporal or inferior sides of the disc (see Plate 4). This atrophy is slowly progressive, and its appearance is pathognomonic of degenerative myopia. In degenerative myopia diffuse pigmentary loss is also found throughout the fundus.

Coloboma of the disc appears as a large pale inferior elongation of the disc (see Plate 5). It is due to a defective closure of the fetal fissure inferiorly. The retinal vessel pattern is distorted, the origin of the inferior vessels being from the peripheral edge of the abnormally large disc.

Shape. In addition to altering the apparent or real size of the disc, degenerative myopia and coloboma change its shape. Because of a nasal overhang of the retina, a myopic disc may be a narrow, vertically oval shape. The downward extension of a coloboma also produces a grossly abnormal, vertically oval shape. If a disc seems at first to be horizontally oval, careful reinspection will usually disclose the presence of a pale area of fundus adjacent to a round or vertically oval disc.

Normal discs are *not* horizontally oval.

Color. Disc pallor suggests some type of *optic atrophy*, whereas hyperemia may indicate *papilledema* or *optic neuritis*. Because of the wide range of normal variation, only the unusually white or extremely red discs permit diagnosis on the basis of color alone. On observing a normal disc critically, the ophthalmoscopist will find its color to be due to a delicate network of perhaps a dozen or so tiny vessels that do *not* extend beyond the disc margins to the retina. Complete absence of these tiny vessels in all or part of the disc periphery permits a definite diagnosis of optic atrophy. Conversely, abnormal dilatation and prominence of these vessels is the earliest definite sign of papilledema (see Plate 24) or optic neuritis. Comparison of the two discs with each other is often helpful in assessing the significance of a normally variable feature such as disc color. Ordinarily the two normal discs are similar. (Refer to Chapter 12.)

Margins. *Edema* of the disc (which may be due to *trauma, inflammation, ischemia,* or *papilledema*) (see Plate 24) causes its margins to become indistinct and fuzzy. Edematous disc or retinal tissue is less transparent and more gray than normal, may appear slightly thickened, and often has a glistening reflecting surface. *Scar tissue* from any cause may overlie and obscure the disc margins. The general blurring of the fundus picture caused by opacities within the clear media of the eye should not be confused with local disease of the disc or any other portion of the fundus. Examination of the red reflex helps identify blurring due to such opacities.

Physiologic blurring of the optic disc is common and is often mistaken for papilledema or optic neuritis. During embryologic life the hyaloid artery extends from the disc to the lens and is accompanied through the vitreous by a sheath of connective tissue. Variable resorption of this connective tissue occurs, resulting in the two extremes of marked physiologic blurring or pronounced physiologic cupping. Physiologic blurring may cause marked indistinctness of the disc margins, which are usually most blurred near the large vessels. Indistinct sheets of connective tissue may cover the disc and sometimes ensheath the vessels overlying the disc. (Vascular sheathing almost always indicates past or present inflammatory or degenerative disease unless it is on the disc, where it is ordinarily a normal variant.) A *glial veil* is a discrete sheet of cellophane-like connective tissue remnant partially covering the disc. *High central branching* refers to a benign variant of development in which the central retinal vessels protrude slightly forward into the vitreous, returning to the normal retinal level at the disc margin. Hemorrhages, exudates, and visible capillary dilatation are *not* caused by normal embryologic variants.

Physiologic depression. A rim of normal disc tissue *always* separates a physiologic depression from the disc margin (see Plate 12). If an excavation drops back into the nerve immediately at the disc margin (see Plate 26), glaucomatous cupping is the most likely diagnosis. Sometimes other types of *optic atrophy* destroy the peripheral disc tissue, causing an excavated appearance. Not only may the physiologic depression be filled up by edematous tissue, but the disc may also protrude forward into the vitreous cavity by as much as several millimeters in *papilledema* and *optic neuritis. Postinflammatory* scar tissue, *diabetic retinitis proliferans* (see Plate 22), or *embryonic remnants* may lie on the inner surface of the disc or obscure its detail and margins.

VESSELS

During examination of the retinal vessels, particular attention should be directed to their size, shape, color, and margins. A systematic approach should be used to ensure that a diseased vascular segment will not be overlooked. A good method is to follow each large vessel from the disc to the periphery, returning to the disc to locate and follow out the next vessel in orderly clockwise sequence. Especially seek out arteriovenous crossings, for the changes of arteriolar sclerosis are most readily recognized at these sites.

Size (caliber). No figure can be given as the standard diameter of retinal arterioles and veins, because size varies inversely with the number of branches. In general, if an arteriole and a vein supply the same tributary area, the arteriole will probably be about two thirds or three fourths the width of the vein. Another guide to proper vessel size is the relationship of the diameters of the vessels to the diameter of the disc, as perceived by experience.

An *increase in vessel diameter* (Fig. 7-1) is seen in diseases that cause more blood to circulate within the eye or that impede the exit of blood from the eye. These diseases include *polycythemia, carotid cavernous fistula, central retinal vein* (or branch) *occlusion* (see Plate 7), and *papilledema*. Both the arterioles and the veins are dilated in the first two conditions; the veins only are dilated in the latter two. Increased blood volume is ordinarily present in polycythemia and may be sufficiently severe to cause dilatation of vessels. A characteristic bruit identifies carotid cavernous fistula. Obvious flame-shaped hemorrhages will be in the portion of the retina tributary to an occluded venous branch. The hemorrhages and edema of papilledema are confined to the area immediately surrounding the disc.

A *decrease in vessel diameter* results from functional constriction of the vessel walls, reduced inflow of blood into the eye, or retinal atrophy. Typical causes are malignant *hypertension* (see Plate 23), *eclampsia, occlusion of the central retinal artery,* and *retinitis pigmentosa*. All these conditions primarily affect the arteriolar caliber, the venous diameter often being virtually unchanged.

The fundamental change of malignant hypertensive retinopathy (grade III) is arteriolar

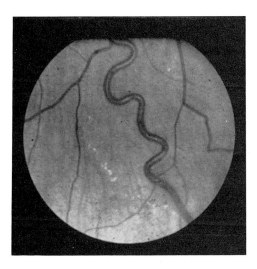

Fig. 7-1. Enormously dilated vessels may lead to a retinal angioma (von Hippel–Lindau disease).

constriction, which may be diffuse or focal. Although conspicuous exudates and hemorrhages are usually also present, these changes are not of value in etiologic diagnosis. Grade IV hypertensive retinopathy is diagnosed by the additional presence of papilledema. Arteriolar attenuation in eclampsia is also associated with hypertension. Renal diseases do not cause retinopathy except through hypertensive changes. (Refer to Chapter 11.)

Occlusion of the central retinal artery is almost the only condition (other than injury) that can cause virtually instantaneous complete monocular loss of vision. Usually, but not always, the occluded arterioles will be recognizably reduced in caliber. A constant finding immediately after occlusion is a gray, edematous discoloration of the area of the retina nourished by the occluded vessel. The gray color is due to dead retinal tissue and therefore is most marked in the posterior part of the eye (where the retina is thicker). In the periphery the retina is so thin that its dead innermost layers may not cause recognizable discoloration or concealment of the underlying choroidal and pigmentary details. Being very thin and nourished mainly by the choroidal circulation, the foveal area remains relatively red (the so-called cherry-red spot). After several weeks the dead inner layers of retinal tissue absorb and disappear, and the fundus may appear normal except for quite variable degrees of arteriolar attenuation and optic atrophy.

Constricted arterioles are typically present in retinitis pigmentosa and a variety of other rare specific retinal degenerations and intoxications. Chorioretinal pigmentary disturbances are usually conspicuous accompaniments of these diseases.

"Nicking" of the arteriovenous crossings refers to a localized apparent or real narrowing of the vein because it is concealed or compressed by the adjacent arteriole. Nicking is a conspicuous and early sign of *arteriolar sclerosis*. Almost all venous branch occlusions occur at an arteriovenous crossing and are due to severe local narrowing of the venous lumen. Generalized arteriolar narrowing is not a diagnostic feature of arteriolar sclerosis.

Emboli are occasionally seen in patients with *cardiac disease* or arise from sites of atherosclerotic degeneration of the internal carotid artery. They appear as glistening gray spots seen within the lumen of an arteriole. Usually the vessel is definitely narrower distal to the embolus. Almost always the embolus will be found at a site of arteriolar bifurcation, a logical location, since the embolus will travel peripherally until it reaches a branch too small to permit further passage.

Shape (distribution and pattern). The greatest distortion of the retinal vessel pattern occurs in *neovascularization*. Newly formed vessels do not follow the orderly branching pattern characteristic of normal retinal vessels. Instead, new vessels follow a tortuous, zigzag course. Such multiple tortuous small vessels often parallel each other or intercommunicate. Newly formed vessels are packed together much more closely than normal vessels, thereby forming localized patches obviously oversupplied with vessels. Neovascularization occurs in *venous occlusion, diabetic retinopathy,* and some types of *chronic chorioretinitis*. The differential diagnosis between these three conditions is easily made by observing the location of the neovascularization and the associated pathologic changes.

Neovascularization due to branch venous occlusion is confined to the region tributary to the occluded branch and is usually greatest near the site of occlusion. The newly formed small veins communicate between the occluded segment and a proximal vein in an obvious attempt to establish a collateral circulation to bypass the block. For many months after the onset of a venous occlusion, large flame-shaped hemorrhages persist in the tributary area of the retina. The occluded venous segment is initially tortuous and distended but may ultimately resemble a gray cord because of changes in the vessel wall and surrounding tissue.

Neovascularization associated with diabetic retinopathy (see Chapter 11) is situated in the posterior portion of the retina and characteristically is much worse in the macular area and near the disc. Its distribution is more diffuse and is not confined to an area tributary to any one venous branch. Neovascularization associated with chronic chorioretinitis is usually in the periphery and is much more localized than the two previously described conditions. Conspicuous gray inflammatory patches are always nearby.

Microaneurysms are commonly present near areas of neovascularization. They appear as tiny discrete red dots in the general range of 20 to 60 μ in diameter (the caliber of a large vessel at the disc is about 100 μ) and represent localized dilatations in the capillary bed (see Plate 21). If no signs of chronic venous occlusion are present, microaneurysms are almost pathognomonic of diabetes.

Beading refers to irregular segmental enlargement of a larger vessel, causing it to assume somewhat the contour of a string of beads. Neovascularization, microaneurysms, and beading occur in venous occlusion, diabetic retinopathy, and some types of chronic chorioretinitis.

Congenital tortuosity of the retinal vessels (see Plate 6) refers to an excessively sinuous course of the large vessels. This differs from the appearance of neovascularization, since the vessels do not intercommunicate and are not packed closely together, and the tortuous pattern is not limited to a small area of the retina. Hemorrhages, microaneurysms, exudates, and other abnormalities are not associated with congenital tortuosity, but it may exist in association with *congenital aneurysms* of the cerebral vessels or *coarctation* of the aorta.

Elevation of vessels anterior to their normal position causes their appearance to become blurred or unrecognizable as the ophthalmoscope follows them peripherally from the disc. Focusing sharply on the rising vessel by adding more plus (black-numbered lenses) to the ophthalmoscope will eliminate the blur (thereby differentiating the condition from the blurring caused by opacities of the media or retinal edema). Elevation of the retinal vessels is caused by *retinal detachment, choroidal melanoma,* or *metastatic tumors* (which characteristically are located in the vascular choroid). A detached retina appears as a translucent gray curtain, behind which is dark and structureless fluid. Melanoma and metastasis cause a solid, fleshy-appearing elevation. *Retinitis proliferans* of diabetes may cause large vessels to grow forward into the vitreous cavity.

Recognizable *displacement* of retinal vessels from their normal position is rare. In *retinopathy of prematurity* (associated with excessive oxygen) shrinkage of connective tissue proliferated on the temporal periphery (which is the last part of the retina to develop) may cause most of the retinal vessels to be pulled over to the temporal side. The majority of vessels are seen to arise from the temporal side of the disc, pass directly across the macula (which is usually avascular), and pursue an unusually straight course toward the temporal periphery. Prolapse of the retina through a *penetrating wound* or *avulsion* of the optic nerve may also displace retinal vessels.

In about 20% of normal persons a *cilioretinal artery* will arise from the temporal side of the disc (see Plate 2). These arteries originate at the edge of the disc from the choroidal circulation and do not communicate with the central retinal artery. The origin of a cilioretinal artery somewhat resembles the disappearance of retinal vessels around the edge of a glaucomatous cup, from which this normal variant must be differentiated.

Color. Critical evaluation will reveal that part of the impression of the ''color'' of a vessel is due to the width of its light reflex. The light reflex is a property of the transparency and reflectiveness of the vessel wall and becomes wider as *arteriolar sclerosis* develops. One of the early and definite signs of arteriolar sclerosis is widening of the arteriolar light reflex to one third or more of the vessel diameter. With progressively increasing severity of arteriolar sclerosis, the color of the retinal vessels will change from red to red-orange, to reddish gray, and finally to dirty gray. Even when the vessel walls are so densely sclerotic that no blood column can be seen, blood may still flow through the lumen. Arteriolar sclerosis causes no visual symptoms unless a secondary vascular occlusion occurs.

Polycythemia causes a dark, cyanotic appearance of both the arteriole and the vein.

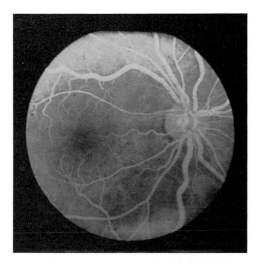

Fig. 7-2. Dilated, cream-colored vessels are seen in lipemia retinalis, the appearance resulting from excessively high blood lipid concentrations, as in diabetic acidosis.

Lipemia retinalis (as seen in severe diabetic acidosis) causes all retinal vessels to assume a creamy pink color (Fig. 7-2).

"Sheathing" of retinal arterioles or veins refers to cellular infiltration of the perivascular spaces. This produces an irregular gray segmental discoloration of the vessel. Causes include *perivasculitis* associated with chorioretinitis, *leukemia*, and sometimes *occlusion* of the vessel.

What we interpret as being the "retinal vessels" is really the blood column. The vessel wall itself is normally transparent and invisible. Loss of the transparency of the arteriolar wall (arteriolar sclerosis) is most easily detected by recognizing the concealment of an underlying vein at an arteriovenous crossing.

Pulsation. During ophthalmoscopy, pulsation of the retinal arterioles is not normally seen. If the intraocular pressure exceeds diastolic blood pressure, the retinal arterioles will collapse during diastole. Such a conspicuous arteriolar collapse may be seen in *glaucoma* or *aortic insufficiency.*

When venous blood flows normally from the eye, the disc ends of the veins usually collapse slightly with each arteriolar systole. Such venous collapse can be perceived in most normal eyes, and in the remainder, gentle external finger pressure on the eye through the lids will cause easily visible venous collapse. Conditions causing venous stasis (*papilledema, optic neuritis,* and *occluded vein*) stop spontaneous venous pulsation and may cause considerable resistance to collapse of the vein by external pressure.

MACULA

Most macular lesions are comparable in appearance and course to the changes of similar etiology that occur throughout the fundus, which are described in the discussion of the periphery. Because of the much higher visual acuity of the fovea, however, a tiny macular lesion may be disabling, in contrast to a considerably larger peripheral lesion that may pass almost unnoticed by the patient. Decreased visual acuity definitely indicates careful ophthalmoscopic examination of the macula. Use of a mydriatic is often necessary for adequate macular visualization.

Having a rich blood supply, the macular region is somewhat more likely than the periphery to be attacked by blood-borne diseases such as metastatic tumors. The infectious agents causing chorioretinitis seem to affect the macula more often than would be expected if localization within the fundus were random.

Heredodegeneration of the macula includes a group of diseases that preferentially affect the posterior pole of the eye. A high proportion of macular lesions found in older patients are heredodegenerative. (Refer to Chapter 9.)

In marked cases of suppression amblyopia associated with strabismus, the fovea of the suppressed eye is not used for fixation. Instead, some adjacent part of the retina is falsely oriented by the brain to have a straight-ahead direction. Fixation may be as much as 2 degrees in error and sometimes more. The higher degrees of eccentricity may be recognized by asking the patient to look at the center of the ophthalmoscope light during fundus examination. If the center of the light now falls on some portion of the retina adjacent to the fovea, nonfoveal fixation is identified. Recognition of eccentric fixation is of great importance because the patient will *not* benefit from occlusion therapy. Many patients have needlessly suffered through months of occlusion of their only good eye in the vain hope of improving vision in the eye with unrecognized eccentric fixation. A special instrument, the Visuscope, permits much more accurate determination of foveal fixation than can be attained with the ordinary ophthalmoscope.

Macular variants. Macular variants may be confusing because the macular area ordinarily is seen very poorly without the aid of a mydriatic. Obstacles to adequate examination are the annoying central corneal light reflections and the maximal light constriction of the pupil occurring with central illumination. Unless a physician uses mydriatics, he may be unfamiliar with the commonly encountered macular appearances. Frequently the macular pigment is clumped into a peculiar granular distribution. A circular reflection, resembling edema, surrounds the macula. Shimmering light reflexes are often most pronounced in this general area temporal to the disc, especially in young patients. Reflections are easily differentiated from exudates or other fixed disorders, because they shift with movement of the ophthalmoscope. The macula will usually be slightly darker than the surrounding retina—either reddish or gray.

PERIPHERY

Throughout their extent, the retina and choroid may be affected by ophthalmoscopically visible disorders. The more common findings include edema, hemorrhage, exudates, drusen, chorioretinitis, myelinated fibers, pigmentary changes, and nevi.

Edema, hemorrhage, and exudates are all rather nonspecific findings that occur in a multitude of different disorders. Contrary to the common impression, an etiologic diagnosis usually *cannot* be made on the basis of these three findings. Diagnosis is usually made on the basis of other findings; for example, flame-shaped hemorrhages of identical appearance are seen in venous branch occlusion and in malignant hypertensive retinopathy. A venous branch occlusion is diagnosed by the distended tortuous appearance of the vein distal to the arteriovenous crossing, which is the site of the block. The flame-shaped hemorrhages will be confined to the area tributary to the involved vein. In hypertension the flame-shaped hemorrhages are scattered throughout the retina, but the diagnostic feature is the marked narrowing of the arterioles.

Even though they are not specific for any given etiology, edema, hemorrhage, and exudates are valuable findings in eye examination, for they are conspicuous signs of disease. They serve as *warning signals* that alert the physician to look more closely for the more subtle features of diagnostic importance.

Edema. An edematous retina is less transparent than normal and hence appears gray. The density of this gray discoloration varies with the amount of edema, ranging from obvious change to an inconspicuous delicate haze that can be recognized only by comparison with the opposite retina. The surface of an edematous retina shows more glistening reflections than normal, although in a young person similar reflections are physiologic. Reflections are identified as such because they move and shimmer as the position of the ophthalmoscope is changed. In contrast, a pathologic finding, such as an exudate, will not move as do reflections.

Edema is present only around recent or continuing lesions and therefore is a sign of active disease. Furthermore, edema is confined to the diseased portion of the retina. In *papilledema* or *optic neuritis,* edema will be confined to the region of the disc. Edema will surround an *active chorioretinitis* but will disappear as the inflammation becomes inactive. Edema is spread diffusely throughout the retina in *hypertensive retinopathy, occlusion of the central retinal artery, ocular contusion,* and so on. When diffuse retinal edema is present, the gray discoloration is always more pronounced posteriorly, since the retina is thickest in the neighborhood of the macula and disc. Edema may transiently occur during certain stages of senile macular degeneration. These diseases are cited as representative examples of conditions causing retinal edema. Edema is present in almost every acute retinal disorder.

Hemorrhage. Almost any red patch found in the retina will be a hemorrhage, and almost all hemorrhages are red. Sometimes a patch of neovascularization is mistaken at first glance for a hemorrhage. Closer inspection will reveal its individual vessels. The large vortex veins of the midperipheral choroid can be seen in blond individuals and may be mistaken for a hemorrhage unless the tributary veins are recognized (see Plate 8). A choroidal hemorrhage underlying normal retinal pigment epithelium will be a dark blue-black color, often with no trace of red color visible.

The retinal structure will shape hemorrhages to conform with tissue planes. The outer retinal neurons run perpendicular to the retina and therefore confine hemorrhages within the deep retina to rather small and rounded shapes. *Diabetes* may cause such small, rounded hemorrhages. They are larger and less sharply outlined than microaneurysms.

Hemorrhages in the nerve fiber layer are oriented radially to the disc and spread out in flattened linear or "flame" shapes. The larger retinal vessels lie in the nerve fiber layer, which is situated on the inner, or vitreous, side of the retina; hence, the hemorrhages of *hypertensive retinopathy* are flame shaped. The preretinal space, between the retina and the vitreous face, is relatively open and permits blood to pool in large, rounded pockets. Gravity causes the red blood cells to sediment inferiorly and the plasma to rise, the two being separated by a more or less sharply defined horizontal line. Rather large preretinal hemorrhages may be found in uncontrolled *blood dyscrasias* (see Plate 9). If hemorrhages break through the vitreous face, red blood cells scatter diffusely throughout the vitreous. Such a distribution of cells obscures fundus details and may even destroy the red reflex. Vitreous hemorrhages are commonly caused by *trauma* and are characteristic of the retinal tears that precede *retinal detachment.*

Intraocular hemorrhages are relatively nonspecific changes and are due to a great variety of ocular and systemic diseases. The preceding examples are meant to indicate that certain types of hemorrhage are more characteristic of some types of disease. However, etiologic diagnosis cannot reliably be based only on the presence of a hemorrhage.

Exudates. Dense, grayish, localized retinal infiltrates are termed exudates. They are of two types, "hard" and "soft." This improbable nomenclature, unverifiable by palpation, is nevertheless useful, for it identifies two distinct types of retinal infiltration. Hard exudates are relatively discrete, with distinct edges and smooth, solid-appearing surfaces. They are *not* translucent. They represent intraretinal lipoid deposits that are gradually formed within diseased retinal areas. Soft retinal exudates are somewhat fuzzy and indistinct gray patches that are usually larger than hard exudates. Soft exudates are microinfarctions of the inner retinal layers and are due to occlusion of tiny arteriolar precapillary branches. Such occlusions can be demonstrated histologically, but the involved vessels are not ophthalmoscopically recognizable. As would be expected, soft exudates may appear rather rapidly, whereas hard exudates require considerable time to develop. Both hard and soft exudates may be caused by the same retinal disease and therefore frequently coexist.

Although exudates are conspicuous signs of disease, they are of absolutely no help in making an etiologic diagnosis. Exudates may occur in all types of *inflammatory* or *degenerative* diseases of the retina and are caused by many *systemic* diseases, including diabetes (see Plate 10), hypertension, and collagen disorders.

Drusen. Drusen (see Plate 11) are commonly seen benign hyaline degenerative deposits on the elastic membrane between the retina and the choroid. They appear as small, rounded, gray or whitish translucent spots, almost always symmetrically located in the two eyes. Drusen are frequently mistaken for hard exudates. This differentiation is important, because the finding of exudates indicates the presence of definite systemic or ocular disease that requires further investigation. The resemblance between these two entities is so close that description of their difference in appearance is difficult. Nevertheless, an experienced ophthalmologist can differentiate them with ease. One of the best gross features is that hard exudates frequently form circular or linear patterns, whereas drusen are haphazardly distributed. Drusen do not signify systemic disease, nor do they interfere with vision (macular exudates usually cause considerable visual disturbance; however, senile macular degeneration is more likely to occur in patients with extensive macular drusen).

Chorioretinitis. Acute focal inflammation of the choroid and retina causes localized infiltration of inflammatory cells. The ophthalmoscopic appearance of this focal infiltration is similar to that of a soft exudate. Accurate differentiation is usually possible on the basis of associated changes. An encircling halo of retinal edema almost invariably surrounds acute chorioretinitis but is not often prominent around exudates. Pigmentation is prominent at the edges of inflammatory lesions after they have been present for a month or so. Exudates lie within the retina and do not affect the retinal pigment epithelium; hence, they *do not* cause pigmentary disturbance. Chorioretinitis has a tendency to recur at a nearby site; hence, the atrophic and pigmented scar typical of old chorioretinitis will often be found adjacent to an acute chorioretinitis. Hemorrhages are often within or immediately adjacent to a focus of chorioretinitis (see Plate 12). Since hemorrhages and exudates often coexist, this feature would seem to be of little diagnostic value; however, the hemorrhages of chorioretinitis are *choroidal* or subretinal, whereas those associated with exudates are intraretinal. Since they are covered by the retinal pigment layer (except in the

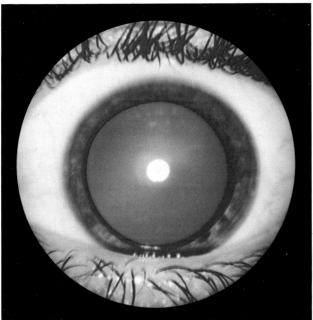

Plate 1. Normal red reflex. The fairly uniform luminous orange reflex visible in all normal eyes gives immediate evidence of the clarity of the media. (The central white disc is the reflection of the photographic light from the cornea and corresponds to the similar, smaller reflection of the ophthalmoscope.) Any opacity of the axial cornea, anterior chamber, lens, or vitreous is conspicuously visible as a dark imperfection in the red reflex.

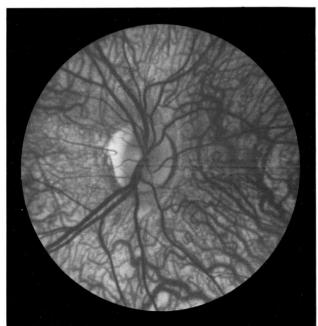

Plate 2. Albinotic fundus. Because of the absence of melanin, the choroidal vessels and the white scleral background are readily seen. A narrow pigment crescent curves around the nasal side of the vertically oval disc. A wider scleral crescent on the temporal side gives, on first glance, the false impression of a round disc with a pale edge. The hook-shaped vessel at the 9:30 position near the disc edge is a cilioretinal artery. The physiologic cup is tiny, giving a C/D ratio of 0.1. Note how much larger normal choroidal vessels are than retinal vessels.

Plate 3. Juxtapapillary chorioretinitis. This is a normal, perfectly healthy, vertically oval disc with a 0.2 C/D ratio. The severe black and white mottling encircling the disc represents old chorioretinitis. An indistinct gray patch about two thirds the size of the disc occupies the macula (to the right side of the disc). Above the macula is an irregular partial halo of subretinal hemorrhage. This appearance is typical of presumed histoplasmic choroiditis. Attention to the size of the disc, with precise recognition of its outside edge, permits accurate classification of this disease as *not* affecting any part of the disc. The disc is neural ectoderm and is *not* affected by mesodermal (identified by the choroidal melanin disturbance) disorders. Histoplasmosis characteristically affects the choroid, the retina suffering only secondary damage.

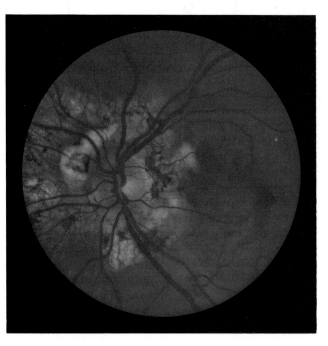

Plate 4. Myopic fundus. The huge temporal scleral crescent, fully as large as the disc itself, is so characteristic as to be termed a "myopic" crescent. The faint pigment granularity remaining on this crescent characterizes a progressively atrophic mechanism of formation, in contrast to the cleaner and more uniform white of a congenital scleral crescent. The disc is vertically oval and slightly tilted, another characteristic feature of myopia. The first false impression, that this is a huge disc, is easily corrected if the ophthalmoscopist first evaluates the *size* of the disc. Almost always a "large" disc is really a normal-sized disc with some type of adjacent pathologic condition.

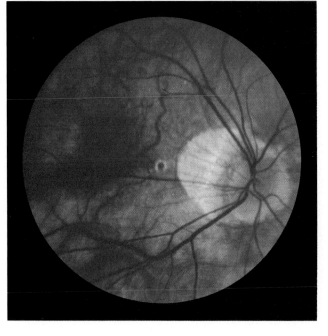

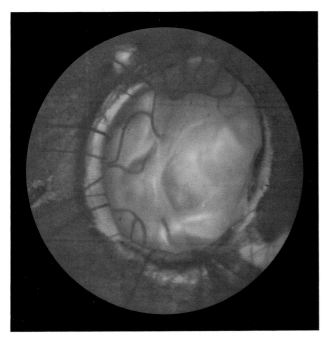

Plate 5. Disc coloboma. Failure of proper closure of the fetal fissure results in a truly enormous "disc," with deeply scalloped excavations. The superior retinal vessels are almost normal in appearance, whereas the remaining vessels are displaced far to the edge, dropping over the edge as in a glaucomatous cup. A glaucomatous cup will not cause enlargement of the disc such as occurs in a coloboma. A rim of sclera of variable width will almost always surround a coloboma. Failure of closure of the fetal fissure may cause islands of white distortion located anywhere on the meridian in the 6 o'clock position, not necessarily continuous with the disc.

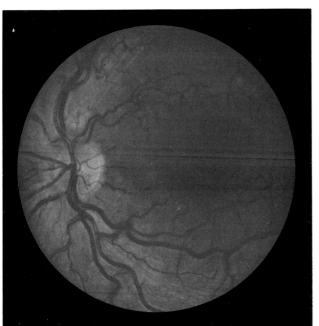

Plate 6. Congenital tortuosity of retinal vessels. The retinal vessels are normally straight or gently curved. Marked angular tortuosity, even if considerably more marked than this, may be entirely physiologic, although it is sometimes associated with intracranial vascular anomalies. Neovascularization is also tortuous, but new-formed vessels are usually of smaller-than-normal caliber and tend to be much more numerous than normal.

Plate 7. Branch retinal vein occlusion. This retinal vein at the 5 o'clock position should have a branch originating about 1 DD below the disc and extending into the hemorrhagic area. Compression from the overlying retinal artery at an arteriovenous crossing has reduced the lumen of the vein sufficiently to cause vascular engorgement and severe intraretinal hemorrhage in the tributary area of this venous branch. Aggregations of hard exudates may be seen above and also to the left of the area of venous stasis. Such discrete lipoidal deposits, forming linear or circular patterns, characteristically surround retinal areas damaged by venous stasis. Masses of intraretinal hemorrhage confined to the tributary area of a vein (shaped roughly like a truncated pyramid) are virtually diagnostic of venous branch occlusion, which may be identified on the basis of the shape alone. The occluded arteriovenous crossing will always be located on the disc side of the hemorrhagic area.

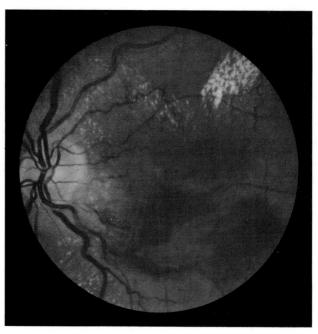

Plate 8. Normal blond periphery. The melanin content of the fundus tends to become more scanty in the periphery; hence, the radial pattern of the numerous choroidal vessels may often be seen in the peripheral fundus (here, inferiorly), especially in blond individuals. The retinal vessels are smaller, more sharply defined, and lie in front of the choroidal vessels.

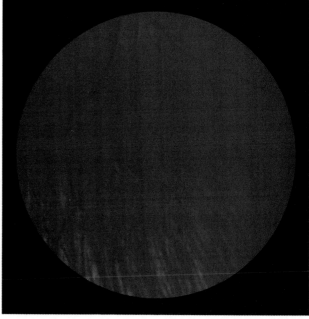

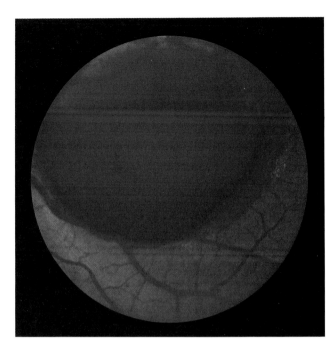

Plate 9. Preretinal hemorrhage. A preretinal hemorrhage is actually confined between the nerve fiber layer and the inner limiting membrane of the retina; hence, it does not extend into the vitreous. Note the sharp and clear fundus details, not in the least obscured by any vitreous hemorrhage. As would be expected, a preretinal hemorrhage covers and conceals the retinal vessels. Red blood cells settle by gravity, leaving a flat top between the blood cells and the overlying pocket of relatively transparent serum. Although red blood appears red when it is in front of the retinal pigment cell layer, preretinal blood may appear black if it is sufficiently dense or is in shadow. Note the progressive darkening of the hemorrhage toward its bottom and the linear dark shadow at its flat top.

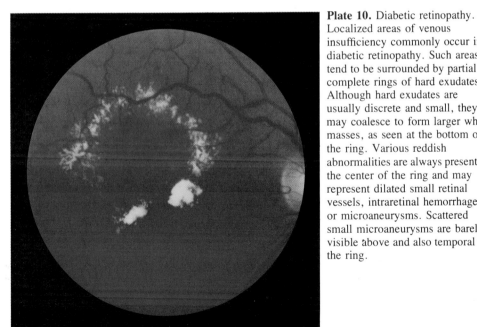

Plate 10. Diabetic retinopathy. Localized areas of venous insufficiency commonly occur in diabetic retinopathy. Such areas tend to be surrounded by partial or complete rings of hard exudates. Although hard exudates are usually discrete and small, they may coalesce to form larger white masses, as seen at the bottom of the ring. Various reddish abnormalities are always present in the center of the ring and may represent dilated small retinal vessels, intraretinal hemorrhages, or microaneurysms. Scattered small microaneurysms are barely visible above and also temporal to the ring.

Plate 11. Drusen of macula. Drusen are small hyaline deposits on the lamina vitrea. Although comparable in size to hard exudates, drusen are relucent and never form circular or linear patterns. As is evident, they may be variable in size and may also become confluent. Drusen may be located in patches in either the macula or the periphery, or they may be scattered randomly throughout the fundus. The distribution in the two eyes is usually strikingly symmetrical. So long as no melanin disturbance is associated with macular drusen, they do not affect vision. A type of senile macular degeneration may develop in some eyes with heavy macular deposits of drusen.

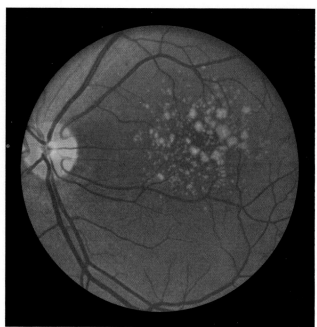

Plate 12. Acute hemorrhagic chorioretinitis. Macular histoplasmosis, a primarily choroidal disease, is characterized by a white central inflammatory focus. Damage to the choroidal vessels and the outer layers of the fundus often causes hemorrhages, which may be either subretinal (red) or beneath the retinal pigment layer (dark). Red subretinal hemorrhages are seen above and below this macular lesion. The indistinct dark area between the disc and the macula represents neovascularization and hemorrhage beneath the retinal pigment layer. The disc is entirely normal, with a C/D ratio of 0.4. The vitreous is perfectly clear in histoplasmosis (in contrast to toxoplasmosis, which is a retinal disease and discharges leukocytes into the vitreous).

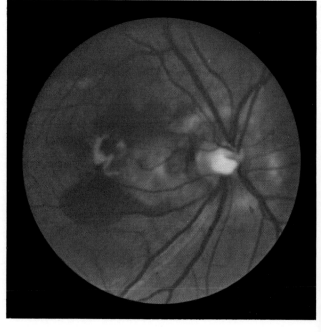

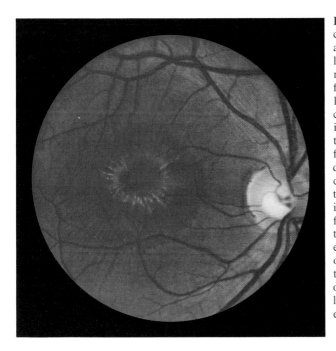

Plate 13. Acute macular chorioretinitis. Inflammatory cells are oriented radially in the nerve layers of the macula. In the macula this radial pattern is formed by the outer molecular layer (between cones and bipolar cells). A small deep hemorrhage in the center of the "star" marks the exact location of the acute focal infection. A faint reddish disc, a little larger than 2 DD in diameter, marks the extent of tissue edema surrounding the inflammatory focus. Note the faint circular reflection outlining the lower nasal edge of the edema. When the ophthalmoscope is positioned so that the angles of incidence and of reflection coincide, a bright line can be seen at the edge of an edematous area.

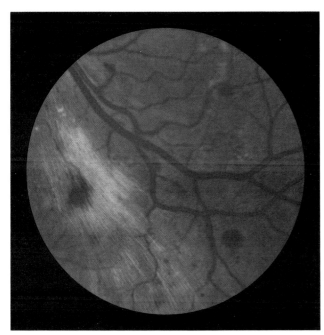

Plate 14. Myelinated nerve fibers, diabetic hemorrhages, and microaneurysms. The feathery, linear white streaks represent developmental myelination of the nerve fiber layer of the retina. The diabetic vasculopathy is purely coincidental, but it stands out conspicuously against the white contrast. Myelinated fibers may or may not adjoin the disc. They must always be oriented in the generally radial (with respect to the disc) direction of the nerve fiber layer. If densely confluent, the center of a myelinated patch may be uniformly white; only the edge farthest from the disc may show an identifiable feathery edge. I repeat, myelination does *not* cause hemorrhage or any other pathologic condition.

Plate 15. Old chorioretinitis. Acute inflammation results in localized tissue disruption, particularly recognizable as a gross granularity of the melanin, which tends to clump within the affected area and to deposit in a peripheral ring of variable density. Choroidal vessels and the sclera become abnormally visible within the area of pigment disruption. A sharp margin usually separates the scar from the adjacent normal fundus.

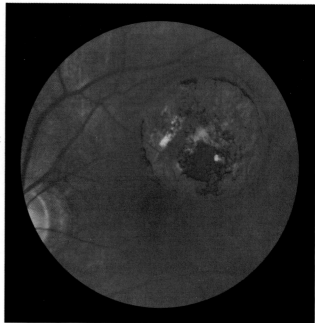

Plate 16. Retinitis pigmentosa. The angular and linear branching pattern (bone corpuscle, chicken track) or perivenous melanin deposition, distributed in a circular pattern in the near periphery of the fundus and bilaterally symmetrical, is characteristic of retinitis pigmentosa. Note the pale and atrophic disc and the severely constricted (threadlike) arterioles—features also typical of retinitis pigmentosa.

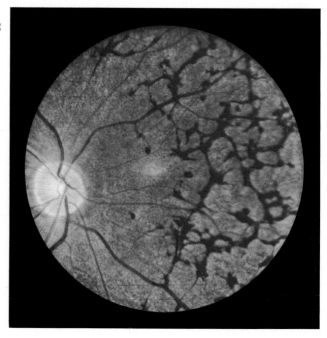

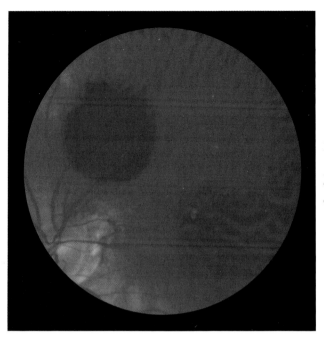

Plate 17. Choroidal nevus. A dark, rounded, circumscribed, not elevated, patch of melanin lies above the disc. This represents a localized, developmental, benign hyperpigmentation of the choroid. Temporal to the disc is another, less dense hyperpigmentation. The choroidal vessels can be seen to course through this temporal lesion, confirming its intrachoroidal location. A scleral crescent is temporal to the disc. The background pattern of visible choroidal vessels is referred to as "tessellated."

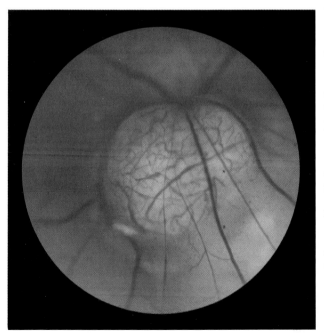

Plate 18. Amelanotic melanoma, retinal detachment. A 4 DD, markedly elevated mass encroaches on the disc from below. Large vessels are present within the tumor and are critically necessary to the diagnosis of the neoplasm. This atypically pale melanoma has been selected because it shows the internal vessels nicely, and it dispels the notion that all melanomas are densely black; most are not. All diagnosable melanomas are elevated, and recognition of any elevated fundus lesion is of serious import. A dependent serous retinal detachment extends downward from the tumor as a gray area through which the normal background pigment and vascular pattern cannot be seen.

Plate 19. Senile macular degeneration. A patch of pigment granularity almost 2 DD in size occupies the macular area. The gross destruction caused by macular chorioretinitis is not present, and the underlying sclera and large choroidal vessels are not grossly visible. A faint choroidal vascular pattern is recognizable on careful scrutiny. The condition tends to be bilateral, although asymmetrical in its intensity.

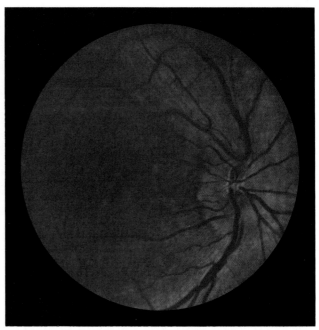

Plate 20. Old disciform macular degeneration, angioid streaks. Degenerative breaks in the lamina vitrea permit subretinal invasion of neovascularization and connective tissue. Acute hemorrhages may occur, with sudden loss of vision and massive dark elevations simulating melanoma of the choroid. With time, the blood absorbs and is replaced by white or irregularly pigmented subretinal scar tissue, as shown here. Faint streaks concentric to the disc and radiating toward the 1 o'clock position are breaks in the lamina vitrea (angioid streaks) that may be associated with pseudoxanthoma elasticum, a generalized heredodegeneration of elastic tissue.

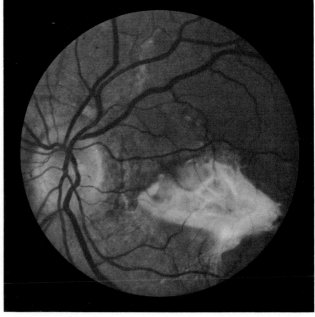

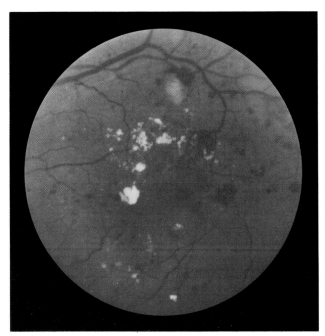

Plate 21. Diabetic retinopathy. Diffusely scattered and bilateral small intraretinal hemorrhages, hard exudates, and microaneurysms are pathognomonic of diabetic retinopathy.

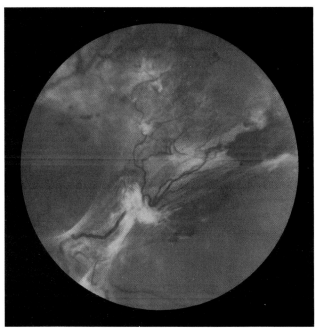

Plate 22. Diabetic retinitis proliferans. Deposition of delicate sheets of connective tissue and new vessels on the anterior surface of the retina may occur in severe diabetic retinopathy. This tissue characteristically shrinks and condenses, forming the heavy linear and curvilinear bands of preretinal tissue shown here. Hemorrhages result when the force of contraction tears vessels. The proliferating tissue lies in front of the retinal vessels, and when dense tissue masses form, they conceal these vessels. Large newly formed vessels may extend into the vitreous cavity and are entirely independent of the retina except at their origin.

Plate 23. Hypertensive retinopathy. The macular star of hard exudates is the most conspicuous abnormality of this photograph, but it is a nonspecific finding of no etiologic diagnostic value. The marked attenuation of the arterioles is the diagnostic feature of malignant hypertension. Incompletely shown in the picture, the margins of the disc are blurred, indicating a grade IV severity of the retinopathy. The pale area beneath the vein near the 12 o'clock position is a soft exudate (microinfarction).

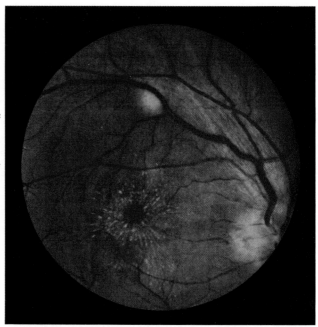

Plate 24. Papilledema. Hyperemia of the disc is the classic consequence of disc venous stasis resulting from increased intracranial pressure. The resultant swelling and edema obscure the disc margins so that no trace of the disc edge is visible here. The disc is slightly elevated, and no physiologic depression is visible. Spontaneous venous pulsations are absent. This disc does not show any nerve fiber layer hemorrhages, but they are often present and appear as tiny radial red streaks on or very near the disc.

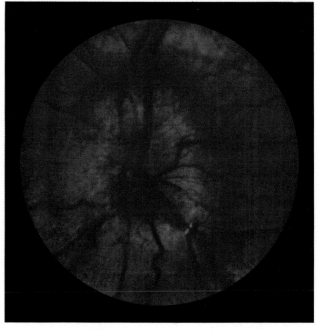

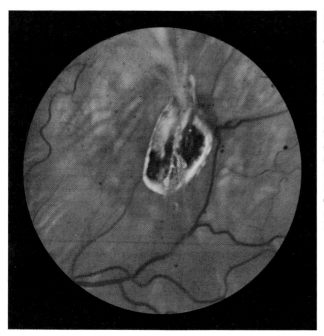

Plate 25. Intraocular foreign body. The discrete dark mass is a chip of steel imbedded in the fundus. A white ring of leukocytes characteristically forms around irritating, infected, or toxic foreign debris. The gray band above the foreign body is the opaque trail left by its transvitreal passage. Recognition of a foreign body is simple—it does not look like any normal structure you have ever seen. On proximal illumination it is entirely opaque. Hemorrhage occurs if vessels are damaged, but is not present in this case.

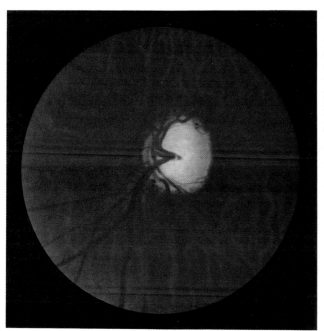

Plate 26. Glaucomatous cup, fundus in a black patient. The C/D ratio is 0.8, and the pale cup extends to the margin of the disc without a rim of normal disc tissue. Dioptric focusing will measure an excavation extending recognizably deeper than the level of the surrounding fundus. The melanin background is intense, a characteristic of the general pigmentation of the individual and not a manifestation of disease.

Plate 27. Acute and old chorioretinitis. A large, densely pigmented scar of old toxoplasmosis is conspicuous. Its inactivity is recognized by the sharp margins and the absence of edema or hemorrhage. Pigmentary hyperplasia occurs only after some weeks of inflammation; initially an acute inflammation is white. At the very top of the pigmented lesion, about 1 DD from the disc at the 5 o'clock position, is a 1/4 DD hazy and indistinct gray spot. This represents an acute recurrence of the lesion. Within several weeks this small spot increased to half the size of the disc and caused such a severe vitreous cellular infiltration as to preclude obtaining a clear fundus picture. During periods of inactivity, *Toxoplasma* organisms encyst and become dormant. Recurrences characteristically are located at the margin of an old lesion.

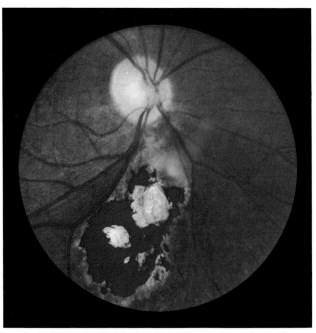

Plate 28. Degenerative myopia. The typical vertically oval, tilted disc of myopia is flanked by a large myopic crescent of sclera, exposed by progressive degeneration. An intensely red hemorrhagic focal macular degeneration is so characteristic of myopic degeneration as to have the eponym, Fuchs' spot. The lower three fourths of the retina is detached, which is recognizable from its gray, homogeneous appearance. Contrast this with the normally visible vascular and pigment markings seen in the upper one fourth. Retinal detachment occurs with much greater frequency in eyes structurally weakened by degenerative myopia.

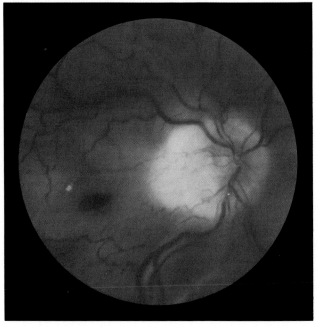

Plate 29. Cup/disc ratios. You should look at these pictures and write down your estimate as to the C/D ratio for each one. My estimate is on p. 280.

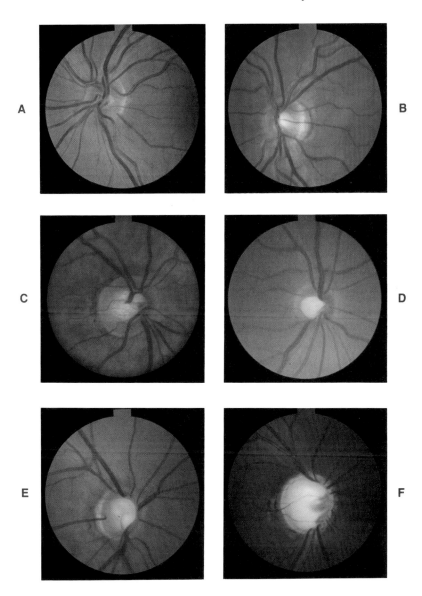

A

B

C

D

E

F

Plate 30. The optic disc is the blurred area just off center. Entirely surrounding it are folds of detached retina. Identification of a detachment is by recognition that it is elevated (dioptric focusing or parallax determination), that transparent fluid is beneath it (translucent appearance rather than the solid structure of a choroidal neoplasm), that it tends to be wrinkled and folded (best seen by proximal illumination), and that it moves gently with eye movements. Also, when detached, the retina obscures the view of underlying choroidal vessel and pigment markings.

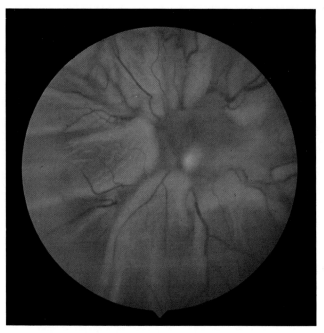

fundi of blond persons), choroidal hemorrhages are much darker, even almost black, in contrast to the red color of intraretinal and subretinal hemorrhages. Finally, acute chorio-retinitis is usually localized in one relatively small area (although disseminated chorio-retinitis with multiple foci rarely occurs), whereas the conditions causing soft exudates ordinarily affect a considerable area of the retina and result in multiple exudates. Severe chorioretinitis may damage the retina sufficiently to cause the formation of exudates (see Plate 13), but these chorioretinal lesions are so conspicuous as to leave little question of the diagnosis.

With time, chorioretinitis subsides, leaving a scar within which the retina and choroid are partially destroyed, the pigment has aggregated into irregular clumps that often line the edge of the lesion, more or less gray scar tissue is deposited, and the sclera may be partially visible. No edema or hemorrhage is found in these completely inactive scars. A white or gray patch of sclera visible within an old atrophic scar may easily be identified because it lies *behind* the large choroidal vessels, a few of which usually persist within the scar or near its edges. A gray patch of proliferated glial tissue may resemble sclera but obviously cannot be, since it lies in *front* of the choroidal vessels.

Myelinated fibers. Myelinated nerve fibers (see Plate 14) occur in about 0.5% of patients and are commonly confused with inflammation, exudates, or papilledema. Their color is a characteristic light gray and often somewhat glistening. Usually, but not always, they adjoin the disc margin. The peripheral edges of a myelin patch often appear frayed, resembling a feather's edge. Myelinated fibers remain unchanged throughout adult life and do not cause pathologic changes such as hemorrhage or edema.

Pigmentary changes. Most disorders of the choroid or outer retina result in some disturbance of the normal pigmentary pattern. These pigmentary changes are more or less nonspecific and may occur after trauma, degeneration, or inflammation. Sometimes the shape of the lesion is of diagnostic value. For instance, a narrow crescent-shaped patch of visible sclera surrounded by pigment represents a choroidal rupture due to trauma. An irregularly rounded patch of chorioretinal atrophy surrounded by pigment is usually in-flammatory if situated behind the equator (see Plate 15) but is usually degenerative if located in the far periphery.

Pigmentary changes may be distributed throughout the fundus rather than in localized areas. The most common such pigmentary disorder is *degenerative myopia* (see Chapter 21). A conspicuous, though rare, type of widespread pigmentary disturbance is retinitis pigmentosa. This slowly progressive, inherited, blinding disorder is recognized by the characteristic angular black pigment clumps found in the midperiphery (see Plate 16).

Nevi. By far the most common pigmentary alteration of the choroid is the benign *nevus* (see Plate 17). Sometimes such nevi are alarming to the ophthalmoscopist and present the problem of differential diagnosis from malignant melanoma. *Choroidal nevi* occur in over 1% of the population. Good mydriasis greatly aids their detection. Size varies from ¼ DD (smaller ones undoubtedly occur but are not readily recognized ophthal-moscopically) to more than 4 DD. They are usually roughly circular or oval. Edges are definite but not sharp because of the overlying retinal pigment. The absence of irregular pigmentary disturbances at their margins aids in differentiation from inflammatory conditions. Naturally, the color and distinctness depend on the density of the overlying retinal pigmentation, whether albinoid, negroid, or intermediate. Choroidal nevi are usually a slate gray color that only partially obscures the choroidal vascular pattern. Jet black, flat, sharply circumscribed lesions are usually congenital retinal pigment layer variations. Rather commonly, drusen are found to overlie a choroidal nevus. The presence of these drusen may be of diagnostic significance inasmuch as they establish beyond question that the given lesion has existed for a considerable length of time. Interference with choriocapillaris nutrition of the outer retinal layers (same mechanism that induces drusen formation?) may result in a relative scotoma (field loss). Such scotomas may frequently be detected with a 1/1000 white test object. This deserves emphasis because of the erroneous popular belief that the presence of a scotoma indicates neoplasm. Benign nevi do not, however, cause dense scotomas or progressive field defects. They are not elevated and do *not* induce neovascularization, edema, exudates, or hemorrhage. Choroidal nevi are of developmental origin.

By means of the characteristics just described, a benign nevus may ordinarily be recognized with confidence. Should doubt exist, a careful drawing, with emphasis on the exact relationship to vessel branching or other landmarks, should be made. Serial fundus photography, if available, is an even better way of detecting possible growth. Serial visual fields are also helpful. Unfortunately, there is no guarantee that a benign nevus will not undergo malignant transformation. Such cases have been reported clinically. Furthermore, the histologic finding of nevus cells at the base of a malignant melanoma is not unusual.

A patient with a benign choroidal nevus should *not* be frightened by having the possibility of a malignancy mentioned to him. A malignant melanoma is recognized by the fact that it is *elevated*, whereas a benign nevus is *flat* (see Plate 18).

SUMMARY

Diagnosis of a disorder causing a given fundus abnormality is best made through systematic observation of the disc, vessels, macula, and periphery. The disc should be evaluated in terms of size, shape, color, margins, and physiologic depression. Important features of the vessels are size, shape, color, and margins (arteriovenous crossings). Changes occurring throughout the retina include edema, hemorrhage, exudates, drusen, chorioretinitis, myelinated fibers, pigmentary degeneration, and nevi. These same changes may also affect the macula, which in addition may be aimed in a faulty direction (eccentric fixation)

Familiarity with these changes is best obtained through careful routine ophthalmoscopic examination performed even if there are no eye complaints. Of necessity, such thorough physical examinations must be performed during the student years or in the early period of establishing a practice, because there will not be time later. The student is advised to use mydriatics for these early examinations in order to avoid discouragement while learning ophthalmoscopy and to permit an excellent view of the normal fundus appearance.

chapter 8 Applied Ophthalmoscopic Technique

Socrates paraphrased: And canst thou teach a student of Hippocrates the technique and interpretation of ophthalmoscopy by stuffing him with knowledge, as a reluctant python is force-fed?

Ophthalmologist: Nay, for he payeth not attention, and his memory of the teacher's efforts fadeth even before he leaveth class.

Socrates paraphrased: If this be so, then how canst the teacher cram the student full of ophthalmoscopy by long and tedious hours of lectures won from the Committee on Medical Curriculum?

Ophthalmologist: Again, I say, the teacher who thinketh he canst cram the student hath partaken of the heady wine of self-delusion.

Socrates paraphrased: Then shall the transmission of knowledge of ophthalmoscopy be impossible?

Ophthalmologist: Nay, for since Helmholtz' invention, textbooks proliferate and ophthalmoscopists abound on the face of the earth.

Socrates paraphrased: And how can this be?

Ophthalmologist: The interested student learneth ophthalmoscopy just as he learneth other things.

Socrates paraphrased: So the teacher of ophthalmoscopy only guideth the student, who learneth effectively through his own cerebration?

Ophthalmologist: Exactly so.

The Socratic method of teaching guides the student to crystallize his own thinking and thereby gain personal insights. The effective Socratic teacher must tantalize the student with provocative questions carefully designed to elicit an appropriate train of thought. Ideally, such an outcome will be the result of thoughtful perusal of this chapter.

• • •

The development of skill in ophthalmoscopy, just as the learning of any other skill, requires guided practice. The illustrations and questions in this chapter have been prepared to convey information of importance in the evaluation of fundus findings. The performance of the student in reasoning through these illustrations and questions will parallel rather closely his future performance during actual ophthalmoscopic examination of the fundus. Hence, this presentation is not simply a novel way of offering information but is designed to coordinate the student's actions and thoughts during ophthalmoscopy.

Just as the principle under consideration in a given illustration is elucidated by an approach of discovery through questioning, so also clinical diagnoses are made by a process of observation, recognition of an abnormality, evaluation of the characteristics of the abnormality, and finally conclusion as to its significance.

The student may expect the answers to the questions he is about to encounter to be shown in the accompanying illustration (or to have been presented in preceding illustrations). Although the answers are summarized after each series of questions, simply reading these answers without first considering the questions and the illustration will defeat the purpose of this chapter. To repeat, its purpose is to simulate the mental processes of ophthalmoscopy, which should be a search guided by pertinent questions. As the ophthalmoscopist again and again examines the media, disc, vessels, macula, and periphery in orderly detail, the proper habit and thought patterns should become almost automatic.

This chapter will be understood much more readily by the student who has already used the ophthalmoscope on at least a few eyes. I strongly recommend that you use the ophthalmoscope, as described in Chapter 5, *before* you read this chapter.

MEDIA

Obviously, the ophthalmoscopist does not see the light leaving his ophthalmoscope, but he does see the light reflected back toward him from the patient's eye. Best observed from a distance of perhaps a foot, this returning light is called the *red reflex*.

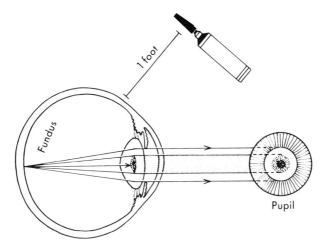

Fig. 8-1

Refer to Fig. 8-1:

1. What reflects the light responsible for the normal red reflex?
2. How will the red reflex be changed by a central opacity of the lens?
3. May similar red reflex changes result from opacities of the cornea or other transparent portions of the eye?

   Finding the red reflex that is reflected from the fundus is the first step in ophthalmoscopy.
   Observation of the red reflex will reveal even small opacities within the clear media (cornea, lens, anterior vitreous) of the eye, provided they are axial.
   Absence of the red reflex immediately identifies the eye as being abnormal (if the pupil is at least several millimeters in diameter).

Diagrammatic representation of the layers of the fundus will be helpful in guiding the consideration of ophthalmoscopic principles. Variations of this basic diagram will repeatedly be presented in future illustrations. Please familiarize yourself with this simplified anatomy at this time.

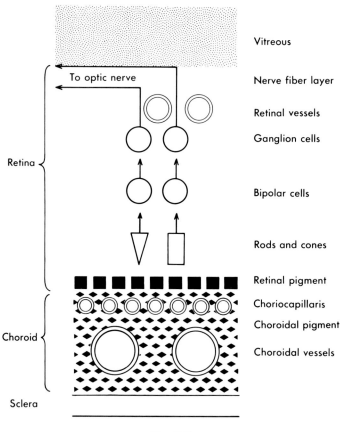

Fig. 8-2

Refer to Fig. 8-2:

1. Which of these layers of the fundus are part of the retina?
2. Is the nerve fiber layer on the vitreous side or on the scleral side of the retina?
3. Are the retinal pigment cells on the vitreous side or on the scleral side of the retina?
4. Which layer of the retina is closest to the ophthalmoscope?
5. What is the first opaque layer encountered as one looks at the fundus with an ophthalmoscope?
6. Which layer is more readily seen with the ophthalmoscope—the rod and cone layer or the retinal pigment layer?
7. Which layer runs to the optic nerve?
8. Where do the nerve fiber layer axons terminate?
9. Does damage to the optic chiasm cause ophthalmoscopically visible atrophy of the optic nerve?
10. What do the double-contoured circles represent?

Since the retina is transparent (except for its pigment layer), the normally visible fundus details are pigment, blood, and reflections (except at the disc, where the light color of its framework is seen).

The nerve fiber layer axons synapse at the lateral geniculate body. Damage to these axons at any point will kill the nerve and result in disc pallor.

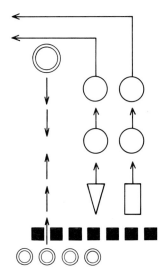

Fig. 8-3

Refer to Fig. 8-3:
1. What do the bottom double-contoured circles represent?
2. What does the top double-contoured circle represent?
3. At what depth within the retina are the retinal vessels?
4. What is the nutritional significance of the lines of arrows?
5. Does the central retinal artery provide the main source of nourishment for the rods and cones?

   Although the nutrition of the outer retinal layers is derived by diffusion from the choroidal capillaries, these vessels do **not** physically extend through the pigment layer and into the retina. Likewise, the central retinal vessels do not extend into the outer layers of the retina.

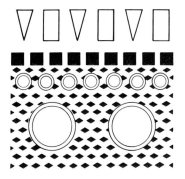

Fig. 8-4

Refer to Fig. 8-4:
1. What does the dark cuboidal layer beneath the rods and cones represent?
2. What do the double-contoured circles represent?
3. Are the large choroidal vessels or are the small capillaries closer to the retina?
4. Does the choroid contain pigment between its vessels?
5. What determines whether the large-vessel pattern of the choroid and the intervening pigment can be seen with the ophthalmoscope?
6. Would the large-vessel pattern of the choroid be seen better in an albino or in a dark brunet?

The color of the fundus is determined mainly by the density of the choroidal pigment and the density of the choroidal vessels. The single layer of retinal pigment cells also contributes recognizable pigmentation.

The irregular background of the fundus, made up of the large choroidal vessels and the pigment of the choroid and retina, is the normal ophthalmoscopic appearance. Concealment of this irregularly mottled background means that an opaque abnormality exists anterior to the retinal pigment layer.

DISC

The lower portion of Fig. 8-5 represents a retinal section at the optic disc. The upper portion represents the disc turned, as it would be viewed with an ophthalmoscope.

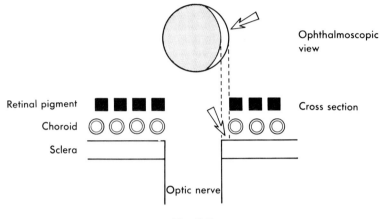

Fig. 8-5

Refer to Fig. 8-5:

1. If, during development of the eye, all layers of the choroid and retina do not extend to the edge of the optic nerve, leaving uncovered sclera adjacent to part of the nerve, what color will this area of uncovered sclera be?
2. If you cannot answer question 1, what color is sclera?
3. If the width of uncovered sclera is greatest temporally and gradually decreases above and below, what shape will the whitish area be?
4. How much of the circle represents the optic disc?

The optic disc is the ophthalmoscopically visible end of the optic nerve. Adjacent portions of the fundus, whether pale or pigmented, are not part of the optic nerve and should not be misinterpreted as being part of the optic disc.

*Specifically, a temporal crescent of sclera, as shown here, is **not** part of the optic disc (see Plate 2).*

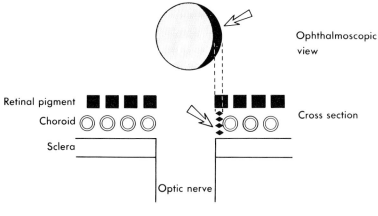

Fig. 8-6

Refer to Fig. 8-6:

1. If irregular hyperpigmentation adjoins the disc, what color will this pigment crescent be?
2. How much of the circle represents the optic disc?

The sharpness of the disc margins is normally quite variable. Especially on the temporal side, crescents of pigment or white sclera are common normal developmental variables. Differentiation of these crescents from the disc area is necessary to recognize the difference between the normal physiologic depression and the typical excavated atrophy caused by glaucoma.

An unusually prominent temporal scleral crescent is part of the characteristic ophthalmoscopic appearance of degenerative myopia.

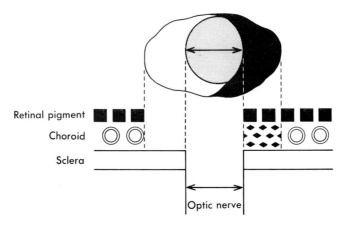

Retinal pigment

Choroid

Sclera

Optic nerve

Fig. 8-7

Refer to Fig. 8-7:

1. Is this a horizontally oval disc with white optic atrophy on its left side and some type of pigmentation of the optic nerve on its right side?
2. Is this optic disc *(span of double-pointed arrow)* larger than the discs shown in Figs. 8-5 and 8-6?
3. When a disc is evaluated, would it be helpful to consider its size?

Abnormalities adjacent to the optic disc are commonly wrongly assumed to represent part of the disc.

*Evaluation of the disc should include conscious study of its **size, shape, color,** and **margins.***

Whatever on first glance appears to be an enlarged disc will almost always be an adjacent abnormality, usually not affecting the optic nerve (see Plates 3 and 4).

Most discs are either vertically oval or almost round.

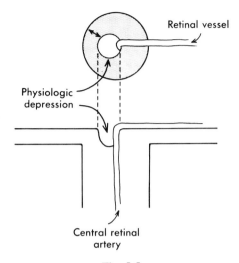

Fig. 8-8

Refer to Fig. 8-8:

1. Is the physiologic depression commonly seen in the temporal central portion of the disc more pale or more hyperemic than the surrounding disc tissue?
2. Does a rim of normal disc tissue *(double-pointed arrow)* exist between the edge of the optic disc and the edge of the physiologic cup throughout its entire circumference?
3. When a vessel descends steeply into a physiologic depression, may it abruptly disappear from ophthalmoscopic view at this point?

*Although the physiologic depression may vary considerably in size, it **never** extends all the way to the disc margin but is always surrounded by at least a narrow rim of disc tissue (nerve fibers). Hence, the vessels can never normally disappear abruptly at the disc edge (except in the case of a cilioretinal artery).*

Pallor within the physiologic depression is normal and should not cause concern as to possible optic atrophy (see Plate 12).

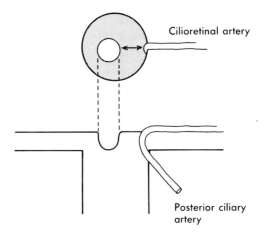

Cilioretinal artery

Posterior ciliary
artery

Fig. 8-9

Refer to Fig. 8-9:
1. Is a cilioretinal artery a branch of the central retinal artery?
2. What is the origin of a cilioretinal artery?
3. Does a cilioretinal artery appear to emerge from the physiologic cup?
4. Does a cilioretinal artery appear abruptly at the disc edge?
5. Does the rim of normal disc tissue exist inside the disc from the point of origin of a cilioretinal artery?

About 20% of eyes have a cilioretinal artery, usually on the temporal side of the disc (see Plate 2). Cilioretinal arteries are important because they simulate the abnormal disappearance of a vessel into a glaucomatous cup.

A cilioretinal artery does not cause disappearance of the rim of normal disc tissue, which always encircles the entire disc circumference.

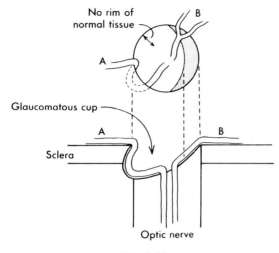

Fig. 8-10

Refer to Fig. 8-10:

1. Is the abruptly disappearing vessel *(A)* a cilioretinal artery or a branch of the central retinal artery?
2. Is the large excavation, extending to the edge of the optic nerve, a physiologic cup?
3. In advanced glaucomatous atrophy, does the abruptly disappearing retinal vessel *(A)* appear continuous with its deeper part within the excavated glaucomatous cup, or may it be displaced to one side?
4. What hides the concealed portion of the abruptly disappearing vessel?
5. When an overhanging scleral edge is not present (as in less severe glaucomatous atrophy, represented by vessel *B*), does a segment of the vessel disappear?
6. Is the normal pink disc color present in the atrophic area of the glaucomatous cup, or is this area pale and whitish?

Unlike a physiologic cup, a glaucomatous excavation begins abruptly at the edge of the optic disc (see Plate 26). The excavation is typical of glaucoma and differentiates it from other types of optic atrophy.

Regardless of the cause of optic atrophy, the portion of the disc that is damaged loses its normal pink color and becomes pale gray or white, the characteristic color of optic atrophy.

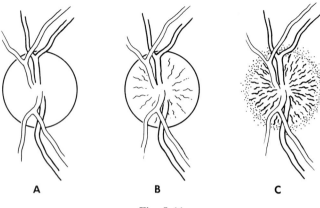

A   B   C

Fig. 8-11

Refer to Fig. 8-11:

1. Which disc has the most capillaries? The fewest?
2. Are the disc capillaries branches of the central retinal vessels?
3. Complete absence of the small capillaries of the disc is characteristic of which of the following: atrophy of the optic nerve or vascular congestion (optic neuritis or papilledema) of the optic nerve?
4. Which condition (optic atrophy or papilledema) characteristically causes increased visibility (and therefore an apparent increase in number) of the disc capillaries?

Because of the wide range of normal color variation, diagnosis on the basis of disc color alone is permissible only if the disc is very white (optic atrophy) or very red (optic neuritis or papilledema). Absence or abnormal prominence of the disc capillaries is the ophthalmoscopic feature of greatest diagnostic importance in the assessment of disc color.

The disc capillaries are independent of the circulation of the retina and are not branches of the central retinal artery or vein.

Papilla is a synonym for optic disc—hence the term papilledema to designate swelling of the disc.

Within the eye there exist three separate circulations, independently nourishing the optic disc, the inner retina, and the choroid and outer retina.

In the condition of papilledema, increased intracranial pressure is transmitted via the meningeal sheaths to compress the veins draining the optic disc. The ophthalmoscopic diagnosis of papilledema is made by consideration of the following.

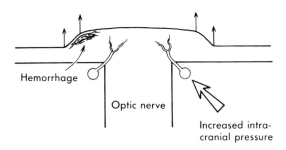

Fig. 8-12

Refer to Fig. 8-12:
1. When their drainage is impeded, what happens to the small vessels on the disc in respect to their size? If they increase in size, what happens to their apparent number?
2. What happens to the color of the disc?
3. Are the disc margins distinct?
4. Is the elevated and edematous disc seen clearly with the same opthalmoscopic lens strength as that by which the surrounding fundus is seen? What dioptric change is necessary?
5. If hemorrhages occur into the nerve fiber layer on or near the disc, will they be superficial or deep in the retina?
6. Note that the peripheral extent of the disc edema is delineated by reflections *(small arrows)* from the curved edges.

The patient with headache or neurologic symptoms requires ophthalmo-scopic examination of both optic discs. Any source of increased intracranial pressure may cause papilledema. Note again that the fundus of the eye has three ***separate*** *circulations that independently supply the retina, the choroid, and the optic disc. The hemorrhages of papilledema originate from the disc vessels and therefore are always within several disc diameters of the optic nerve. More distant retinal hemorrhages cannot be caused by papilledema.*

To remember the appearance of papilledema, one need only recall the con-sequences of venous stasis affecting the disc circulation (see Plate 24).

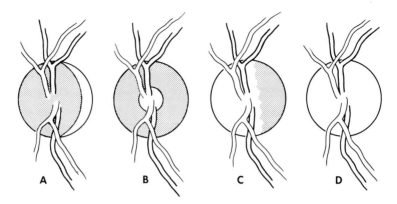

Fig. 8-13

Refer to Fig. 8-13:

1. If a crescent-shaped pale area exists adjacent to the optic disc *(A)*, does this area represent a type of optic atrophy, or is it simply a normal variant (scleral crescent)?
2. If a pale, slightly excavated area exists centrally within the disc *(B)* but does *not* extend to the disc margins, does this area represent a type of optic atrophy, or is it simply a normal variant (physiologic depression)?
3. If a sector of the disc is recognizably pale, extending from center to edge *(C)*, does this paleness represent death of part of the disc (optic atrophy), or is it simply a normal variant?
4. If the entire disc is recognizably pale *(D)*, does this paleness represent death of the optic nerve (optic atrophy), or is it simply a normal variant?

Definite pallor of the optic disc extending from center to edge represents optic atrophy. It may involve the entire disc or only a sector.

The temporal part of a disc is normally slightly paler than the nasal part.

Comparison of the two optic discs will permit earlier recognition of abnormal changes, since the two discs of the same person are normally of comparable appearance.

Optic atrophy may result from damage to any part of the ganglion cells and their axons, whether the damage occurs in the retina, optic nerve, optic chiasm, or optic tract.

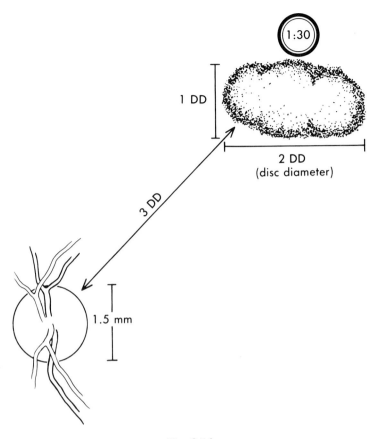

1 DD

1:30

2 DD
(disc diameter)

3 DD

1.5 mm

Fig. 8-14

Refer to Fig. 8-14:
1. What is the diameter of the normal disc?
2. In recording or verbally describing a fundus lesion, what units may be conveniently used to state its size and its distance from the disc?
3. In what units can you conveniently designate the direction of a lesion from the
   disc?

   *Size and distance are easily stated in terms of disc diameters (DD). Direc-
tions are expressed as time o' clock positions as a clock face is viewed.*
   Use the disc as a reference standard for size.

VESSELS

The sequence of examination is media, disc (size, shape, color, margins), vessels (size [diameter], shape, color [light reflex], margins [arteriovenous crossings]), macula, and periphery. When the disc has been thoroughly studied, proceed to examine the vessels in an orderly manner.

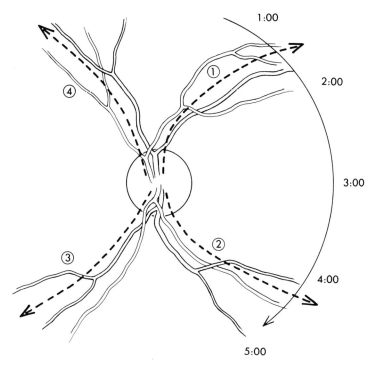

Fig. 8-15

Refer to Fig. 8-15:
1. When surveying the retinal vessels for the presence of abnormality, is the physician more likely to observe all the vessels by haphazard and random movements of the ophthalmoscope or by methodical following of the vessels?
2. Describe a sequence of ophthalmoscopic examination (arrows) that would ensure observation of all the major vessels of the fundus.

   In studying the major retinal vessels, follow them from disc to periphery in a clockwise sequence.
   Observation of the entire extent of the retinal vessels is important in the study of the fundus and in the evaluation of the vascular status of the patient.

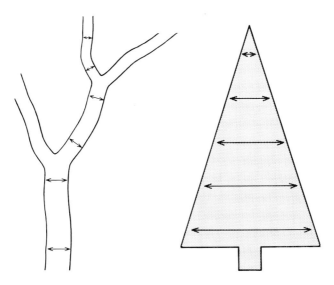

Fig. 8-16

Refer to Fig. 8-16:

1. Does the diameter of a retinal vessel gradually diminish as it extends to the retinal periphery, just as a fir tree tapers gradually to its top?
2. Does the diameter of a retinal vessel normally remain essentially unchanged except when branching occurs?
3. Is a more peripheral segment of a retinal vessel normally of larger diameter than a more central segment?

*When studying retinal vessels, note their **diameter, shape (lack of tortuosity), color,** and **arteriovenous crossings (margins).***

Especially note that a vessel segment between branching points is of uniform diameter through its entire length, and that a more peripheral vessel branch is always smaller than a more central segment of the vessel. Deviations from these appearances always indicate disease.

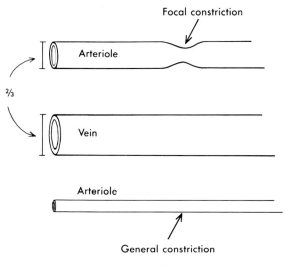

Fig. 8-17

Refer to Fig. 8-17:
1. Which is normally of larger diameter, a retinal arteriole or a retinal vein?
2. What is the normal approximate ratio of the diameters of corresponding retinal arterioles and veins?
3. If a localized portion of an arteriole is constricted, what name may be used to describe this change?
4. If an extensive portion of an arteriole is constricted, what name may be used to describe this change?

Arteriolar constriction, either focal or general, is the basic abnormality present in hypertensive retinopathy and hence should be looked for as the most important ophthalmoscopic sign of hypertension (see Plate 23).

The ratio of arteriole diameter to vein diameter (normally 2:3) may be of help in evaluating vessel caliber, provided vessels serving a comparable retinal area are selected.

Arteriole

Vein

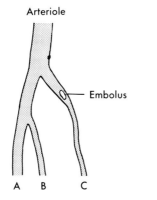
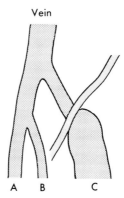

Embolus

A   B   C

A   B   C

Fig. 8-18

Refer to Fig. 8-18:
1. Why is arteriole *A* of larger caliber than arteriole *B?*
2. Why is arteriole *A* of larger caliber than vein *B?*
3. Why is arteriole *C* of smaller caliber than arteriole *A?*
4. Why is arteriole *C* of smaller caliber than vein *A?*
5. Why is vein *C* of larger caliber than vein *A?*
6. Why is vein *C* of larger caliber than arteriole *A?*
7. Why is vein *A* of larger caliber than arteriole *A?*
8. Does an arteriole become larger or smaller peripheral to a site of occlusion?
9. Does a vein become larger or smaller peripheral to a site of occlusion?

The normal diameter of a retinal arteriole or vein is determined by the size of the retinal area it serves. Depending on the area served by a given vessel, it may be larger or smaller than a nearby vessel (which does not necessarily serve an area of the same size). Hence, although a representative artery is smaller (perhaps two thirds or three fourths the size of a comparable vein), branching and distribution differences preclude rigid comparisons. Ophthalmoscopic diagnosis requires recognition of a pathologic increase or decrease in diameter of vessels that supply a comparable retinal area.

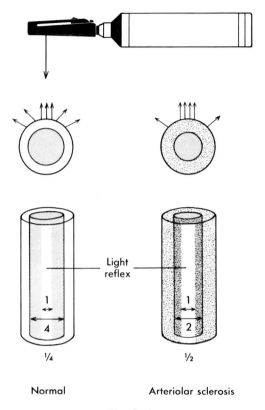

Normal   Arteriolar sclerosis

Fig. 8-19

Refer to Fig. 8-19:

1. Is a normal retinal arteriolar wall ophthalmoscopically visible, or does the examiner simply see the red column of blood itself?
2. Is the reflection of light (light reflex) from the surface of a normal arteriolar wall visible from the entire width of the vessel wall? Why not?
3. When early arteriolar sclerosis causes the vessel walls to lose their transparency, what happens to the width of the light reflection from the arteriolar wall?
4. In *severe* arteriolar sclerosis, what happens to the diameter of the visible blood column?
5. What is the normal ratio of width of arteriolar light reflex to width of visible blood column?
6. In arteriolar sclerosis, what happens to the ratio of width of arteriolar light reflex to width of visible blood column?
7. With progressive opacification of the sclerotic arteriolar wall, what happens to the red color of the blood within the vessel?

The normal vessel wall is invisible except for the reflections arising from its surface. The ophthalmoscopist sees only the blood column.

Widening of the arteriolar light reflex to one half or more of the diameter of the blood column is a definite sign of early arteriolar sclerosis.

With progressive sclerosis, the red column of blood becomes discolored — becoming at first somewhat orange, ultimately perhaps becoming completely obscured by the gray sclerotic walls.

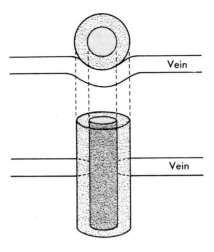

Fig. 8-20

Refer to Fig. 8-20:
1. When an arteriole develops arteriolar sclerosis, what happens to the transparency of its walls?
2. What happens to a vein when it encounters the abnormally rigid walls of a sclerotic arteriole?
3. How is the appearance of a retinal vein altered where it is crossed by an arteriole suffering from the decreased transparency and increased rigidity of arteriolar sclerosis?
4. What portion of the retinal vascular tree should be sought out particularly when one is trying to evaluate the status of the retinal arteriolar walls?

Displacement of the veins at arteriovenous crossings is a characteristic abnormality found in moderately severe arteriolar sclerosis. Ophthalmoscopically, the column of venous blood is hidden and appears to be constricted where the vein is crossed by the arteriole. This apparent constriction is commonly termed "nicking" of the vein.

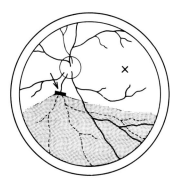

Fig. 8-21

Refer to Fig. 8-21:

1. If an embolus *(arrow)* blocks this branch of the central retinal artery, of what will the patient complain?
2. At what anatomic site will an embolus lodge?
3. Is the caliber of the arteriole peripheral to the occlusion likely to be larger or smaller than normal?
4. If the arterial circulation is blocked, will the involved peripheral portion of the retina be likely to contain hemorrhages?
5. Is living retina more transparent than dead retina?
6. Will the choroidal pigmentary and vascular markings be normally visible through opaque, recently dead retina?

Prompt and usually permanent blindness of the affected portion of the retina follows arteriolar occlusion.

Emboli arising from the carotid artery or heart are the usual cause of retinal arteriolar occlusion, which is therefore a manifestation of serious systemic disease rather than simply an eye problem. Emboli lodge at arteriolar bifurcations.

During the first few weeks after arteriolar occlusion, the dead inner retina is a dense gray color, obscuring the view of the normally apparent choroidal pigmentary and vascular markings. Hemorrhages are not usually present.

Since the peripheral retina is much thinner than the central retina, the typical gray retinal opacity of recent arteriolar occlusion is relatively inconspicuous in the periphery.

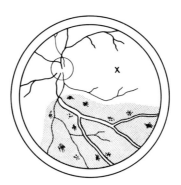

Fig. 8-22

Refer to Fig. 8-22:
1. If thrombosis occludes this branch of the central retinal vein, will the involved portion of the retina be likely to contain hemorrhages?
2. Peripheral to the occlusion, is the caliber of the occluded vein likely to be larger or smaller than normal?
3. At what anatomic site is venous branch occlusion likely to occur?

Extensive hemorrhagic infiltration coextensive with the tributary area of a retinal vein is virtually diagnostic of partial occlusion of that vein. Such partial occlusions are almost always due to compression by an arteriosclerotic arteriole at an arteriovenous crossing. With time, vascular proliferation (neovascularization, microaneurysms) occurs within the area of venous stasis (see Plate 7).

The changes (small hemorhages, microaneurysms, neovascularization) of old venous branch occlusion are virtually identical to those of diabetic retinopathy, except that the venous changes of the former are limited to the tributary area of the occluded vein. Diabetic retinopathy is mostly in the posterior retina; it is not limited to the area of a single vessel.

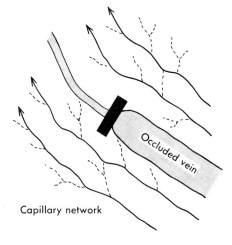

Fig. 8-23

Refer to Fig. 8-23:
1. After venous occlusion, the retina attempts to reestablish its circulation. What is the origin of such a compensatory circulation?
2. Arising from the capillary bed, will the new vessels be straighter or more tortuous than normal retinal vessels?
3. How does the caliber of new vessels compare with that of normal retinal vessels? How about their number?
4. What is the significance of a patch of retinal vessels that are tortuous, narrow, and numerous?

Neovascularization is a typical retinal response to venous stasis.

Diabetes and occlusion of a retinal vein are the two most common causes of neovascularization of the retina.

Newly formed vessels may be differentiated from normally existing vessels because such abnormal vessels are tortuous, narrow, and numerous.

MACULA

The sequence of examination is media, disc (size, shape, color, margins), vessels (diameter, lack of tortuosity, color, arteriovenous crossings), macula, and periphery. When the disc and vessels have been thoroughly studied, proceed to examine the macula carefully.

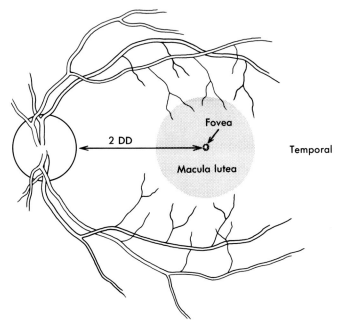

Fig. 8-24

Refer to Fig. 8-24:
1. What is the name of the center of the macula?
2. How far from the disc is the fovea?
3. In which direction from the disc is the macula?
4. If a patient complained of blurred vision in the very central part of his visual field, what part of the fundus would you particularly wish to examine with the ophthalmoscope?
5. Do retinal blood vessels extend to the center of the macula?

Because of the acute vision of the macula, patients tend to move the eye away from the ophthalmoscope light during macular examination. Correct this problem by requesting the patient to hold his eye steadily fixed in the direction of some known object.

Examine the macula after the patient's eye has become partially accustomed to the light during the prior examination of the disc and vessels.

The glistening pinpoint reflection of the fovea is always normally visible in a young eye (at least for 20 or 30 years) but may normally be absent in the older eye (50 years or older).

Although the macula may be generally darker than the adjacent retina, marked clumping or disruption of its pigment is characteristic of disease.

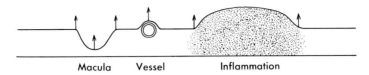

Macula   Vessel   Inflammation

Fig. 8-25

Refer to 8-25:
1. Although light reflections *(arrows)* may be seen throughout the retinal surface, especially in younger persons, they are most pronounced at certain sites. What feature do these sites of increased reflection have in common?
2. Will the reflection from the center of the macula be linear or pinpoint? What about the reflection from a vessel?
3. What ophthalmoscopic finding characteristically is found about the periphery of an edematous area (such as might be found with acute inflammation)?

Abnormally prominent reflections characteristically encircle edematous areas and are helpful in the diagnosis of acute chorioretinitis, papilledema, retinal contusion, nutritional defect, and so on. Delicate scar tissue on the retinal surface (as in early diabetic retinitis proliferans) causes increased reflections, simulating the appearance of irregularly wrinkled cellophane.

Prominent reflections are found throughout the retina of a healthy young eye and are especially pronounced in the macular area.

Convex or concave curvatures are responsible for reflecting light seen from the retinal surfaces.

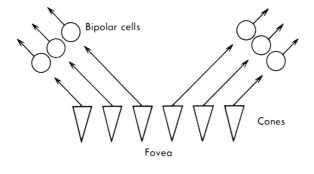

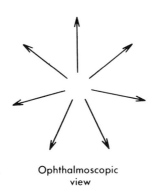

Ophthalmoscopic
view

Fig. 8-26

Refer to Fig. 8-26:
1. Is the fovea composed primarily of rods or cones?
2. In order to achieve the clearest central vision, what is the structural arrangement of the retinal layers at and immediately surrounding the fovea?
3. Viewed from straight ahead with the ophthalmoscope, what is the configuration of the nerve layers immediately surrounding the fovea?

Note that in the macular area (only), the outer layers of the retina are arranged radially with respect to the macula. This is the anatomic basis for the radial arrangement of the potential spaces between the nerve structures (which may become evident in disease).

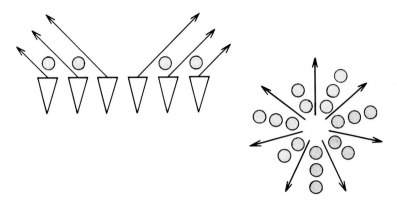

Fig. 8-27

Refer to Fig. 8-27:

1. If nutritional damage or inflammation results in deposits of fatty debris within the retina in the macular area, what pattern will this debris form?

2. If an abnormality of the macula assumes a radial, or "star," pattern, is this disorder situated primarily in the vitreous? In the choroid? In the sclera? Where is it?

Discrete, small, pale deposits within the retina in the macular area usually form a radial pattern (star or fan). Such a radial appearance usually is caused by hard exudates, which are commonly due to the nutritional damage of systemic disease (for example, diabetes and hypertension) (see Plates 13 and 23).

Localized degenerative changes (senile macular degeneration) may also result in deposition of whitish debris, but this debris is ordinarily subretinal and arranged in circular or semicircular patterns, rather than radially.

Pigmentary irregularity of the macula is a sign of macular damage from degeneration or inflammation. Pigmentary changes are in the choroid or retinal pigment layer, rather than within the retina, and hence do not form radial patterns. Diabetes and hypertension do not ordinarily cause pigmentary changes.

The radial pattern surrounding the macula exists in the deep layers of the retina, which do not usually contain blood vessels. Hence, radial hemorrhages surrounding the macula are not often encountered clinically.

PERIPHERY

(If you do not remember the names of the various layers represented in this diagrammatic cross section, refer to Fig. 8-2).

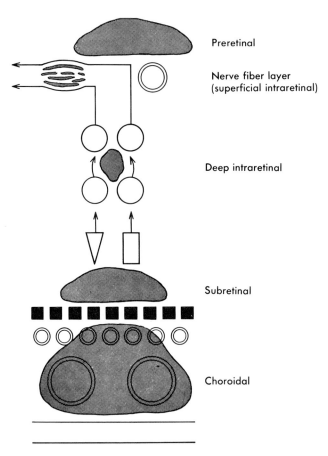

Preretinal

Nerve fiber layer
(superficial intraretinal)

Deep intraretinal

Subretinal

Choroidal

Fig. 8-28

Refer to Fig. 8-28:

1. What term designates a hemorrhage situated between the vitreous and the retina?
2. What is the name of the hemorrhage between the retina and the sclera?
3. What is the name of the hemorrhage between the rods and cones and the retinal pigment epithelium? (Note that this name is not anatomically strictly correct.)
4. What is the name of the hemorrhage deep within the retina itself?
5. What is the name of the hemorrhage that occurs very superficially in the retina?
6. Which three of these hemorrhages are large?
7. Which two of these hemorrhages are small?
8. State a reason why a hemorrhage in one anatomic location might characteristically be larger than a hemorrhage in another anatomic location.

The depth of a lesion within the fundus has etiologic significance and hence is important to determine. For example, choroidal and subretinal hemorrhages are usually of inflammatory or degenerative origin, intraretinal hemorrhages are usually due to systemic disorders such as hypertension or diabetes, and pre-retinal hemorrhages characteristically suggest blood dyscrasia.

The size and shape of a space-occupying lesion, such as a hemorrhage, are partially determined by the space within which it is confined. Within the fundus, large potential spaces exist in preretinal, subretinal, and choroidal locations. The retinal structure itself is compact and will not permit space for large hemor-rhages.

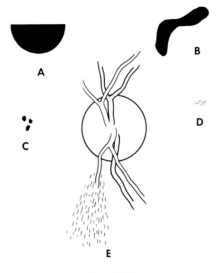

Fig. 8-29

Refer to Fig. 8-29:

1. Are *A* and *B* large hemorrhages or small ones?
2. Are *C* and *D* large hemorrhages or small ones?
3. Is *E* a large hemorrhage, or is it an aggregate of many small hemorrhages?

Intraretinal hemorrhages are tiny—comparable in size to the diameter of a retinal vessel.

Preretinal, subretinal, and choroidal hemorrhages exist in large potential spaces and can be much larger than the disc in size, or smaller, depending on the amount of hemorrhage.

Many intraretinal hemorrhages located close together may simulate a large hemorrhage; however, careful observation will ordinarily disclose the discontinuous nature of the hemorrhagic area, especially near the edges.

The size of a hemorrhage is an easily observed criterion, which is helpful in determining its depth within the fundus.

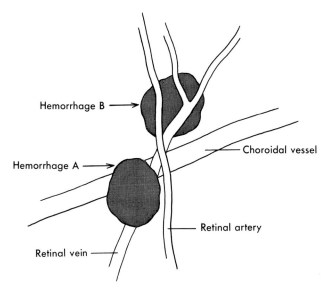

Hemorrhage B

Choroidal vessel

Hemorrhage A

Retinal artery

Retinal vein

Fig. 8-30

Refer to Fig. 8-30:

1. In Fig. 8-30, which vessel is closest to the ophthalmoscope?
2. How do you know?
3. State a general principle that helps determine the relative depth of a fundus detai
4. Using this principle, can you determine whether hemorrhage *A* (a large hemoı rhage) is in a preretinal or a subretinal location?
5. Using this principle, you can determine whether hemorrhage *B* (a large hemor rhage) is in a subretinal or a choroidal location?

To determine the depth of a fundus detail, seek a structure of known depth (for example, a retinal vessel) and ascertain whether it conceals or is concealed by the detail of unknown depth.

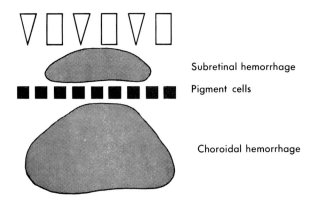

Fig. 8-31

Refer to Fig. 8-31:

1. What layer is in front of a choroidal hemorrhage (a large hemorrhage, deep to the retinal vessels), partially obscuring it from ophthalmoscopic view, but is not in front of a subretinal hemorrhage (also a large hemorrhage, deep to the retinal vessels)?

2. What color is a hemorrhage not obscured by any opaque layers (for example, a subretinal hemorrhage)? If you cannot answer this question, what color is a red barn?

3. Would the color of a hemorrhage covered by a layer of pigmented cells (for example, a choroidal hemorrhage) be as bright red as one not so covered (for example, a subretinal hemorrhage)?

4. Do all individuals have equally dense body pigmentation?

Covered by retinal pigment of variable density, a choroidal hemorrhage will not usually appear bright red but will be darkly shaded, sometimes approaching black in a heavily pigmented fundus. This color change differentiates choroidal hemorrhages from fundus hemorrhages anterior to the retinal pigment layer.

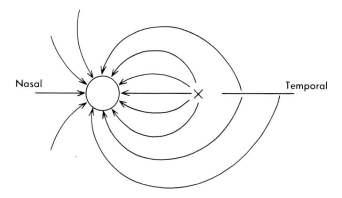

Fig. 8-32

Refer to Fig. 8-32:
1. In what layer of the retina do nerve axons run as they pass from the ganglion cells toward the optic nerve *(circle)?*
2. Do the nerve fiber layer axons from the temporal retina run straight to the disc, or are they displaced by the fibers from the macula (represented by *X*)?
3. What is the configuration of the nerve fiber layer axons with respect to the disc?

This pattern represents the course of the axons in the nerve fiber layer of the retina. This pattern is significant because it determines the anatomic shape of changes in the nerve fiber layer.

Note that the nerve fiber is oriented approximately radially in respect to the disc. Do not confuse this pattern with the radial pattern of the outer retinal layers surrounding the macula (Fig. 8-26). The nerve fiber layer arches above and below the macula.

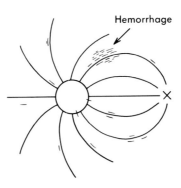

Hemorrhage

Fig. 8-33

Refer to Fig. 8-33:

1. If hemorrhages exist between the axons of the nerve fiber layer of the retina, into what shape will the small hemorrhages be formed by the parallel, closely packed axons?
2. How are the linear nerve fiber layer hemorrhages oriented?
3. Are nerve fiber layer hemorrhages large or small?
4. Do small linear spaces oriented parallel to the nerve fiber layer pattern exist in the choroid? In the vitreous? In other layers of the retina?
5. Since such spaces exist only in the nerve fiber layer of the retina, at what depth in the fundus must all small linear hemorrhages be that are oriented more or less radially from the disc?

The presence of small linear hemorrhages identifies the disorders as affecting the nerve fiber layer of the retina.

By clinical custom, groups of small linear hemorrhages of the nerve fiber layer have been termed ''flame-shaped'' hemorrhages.

Blood does not have a configuration but assumes the shape of the cavity containing it.

Nerve fiber layer hemorrhages are found in hypertension, papilledema, and retinal vein occlusion.

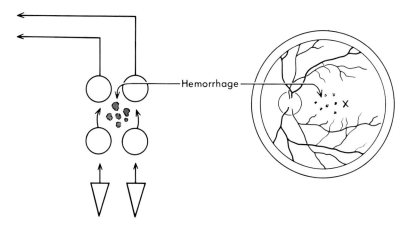

Fig. 8-34

Refer to Fig. 8-34:

1. Are these hemorrhages large or small?
2. Are these hemorrhages anterior or posterior to the retinal pigment layer?
3. Are these hemorrhages preretinal, subretinal, or intraretinal?
4. Are these hemorrhages nerve fiber layer hemorrhages or deep intraretinal hemorrhages?
5. Describe the identifying characteristics of deep intraretinal hemorrhages.

Small, more or less rounded hemorrhages are located in the inner layers of the retina (but are deep to the nerve fiber layer).

Such deep intraretinal hemorrhages are characteristic of diabetes or retinal vein occlusion.

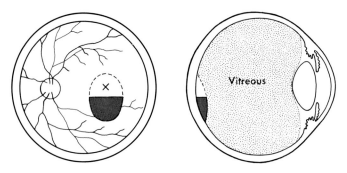

Fig. 8-35

Refer to Fig. 8-35:

1. Is this hemorrhage in the nerve fiber layer of the retina? Why?
2. Is this hemorrhage between the choroid and the sclera? Why?
3. What is the significance of the concealment of the retinal vessel by the hemorrhage?
4. What is the significance of the horizontal flat top of the hemorrhage?
5. Is this hemorrhage freely scattered within the vitreous cavity?
6. Where is the hemorrhage?
7. If an unclotted preretinal hemorrhage is confined between the retina and the vitreous, what shape is the top of the layer of red blood cells?
8. Can a preretinal hemorrhage be seen clearly with the ophthalmoscope?
9. Does the fundus picture differ if the vitreous is healthy and solid or if it is thin and partially liquefied?

Typically, a preretinal hemorrhage has a flat top, caused by gravity (see Plate 9).

The formation of a preretinal hemorrhage requires a moderately large amount of bleeding from a retinal vessel in a young eye (with a healthy vitreous). Spontaneous preretinal hemorrhages are uncommon except in blood dyscrasias.

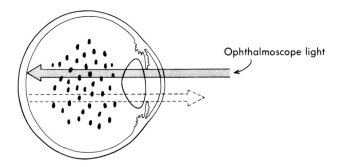

Fig. 8-36

Refer to Fig. 8-36:
1. When many red blood cells are suspended in the vitreous, will this suspension transmit light clearly, or will its density scatter and absorb the light?
2. Since the red reflex seen in the pupil with the ophthalmoscope is caused by light reflected from the fundus, what happens to the red reflex in the presence of a dense vitreous hemorrhage?
3. Therefore, what color are red blood cells suspended in the vitreous when observed with an ophthalmoscope?
4. Can fundus details be observed with the ophthalmoscope in the presence of a dense vitreous hemorrhage?

   Depending on its amount, a vitreous hemorrhage darkens or obliterates the red reflex and conceals fundus details.

HEMORRHAGE

Hemorrhages are conspicuous fundus abnormalities and hence are useful to the ophthalmoscopist because they readily identify the presence of disease. In addition, hemorrhages have different characteristics depending on their depth within the fundus, thereby permitting recognition of the exact depth of the disorder. The depth of a hemorrhage may be determined by its size and shape and by its relationship to retinal vessels and to the retinal pigment layer. Finally, the extent of the hemorrhage helps define the damaged area, another fact of great diagnostic significance.

Hemorrhages exist *near* the vessels from which they originate. This feature will differentiate whether a hemorrhage originates from the disc vessels, the retinal vessels, or the choroidal vessels. Disc vessels are affected by neurologic diseases. Retinal vessels are affected by systemic diseases. Choroidal vessels are affected by degenerative or inflammatory diseases (see Fig. 8-61).

MICROANEURYSM

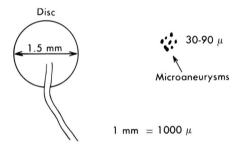

Fig. 8-37

Refer to Fig. 8-37:
1. The optic disc measures 1.5 mm. What is this measurement in microns?
2. If a moderately large vessel at the disc margin is one fifteenth the diameter of the disc, how many microns wide is the vessel?
3. In diabetic retinopathy or in *old* venous occlusion, the typical change is the microaneurysm—a small venous capillary dilatation. How large are microaneurysms?
4. Can the ophthalmoscopist see a 100 μ retinal vessel as it leaves the disc and runs across the retina?
5. Can the ophthalmoscopist see a detail as small as a microaneurysm?

The dioptric power of the eye is capable of remarkable magnification. Details as small as large pigment cells can be resolved by ophthalmoscopy and biomicroscopy.

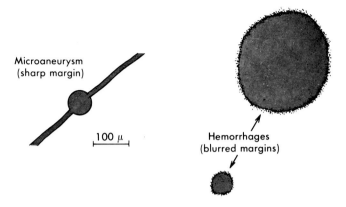

Fig. 8-38

Refer to Fig. 8-38:
1. Since both hemorrhages and microaneurysms contain red blood cells, what color are both?
2. Is color a criterion of value in differentiating hemorrhages from microaneurysms?
3. Can the size of a red lesion be helpful in differentiating small hemorrhages from microaneurysms?
4. Can the sharpness of the margins of a *small* red lesion help differentiate hemorrhages from microaneurysms?

Although on first glance it resembles a small hemorrhage, a microaneurysm (a lesion smaller than the diameter of a large retinal vessel) may be recognized because of its sharp borders (red blood cells confined within the dilated vessel wall, not free in the tissue).

The presence of microaneurysms signifies chronic venous nutritional insufficiency within the retina. They occur in diabetes and venous occlusion and are of great diagnostic value (see Plate 21).

Microaneurysms and neovascularization (see Fig. 8-23) commonly occur together and have the same causes. Both of these red lesions should be distinguished from hemorrhages, since they have much greater specific diagnostic value.

LIGHT-COLORED PATHOLOGY

A variety of unrelated light-colored disorders occur in the fundus. In Figs. 8-39 to 8-51 are illustrations of the basis for the common changes that cause a lighter-than-normal fundus appearance.

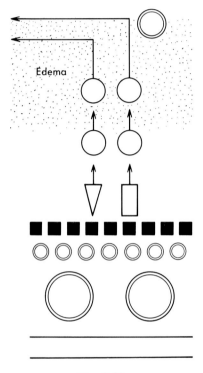

Fig. 8-39

Refer to Fig. 8-39:

1. Is the normal retina transparent?
2. Therefore, can the ophthalmoscopist normally see the irregularly pigmented background composed of retinal and choroidal pigment and the choroidal vessels?
3. If the *inner* retinal layers lose their transparency and become gray or white because of edema, can the ophthalmoscopist still see the pigmented background? Can he still see the *retinal* vessels?

Loss of retinal transparency will block the view of the normal pigment and choroidal vessel details of the fundus background but will not conceal the retinal vessels, because they lie very superficially in the retina.

*The white or gray discoloration of retinal edema will extend as far as the diseased area. Such large gray areas affecting the **inner** retina are due to such disorders as occlusion of a retinal arteriole (see Fig. 8-21) and contusions of the eye.*

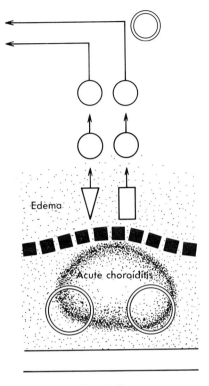

Fig. 8-40

Refer to Fig. 8-40:
1. If the *outer* retinal layers become edematous and opaque because of acute inflammation of the choroid, will the normal pigment and choroidal vessel background be visible in the affected area?
2. Will the retinal vessels be visible in the affected area?
3. Is it possible to differentiate between *outer* and *inner* retinal edema on the basis of visibility of choroidal vessels and the pigment background?

   Opacity of the retina itself, whether due to inflammation, trauma, or nutritional defect, will be recognized as a gray or white area concealing the choroidal vessels and the pigmented background but not concealing the anteriorly located retinal vessels.
   *Choroiditis causes opacity of the **outer** retina.*

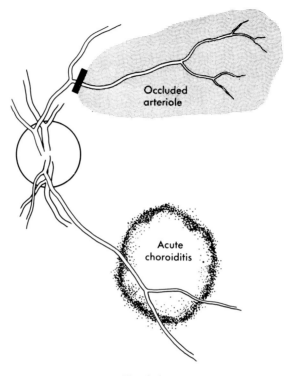

Occluded
arteriole

Acute
choroiditis

Fig. 8-41

Refer to Fig. 8-41:

1. Since both acute arteriolar occlusion and acute choroiditis cause gray opacification of the involved area and conceal the underlying background fundus detail, can these two conditions be differentiated on the basis of the gray color of the lesion? On the basis of the concealment of choroidal vessels and fundus pigment?

2. Is a gray patch that is coextensive with the nutritional area of a retinal arteriole likely to be due to acute choroiditis?

3. Is a roughly circular, moderately large gray patch likely to be due to occlusion of a large retinal arteriole?

Ophthalmoscopic diagnosis is not made only on the basis of the color of a lesion; its distribution and shape are also important, as well as its relationship to anatomic structures such as retinal vessels.

Retinal opacity due to occlusion of a retinal arteriole will extend throughout the area nourished by the vessel (but will be more dense posteriorly because the retina is thicker there than in the periphery).

Retinal opacity due to a focal inflammation will naturally be more severe near the lesion.

Located in the heavily pigmented and vascularized choroid, choroiditis tends to cause pigment disruption and proliferation, as well as hemorrhage.

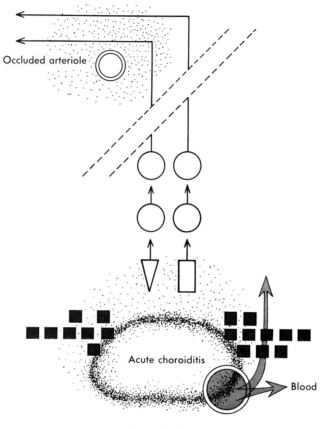

Fig. 8-42

Refer to Fig. 8-42:
1. Would subretinal or choroidal hemorrhage adjacent to a gray lesion help make the differential diagnosis between retinal arteriolar occlusion and acute choroiditis?
2. Would conspicuous hyperpigmentation surrounding a gray lesion be helpful in this differential diagnosis?

Ophthalmoscopic diagnosis is not made only on the basis of color and distribution of a lesion; it is also aided by the interpretation of associated abnormalities.

Anatomic knowledge is helpful. For example, the retinal vessels are distant from the retinal pigment and do not nourish it; hence disorders of the retinal vessels do not change the appearance of the pigment. However, changes in the choroidal vessels may cause atrophy and disappearance of the pigment, which they do nourish.

Hemorrhage originates from blood vessels. Recall that three separate vascular sources nourish the fundus: the vessels of the choroid, those of the retina, and those of the disc. Hemorrhage from each of these three sets of vessels will be located near the bleeding vessel.

After choroiditis, a certain amount of permanent tissue loss occurs.

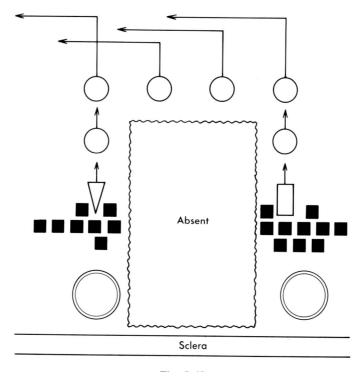

Fig. 8-43

Refer to Fig. 8-43:
1. If this tissue loss includes a substantial area of retinal and choroidal pigment and the choroidal vessels, will the underlying sclera be more or less visible than it is normally?
2. What color is the sclera?
3. Therefore, what color is a fundus area devoid of its normal pigment and choroidal vessels?
4. May hyperpigmentation be expected adjacent to the white center of an old inactive scar of choroiditis?

White or gray areas may be due to exposure of the underlying sclera through loss of normal pigment and vessels. Inflammatory loss of pigment usually causes adjacent hyperpigmentation, whereas nutritional damage to pigment (choroidal vessel failure) usually causes no conspicuous hyperpigmentation surrounding the defect (see Plate 27).

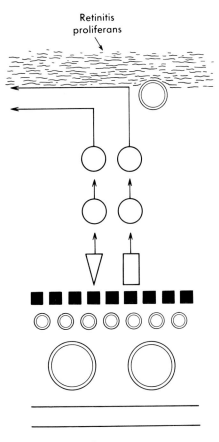

Fig. 8-44

Refer to Fig. 8-44:

1. If a light-colored sheet of opaque connective tissue proliferates on the inner surface of the retina, will it conceal the ophthalmoscopic view of the normal pigment and choroidal vessel background?

2. Will such a sheet of tissue (retinitis proliferans) conceal the retinal vessels also?

Retinitis proliferans is the growth of a sheet of light-colored opaque connective tissue on the inner retinal surface (see Plate 22). If sufficiently dense, this tissue conceals all underlying details. Markedly tortuous new vessels characteristically accompany the growth of connective tissue and are distinguished from normal retinal vessels because they are so tortuous and because they grow forward into the vitreous space.

Advanced diabetes is the most common cause of retinitis proliferans. It may follow severe trauma.

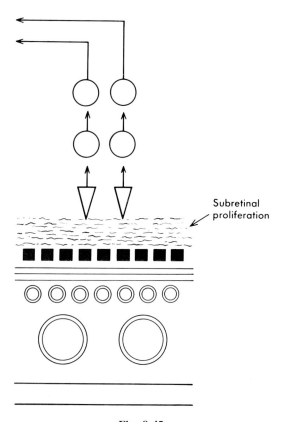

Subretinal
proliferation

Fig. 8-45

Refer to Fig. 8-45:
1. If a light-colored sheet of opaque connective tissue proliferates between the cones and the retinal pigment layer, will it conceal the ophthalmoscopic view of the normal pigment and choroidal vessel background?
2. Will such a sheet of tissue conceal the retinal vessels also?

Abnormal tissue proliferation may also occur in the subretinal space. Here it is almost always due to a degenerative or inflammatory etiology. Degenerative subretinal tissue proliferation almost always occurs in the macular area (see Plate 20). Such changes due to inflammation may occur in any part of the fundus, including the macula, and are commonly multiple in number.

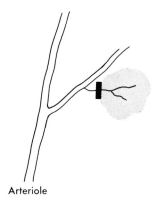

Arteriole

Fig. 8-46

Refer to Fig. 8-46:

1. If a *very tiny* arteriole is occluded, will the inner retinal area nourished by it be more or less transparent than normal?
2. Will the small gray patch (soft exudate) at the site of a retinal microinfarction have adjacent hyperpigmentation?
3. Will subretinal or choroidal hemorrhages (or any other hemorrhages) be associated with the soft exudate resulting from arteriolar microinfarction?

"Exudate" is the term applied to small gray intraretinal lesions caused by retinal nutritional disturbances of many different etiologies.

*A "soft" exudate (cotton-wool exudate) is caused by arteriolar microinfarction and hence may appear rapidly. Although homogeneous and fairly well defined, a soft exudate tends to have relatively fuzzy and indistinct edges. The responsible arteriole is **too small** to identify with the ophthalmoscope.*

Although acute chorioretinitis somewhat resembles a soft exudate, such a deep inflammatory change ordinarily is soon surrounded with sufficient immediately adjacent hemorrhage and hyperpigmentation to make the differential diagnosis easy.

*The various causes (for example, malignant hypertension) of soft exudates may also cause intraretinal hemorrhages, but these hemorrhages will be scattered about the fundus and will have no direct relationship to the soft exudate. A soft exudate is **not** an old, decolorized hemorrhage.*

With time, soft exudates gradually disappear, leaving no visible trace.

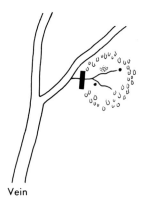

Vein

Fig. 8-47

Refer to Fig. 8-47:

1. If a *very tiny* vein has been occluded for some time, discrete lipoid deposits (hard exudates) gradually occur about the periphery of the area of venous stasis. In what pattern will these hard exudates tend to appear?

2. What two small red abnormalities (with which you are already familiar) characteristically occur in an area of chronic venous stasis (see Fig. 8-38)?

    *A "hard" exudate is a lipoidal intraretinal deposit resulting from chronic partial occlusion of a small retinal vein. Hard exudates have distinct edges (although they may become confluent) and smooth, solid-appearing surfaces. Hard exudates characteristically form incomplete **circular** or **fan-shaped** figures, a distribution of value in making the diagnosis of hard exudates. The dilated tiny vein is usually barely visible in the center of the ring of exudates.*

    Hard and soft exudates are valuable to the ophthalmoscopist because they are an easily recognizable and conspicuous sign of disease. However, both hard and soft exudates may be caused by a wide variety of systemic and ocular diseases and hence are of no help in making an etiologic diagnosis.

    Microaneurysms and small intraretinal hemorrhages commonly occur within the center of a ring of hard exudates (see Plate 10).

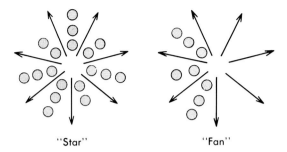

"Star"   "Fan"

Fig. 8-48

Refer to Fig. 8-48:

1. The arrows represent the unique anatomic pattern of the retinal structure in the macular area of the retina. Are the anatomic spaces in the macula oriented horizontally, vertically, circularly, or radially (see Figs. 8-26 and 8-27)?

2. If hard intraretinal exudates are deposited in the macular area, will they assume the circular pattern characteristic of hard exudates elsewhere in the retina?

3. What two patterns may be assumed by hard exudates deposited in the macular area?

Because of the radial configuration of the molecular layers of the retina in the macula, intraretinal deposits (such as hard exudates) immediately adjacent to the fovea do not form circular figures but are forced to assume radial "star" or "fan" patterns (see Plate 23).

Being of nutritional origin, such star patterns signify the presence of diseases such as hypertension.

(Circular patterns of small light-colored deposits rarely surround the macula in some forms of senile macular degeneration. Such circular debris around the macula is deposited in the subretinal space, is not intraretinal, and is not due to systemic disease such as hypertension or diabetes.)

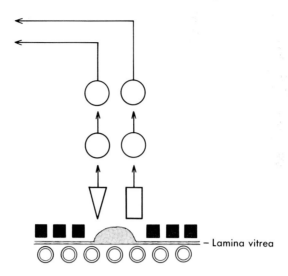

– Lamina vitrea

Fig. 8-49

Refer to Fig. 8-49:

1. If a hyaline nodule develops on the elastic layer (lamina vitrea) that separates the retina from the choroid, what does the nodule do to the retinal pigment layer?
2. How would such a pigment layer fault appear to the ophthalmoscopist?
3. If numerous such hyaline nodules (drusen) were present in chance distribution on the elastic membrane behind the retina, would they be irregularly arranged or would they form the circular, star, or fan patterns characteristic of hard exudates within the retinal structure?
4. Both drusen and hard exudates appear as discrete, small, rounded pale areas of similar appearance. An experienced observer can usually differentiate these lesions by the appearance of the individual lesions. Can you state a way in which a beginner may differentiate between drusen and hard exudates?

*Drusen are common, essentially asymptomatic, small light-colored degenerative changes (see Plate 11). Drusen may be relatively concentrated in the macular area or may be scattered throughout the periphery. Drusen should not be confused with hard exudates, which signify serious general disease, often requiring medical treatment (for example, diabetes or hypertension). **Drusen do not form patterns,** as hard exudates commonly do.*

Differentiation between drusen and hard exudates is most easily made by noting whether or not the lesions occur in a pattern (radial or circular) distribution or haphazardly.

The myelin sheaths of the nerve axons within the optic nerve normally stop just behind the eye and do not enter the retina.

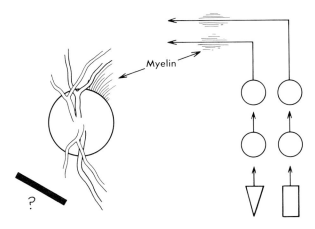

Fig. 8-50

Refer to Fig. 8-50:
1. When the myelin sheaths extend into the retina, what layer of the retina is involved?
2. Therefore, in what direction will a myelinated nerve fiber run?
3. If a linear lesion is oriented as is the heavy line, can it be myelinated nerve fibers? Why or why not?

Myelinated nerve fibers are congenital, nonprogressive, and asymptomatic. They are commonly confused with inflammation, exudates, or papilledema. They are almost white, are often somewhat glistening, usually begin at the disc margin, and always run radially from the disc in the anatomic direction of the nerve fiber layer distribution. Since the myelin sheaths do not all end simultaneously, some being longer than others, the peripheral edge of a myelin patch is often irregularly frayed, somewhat like a rough feather edge (see Plate 14).

Myelination does not cause pathologic changes such as hemorrhage, pigment disturbance, or edema, which are commonly associated with exudates, inflammations, or papilledema.

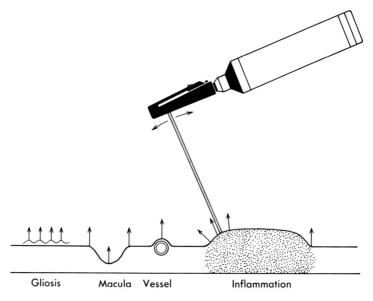

Gliosis   Macula   Vessel   Inflammation

Fig. 8-51

Refer to Fig. 8-51:

1. Are reflections *(arrows)* from the retinal surface more apt to be noticeable in areas where the surface is flat or where it is curved?
2. Identify several situations in which the retinal surface will be curved and therefore produce more conspicuous reflections.
3. Will movement of the ophthalmoscope, thereby changing the incidence of light, cause apparent shifting of the retinal reflections?
4. If the answer to question 3 is affirmative, what can the ophthalmoscopist do to differentiate reflections from structural abnormalities as the cause of a light-colored fundus appearance?

Reflections may be identified as such because they move as the position of the ophthalmoscope is changed. Reflections are always present at the edge of an area of retinal edema and are essential to this diagnosis. The corrugated contour of delicate scar tissue on the inner retinal surface causes exaggerated reflections. Reflections are universally present in healthy young fundi and are particularly conspicuous where curvatures change (for example, in the vessels and macula).

Study of the pattern of reflections will reveal the contour of a transparent interface such as the retinal surface. Distortion of the interfaces within the eye occurs characteristically with a variety of relatively uncommon ocular diseases.

PIGMENTARY CHANGES

Changes in the melanin of the fundus affect, of course, only the choroid and the retinal pigment layer. This pigment may disappear or proliferate in response to injury, inflammation, or degenerative change (see Figs. 8-42 and 8-43). Choroidal hemorrhage appears dark (see Fig. 8-31).

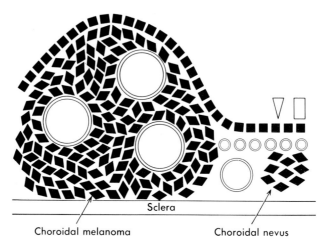

Fig. 8-52

Refer to Fig. 8-52:
1. If a localized benign hyperpigmentation (nevus) occurs in the choroid, will this area appear lighter or darker than the normal adjacent fundus?
2. Will a benign hyperpigmentation of the choroid (nevus) cause a thickening of the choroid and therefore an ophthalmoscopically recognizable elevation of the area?
3. Will growth of a malignant melanoma in the choroid cause an ophthalmoscopically recognizable elevation of the area?
4. Would differentiation between a choroidal nevus and a choroidal melanoma be made on the basis of the color of the lesion or the elevation of the lesion?

*Benign nevi of the choroid are commonly seen, rounded, dark areas, of size varying from smaller than the disc to many disc diameters (see Plate 17). Benign nevi are **never** elevated, whereas malignant melanomas **must** be elevated before diagnosis is possible (see Plate 18).*

Localized hyperpigmentation or pigment loss may occur developmentally (see Fig. 8-6), as a result of inflammation (see Figs. 8-8, 8-42, and 8-43), or because of injury or spontaneous degeneration.

Pigmentary changes result, of course, only when the pigmented layers (retinal pigment layer, choroid) of the fundus are affected, and they do not accompany changes of the inner retina only. For example, papilledema, occlusion of the central retinal vein, and occlusion of the central retinal artery do not cause pigmentary changes.

In retinitis pigmentosa (a rare hereditary degenerative eye disorder) and in ocular syphilis, the retinal pigment layer and the retina itself deteriorate. This results in a unique fundus hyperpigmentation.

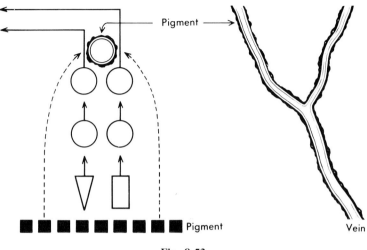

Fig. 8-53

Refer to Fig. 8-53:
1. Around what normally unpigmented structure in the inner retina does the migrating pigment debris accumulate?
2. When the retinal vein is sheathed with melanin pigment, what color does the ophthalmoscopist perceive surrounding and paralleling the course of the retinal veins?
3. In frontal ophthalmoscopic view, is the shape of pigment sheathing of small venous branches rounded, or is it linear, angular, and branching?

Densely black or very dark pigment in linear or angular distribution is characteristic of deposition along retinal veins. This unusual finding (called "bone corpuscle" pigmentation) is almost pathognomonic of syphilis or of retinitis pigmentosa (see Plate 16).

Characteristically, in retinitis pigmentosa such bone corpuscle pigmentation occurs just posterior to the equator and is associated with a marked narrowing of the arteriolar diameter.

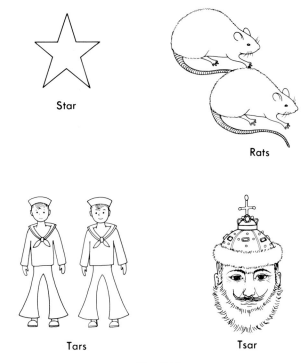

Star

Rats

Tars

Tsar

Fig. 8-54

Refer to Fig. 8-54:
1. What common feature unites a star, a pair of rodents, several sailors, and the imperial ruler of old Russia?
2. What differs in regard to these four letters as they designate these various things?

In our language, a word is identified not only by the letters it contains but also by the arrangement of these letters.

So also, the diagnosis of a fundus disorder is made not only by the kinds of abnormalities present but also by their arrangement.

GENERAL REVIEW

In the preceding figures you have been introduced to most of the basic types of abnormalities that may be found in the fundus. These abnormalities include the following:

Arteriolar constriction	(Figs. 8-17 to 8-19, 8-21)
Venous dilatation	(Figs. 8-18, 8-22)
Hemorrhages	
Preretinal	(Figs. 8-28 to 8-30, 8-35)
Nerve fiber layer	(Figs. 8-28, 8-29, 8-33)
Deep intraretinal	(Figs. 8-28, 8-29, 8-34, 8-38)
Subretinal	(Figs. 8-28, 8-30, 8-31)
Choroidal	(Figs. 8-28, 8-30, 8-31)
Microaneurysms	(Figs. 8-22, 8-37, 8-38, 8-47)
Neovascularization	(Figs. 8-22, 8-44, 8-47)
Exudates	
Hard	(Figs. 8-27, 8-47, 8-48)
Soft	(Fig. 8-46)
Drusen	(Fig. 8-49)
Edema	(Figs. 8-25, 8-29 to 8-42, 8-46, 8-51)
Newly formed tissue	(Figs. 8-44, 8-45)
Myelin	(Fig. 8-50)
Hyperpigmentation	(Figs. 8-6, 8-7, 8-40, 8-42, 8-52, 8-53)
Pigment loss	(Figs. 8-5, 8-7, 8-43)
Elevation	(Figs. 8-12, 8-25, 8-52, 8-58 to 8-60)

The ophthalmoscopist should seek to recognize these various types of abnormalities *and* their distribution within the fundus, for this information is required for etiologic diagnosis.

CHARACTERISTICS OF SOME COMMON DISEASES

For illustrative purposes, the findings and the distribution of the findings in some representative fundus disorders will be listed. Obviously, to diagnose the cause of a fundus abnormality, the physician needs to recognize all the varieties of fundus change present and also the area involved by the changes.

Diabetes

Findings of primary significance
   Microaneurysms (early)
   Neovascularization (moderately advanced)
   Retinitis proliferans (far advanced)
Distribution
   Rather uniformly about posterior fundus
   (*Not* in venous tributary area)
Secondary findings
   Hard exudates
   Deep intraretinal hemorrhages
   Small retinal venous occlusions

Hypertension

Findings of primary significance
  Arteriolar narrowing, focal or generalized
  Nerve fiber layer hemorrhages
Distribution
  Throughout fundus
  (*Not* in single-vessel tributary area, except in early stages)
Secondary findings
  Soft exudates
  Hard exudates
  Retinal venous branch occlusions

Papilledema

Findings of primary significance
  Hyperemia
  Edema
  Nerve fiber layer hemorrhages
  Elevation of disc
Distribution
  Confined to area within several disc diameters of disc
Secondary findings
  Hard exudates

Arteriolar sclerosis

Findings of primary significance
  Widening of arteriolar light reflex
  Nicking at arteriovenous crossings
  Orange or gray discoloration of arterioles
Distribution
  Throughout larger arterioles
Secondary findings
  Disappearance of retinal pigment (because of choroidal sclerosis)

Blood dyscrasia

Findings of primary significance
  Hemorrhages of retina, especially preretinal
Distribution
  Throughout fundus
Secondary findings
  White centers in intraretinal hemorrhages
  White sheathing of vessels

Occluded retinal arteriole

Findings of primary significance
   Gray discoloration (loss of transparency) of affected retina
   Reduced caliber of arteriole (not always present)
   Embolus may be visible at site of occluded bifurcation
Distribution
   In area nourished by affected vessel
   Does not extend to periphery of retina (too thin to show discoloration)
Secondary findings
   Late optic atrophy (after 1 month)

Occluded retinal vein

Findings of primary significance
   Hemorrhages
     Nerve fiber layer
     Deep intraretinal
   Neovascularization
   Compression of affected vein at arteriovenous crossing
Distribution
   Confined to tributary area of affected vein
   Numerous hemorrhages throughout affected area
Secondary findings
   White sheathing of venous walls, late
   Proliferation of glistening delicate layer of connective tissue on inner retinal surface,
     especially in macular area, late

Chorioretinitis

Findings of primary significance
   White choroidal infiltrate (leukocytes)
   Pigment proliferation about periphery of lesion
   Subretinal or choroidal hemorrhages
Distribution
   Localized rounded lesion anywhere in fundus
Secondary findings
   Late exposure of sclera through atrophic center of lesion

Retinal detachment

Findings of primary significance
   Uneven elevation of retina
   Disappearance of normal pigment and vessel background (concealed by subretinal
     fluid)
   Retinal hole (the beginner cannot find this detail)
Distribution
   Any part of retina may be affected, usually the periphery first
Secondary findings
   Cystic degeneration of retina
   Pigmented subretinal demarcation lines

Senile macular degeneration

Findings of primary significance
  Pigment disturbances
  Choroidal and subretinal hemorrhages
Distribution
  Confined to macular area
Secondary findings
  Cystic retinal deterioration

Ocular contusion

Findings of primary significance
  Gray discoloration of affected retina
  Hemorrhages (usually subretinal or choroidal)
  Crescentic ruptures of retinal pigment epithelium
Distribution
  Especially in posterior portion of fundus
  May be directly internal to site of contusion
Secondary findings
  Vitreous hemorrhage
  Retinal detachment

TECHNIQUES OF OPHTHALMOSCOPE USE

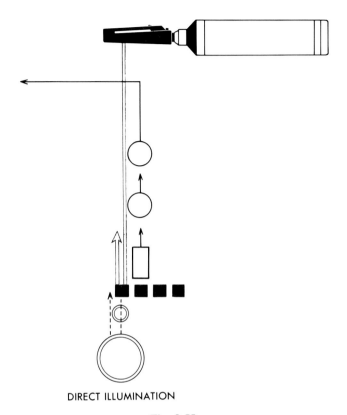

DIRECT ILLUMINATION

Fig. 8-55

Refer to Fig. 8-55:
1. When the ophthalmoscope light is positioned directly on the detail being observed (direct illumination), does the entering light first encounter the retinal pigment epithelium or the underlying choroidal details?
2. If the retinal pigment epithelium is normally dense, will more returning light (visible detail) come from the pigment epithelium or from the choroidal structures?
3. With direct illumination, is the normal pigment epithelium more clearly visible than the underlying choroid?

   With direct illumination (ophthalmoscope light directed on the detail under study), the retinal pigment epithelium and all details internal to it (for example, retinal vessels) are clearly visible. However, details external to the retinal pigment epithelium (for example, choroidal vessels) are relatively indistinct or concealed completely.

As defined in Fig. 8-55, the light returning from the illuminated site is termed "direct illumination." A lesser amount of light scatters deep to the pigment epithelium and is reflected forward to become visible as a dim illumination of the adjacent areas. This is called "proximal illumination."

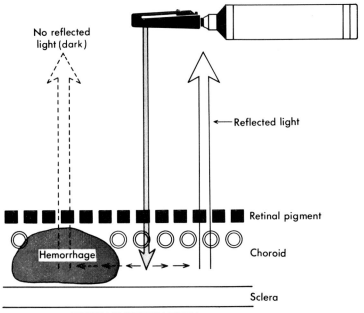

PROXIMAL ILLUMINATION

Fig. 8-56

Refer to Fig. 8-56:
1. If the light scattering through the choroid is blocked by a light-absorbing mass such as a hemorrhage or a benign nevus, will the observer see more or less light returning from the area of the deep hemorrhage as compared with an adjacent normal area?
2. Therefore, will the area of choroidal hemorrhage appear darker or lighter than the adjacent fundus when studied by proximal illumination?
3. If the ophthalmoscope light is directed *beside* rather than *on* a fundus detail (especially a detail deep to the retinal pigment epithelium), will this technique help determine whether the detail is opaque or translucent?

*Proximal illumination (ophthalmoscope light directed adjacent to the detail under study) enhances the study of all details deep to the retinal pigment epithelium. In evaluation of **all** fundus abnormalities, the ophthalmoscopist should employ **both** direct and proximal illumination.*

Proximal illumination is most effective when the smallest white light aperture of the ophthalmoscope is used. The light should be directed immediately adjacent to the lesion, on the same side of the lesion at which the handle of the ophthalmoscope is positioned (for example, the bottom of the lesion, if the ophthalmoscope is being held exactly vertical).

Because degenerative and inflammatory changes selectively affect the choroid and the outer layers of the retina, the technique of proximal illumination will be especially rewarding in the study of these lesions.

●   ●   ●

IMPORTANT: *Everyone (you included) thinks the ophthalmoscope light should be aimed directly at the detail being studied.* **This is not always true!** *Also use proximal illumination during your examination of every eye (look adjacent to the light, as well as directly at it).*

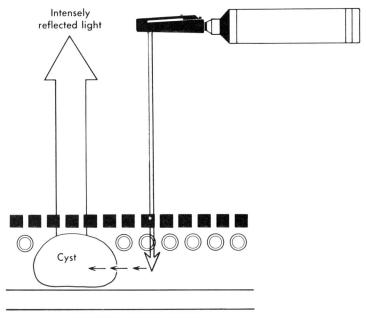

PROXIMAL ILLUMINATION

Fig. 8-57

Refer to Fig. 8-57:
1. If the light scattering through the choroid by proximal illumination encounters an abnormally translucent area such as a cyst, will the observer see more or less light returning from the area of the cyst, as compared with an adjacent normally pigmented area?
2. Therefore, is the technique of proximal illumination useful in recognizing abnormally translucent areas as well as opaque areas?

Proximal illumination will reveal whether a fundus lesion is translucent or opaque. This knowledge is of obvious value in differential diagnosis.

The usually employed direct illumination will often not disclose whether a fundus lesion is translucent or opaque.

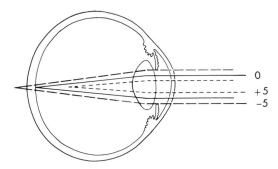

Fig. 8-58

Refer to Fig. 8-58:

1. What ophthalmoscopic lens power will focus on the emmetropic fundus (excluding accommodation by observer and patient)?
2. Are plus or minus lenses required to focus anteriorly within the eye?
3. Are plus or minus lenses required to focus farther back into a long myopic eye?
4. State a general principle of help in determining the amount of elevation of an intraocular detail.

Focusing with the lens wheel will help in judging depth (elevation or excavation) within the eye. Three diopters of lens focusing corresonds to 1 mm of elevation.

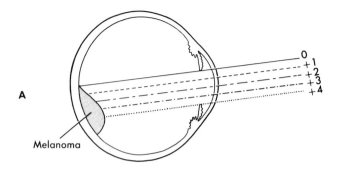

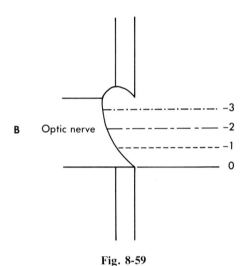

Fig. 8-59

Refer to Fig. 8-59:
1. Is greater plus or minus lens power required to focus forward within the eye on an elevated object such as a choroidal melanoma?
2. Can the bottom of a deeply excavated glaucomatous cup be clearly seen with the same ophthalmoscopic setting used to view the surrounding fundus?
3. Should the ophthalmoscope be changed in a plus or minus direction to focus from the fundus to the bottom of a glaucomatous cup?

   Recognition of elevation identifies the presence of an abnormality within the eye. Examples of elevated abnormalities include neoplasms, retinal detachment, and retinitis proliferans.
   If a given detail is extremely blurred, it may simply be elevated out of focus. In evaluation of such a blur, turn the lens wheel in an attempt to focus it more clearly.

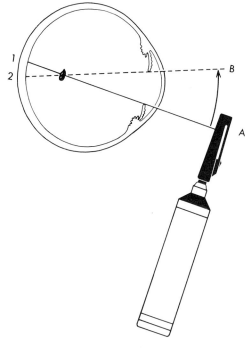

Fig. 8-60

Refer to Fig. 8-60:

1. If, as the ophthalmoscope is moved from *A* to *B*, the background of an object changes from *1* to *2*, what is indicated in regard to the level of the object within the eye?
2. Can parallax movements of the fundus background be observed if the object is situated directly on the retina?
3. What limits the excursions of the ophthalmoscope during the use of the technique of parallax to determine if a given object is elevated above the retinal surface?
4. Would mydriasis help in the parallax estimation of intraocular depth?
5. State a general principle of help in determining the depth of an object suspended within the transparent media.

   Depth within the eye can be determined by the following:
   1. *Concealment. The most anterior of several structures will lie in front of, and conceal, deeper details.*
   2. *Focusing. Changing the dioptric lens strength of the ophthalmoscope is required to focus clearly details at different depths within the eye.*
   3. *Parallax. Lateral movement of the ophthalmoscope will cause apparent displacement of an object against its background—if it is in front of the background.*

ANALYTICAL SEQUENCES

Why do you use the ophthalmoscope? To detect the presence of disease and to diagnose its cause. How do you do this? In Chapter 5, introducing you to physical examination of the eye, I indicated that you must follow the orderly sequence of observing the disc, vessels, macula, and periphery. In general terms, the size, shape, color, margins, and relationship to blood vessels are the details that should be ascertained when you analyze normal fundus structures or pathologic foci.

In Chapter 7 we discussed the clinical characteristics of various types of fundus pathology, again in the orderly sequence of disc, vessels, macula, and periphery. In this chapter the same sequence is followed, this time with the intent of simulating the thoughts that should occur to you as you methodically use an ophthalmoscope and try to interpret what you see.

As you scan the fundus, you will encounter abnormalities that must be interpreted. How do you do this? Are you supposed to recognize a given disease just as you recognize your Aunt Minnie—just because you have seen her before? Or can you follow some orderly differential sequence that will force all the scattered data to make sense? My purpose is to show you just such orderly and logical sequences that will transform your scattered observations into definite diagnostic data.

When you discover a fundus lesion, analyze its color. Is it *red, white,* or *black?* Immediately concede that these colors are all mixed up throughout both the normal and the abnormal fundus. Still, try to decide whether the disorder has red, white, or black components. Although there is an analytical sequence for red (see Table 6), white (see Table 7), and black (see Table 8), the red sequence is usually the most helpful and the black sequence the least helpful in determining an etiologic diagnosis. Therefore, if a lesion has a recognizable hemorrhagic component, first process it through the red sequence. Next, reprocess the lesion through the white sequence (assuming it also has a white component), and finally through the black sequence (if black is also present). The conclusions you reach with each of the color sequences can then be combined to form a sensible diagnosis. With experience, you will find that your mind will automatically

---

RECOGNITION OF LESION

Your first step on recognition of the existence of a fundus lesion is to attempt its classification as primarily red, white, or black.

Is it:

Fundus lesion ——————— Red
——————— White
——————— Black

process your ophthalmoscopic findings, permitting you to diagnose an old chorioretinitis as easily as you recognize Aunt Minnie. But first, you should understand the red, white, and black sequences.

Red sequence. The basic facts about red lesions are that fundus hemorrhage may originate from one of three vessel groups, that each of these three vessel groups suffers uniquely from specific disorders, that each of the three groups bleeds into recognizably different potential spaces within the fundus, and hence that your recognition of the location of a fundus hemorrhage permits identification of its cause.

The fundus is nourished by these three entirely separate vessel groups. Empirically, each vessel group suffers from its own type of diseases (Table 3).

As you learned from Fig. 8-28, there are five potential fundus spaces into which bleeding may enter. Access to these spaces will be possible only from vessels located at the given space. Table 4 indicates the vessels from which bleeding can enter the potential spaces. Fig. 8-61 illustrates the relationships of the vessels to the spaces.

It is evident, therefore, that the ophthalmoscopic recognition of a given hemorrhage will permit the physician to make an etiologic diagnosis of the type of disease, which is the reason why he is using his ophthalmoscope. Table 5, specifying etiology, is derived by combining Tables 3 and 4. *Neurologic* implies that disorders of the central nervous system affect the disc vessels. *Systemic* means the general diseases, such as diabetes, hypertension, or blood dyscrasia. *Degenerative* and *inflammatory* refer to purely ocular diseases.

Note that preretinal and nerve fiber layer hemorrhages may originate from either disc or retinal vessels; therefore, they may have either a neurologic or a systemic origin. The distinction between these vessels of origin may be made by nearness to the disc. Hemor-

Table 3. Usual etiology of disease affecting the various groups of fundus vessels

Affected vessel	Etiology
Disc	Neurologic
Retinal	Systemic
Choroidal	Inflammatory or degenerative

Table 4. Correlation between vessel groups and the types of fundus hemorrhage

Hemorrhage	Vessel(s) or origin
Preretinal	Disc and retinal
Nerve fiber layer	Disc and retinal
Deep intraretinal	Retinal
Subretinal	Choroidal
Choroidal	Choroidal

THREE VESSEL SYSTEMS

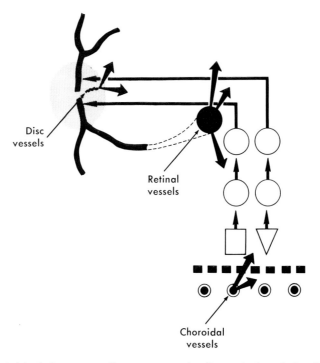

Fig. 8-61. Located in their corresponding structures, the disc, retinal, and choroidal vessels can bleed only into contiguous spaces, as shown by the arrows.

Table 5. Correlation between type of hemorrhage and etiology

Hemorrhage	Etiology
Preretinal	Neurologic or systemic
Nerve fiber layer	Neurologic or systemic
Deep intraretinal	Systemic
Subretinal	Degenerative or inflammatory
Choroidal	Degenerative or inflammatory

Table 6. Red differential sequence—flow chart for localization of fundus hemorrhages

Size	Shape/color		Differential diagnosis
Small	Linear		Nerve fiber layer
	Rounded		Deep intraretinal
Large	Dark		Choroidal
	Red	Vessel concealed	Preretinal
		Hemorrhage concealed	Subretinal

"WHITE" PATHOLOGY

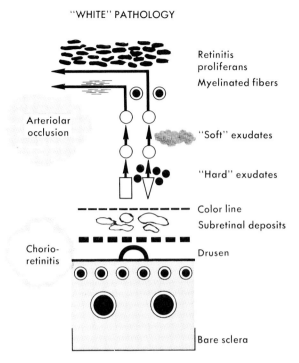

Fig. 8-62. Locations of nine common "white" fundus lesions.

rhages from disc vessels must be within a few disc diameters of the disc, whereas hemorrhages from retinal vessels may be anywhere in the area of the retina.

In order to diagnose the type of fundus hemorrhage, the physician should follow the red sequence (Table 6). A *small* (less than 100 μ, which is the size of a retinal vessel at the disc) hemorrhage (see Figs. 8-28 and 8-29) will be in the nerve fiber layer or deep intraretinal spaces. Distinguish these by *shape*, since nerve fiber hemorrhages are *linear* (see Figs. 8-32 and 8-33) and deep intraretinal hemorrhages are *rounded* (see Fig. 8-34).

Distinguish *large* hemorrhages (usually ½ DD or larger) by their *color*. If *dark*, they are beneath the retinal pigment layer (see Fig. 8-31) and hence are choroidal. If *red*, determine the relationship of the retinal vessels to the hemorrhage (see Fig. 8-30). A preretinal hemorrhage will conceal the retinal vessels, whereas the retinal vessels overlie a subretinal hemorrhage.

White sequence. Unfortunately, a myriad of "white" fundus lesions exist that are not conveniently confined within potential spaces and do not permit neat differentiation, as is possible with hemorrhages. Our approach will be to select the nine most common white changes, shown in Fig. 8-62. Obviously, other rarer white lesions will not fit neatly into this differential sequence; however, there are not many retinoblastomas or other rare lesions.

Table 7. White differential sequence—flow chart for differential diagnosis of "white" fundus lesions

Size			Differential diagnosis
	Shape		
	No pattern (refractile)		Drusen
Small			
	Circle or star pattern (nonrefractile)		Hard exudate
	Relation to vessels		
	Conceals retinal vessels		Retinitis proliferans
Large	Below choroidal vessels		Sclera
	Tributary to retinal arteriole		Occluded arteriole
	Color	*Shape*	
		Rounded	Soft exudate
	No melanin change		
Medium		Striated	Myelinated fibers
		Other findings	
		Inflammatory	Chorioretinitis
	Melanin change		
		Atrophic	Degenerative

The white sequence is shown in Table 7. *Small* designates a size of 100 μ or so, comparable to the size already described as a small hemorrhage. Inspection of small lesions by proximal illumination will disclose whether they do or do not transmit light (refractility). Although an experienced observer can make such a distinction, the beginner is usually unable to do so and should therefore determine whether the small white lesions do or do not form patterns. Drusen (see Fig. 8-49) occur haphazardly, in contrast to hard exudates, which form circular (see Fig. 8-47) or star (see Fig. 8-48) patterns.

If the white defect is *large,* determine its relationship to vessels. A large white lesion that conceals the retinal vessels must be a proliferating membrane (see Fig. 8-44) on the retinal surface. A white structure beneath the choroidal vessels must represent sclera that has been exposed by damage to the overlying pigment (see Fig. 8-43). A white area corresponding to the distribution of a retinal arteriole (see Figs. 8-39 and 8-41) represents retinal infarction. Already we have identified five of the nine common white defects.

Medium-sized (perhaps 1 DD, more or less) white lesions are evaluated as to the presence or absence of melanin disruption. A medium-sized white lesion not associated with a black component is evaluated for shape—if rounded, it is a soft exudate (see Fig. 8-46); if striated, it is a patch of myelinated fibers (see Fig. 8-50).

Note the "color line" in Fig. 8-62. This indicates that melanin disturbance will occur in association with lesions affecting the choroid and the retinal pigment cell layer but will not occur with lesions anterior to these pigmented layers. Medium-sized white lesions with associated melanin disruption are usually chorioretinitis or degenerative changes. Their differential diagnosis is not easy and usually requires a search for other manifesta-

Table 8. Black differential sequence—flow chart for differential diagnosis of "black" fundus lesions

Shape	Elevation	Differential diagnosis
Angular		Retinitis pigmentosa
Doughnut		Old chorioretinitis
	Elevated	Melanoma
Disc		
	Flat	Choroidal nevus
Diffuse		Degenerative

tions of inflammation or of atrophy. Not infrequently, a group of ophthalmologists will not agree on this differential in a given patient.

Please remember that other white lesions exist. For example, some neoplasms are "white." Such neoplasms will usually be elevated and possess increased vascularity—two obvious signs. Deal with atypical white lesions by asking an ophthalmologist to interpret and explain the problem to you.

Black sequence. Normally, melanin is found only in two layers of the fundus: the choroid and the retinal pigment layer. Although a variety of diseases may damage melanin, it can respond in only two ways: *addition* or *subtraction* (more melanin, or less). Commonly, both changes exist, since disruption and rearrangement of melanin by disease cause some areas to be hyperpigmented and others to be hypopigmented.

The black differential sequence is shown in Table 8. It is far simpler than the red and white sequences, because only the melanin containing part of the fundus requires consideration. In most cases you need consider only the shape of the pigment change.

Angular hyperpigmentation (bone corpuscle, chicken track) is a unique and uncommon change occurring when both the pigment epithelium and the retina have been damaged in such a way as to permit pigment migration forward to ensheath the retinal veins and capillaries (see Fig. 8-53). If the hyperpigmentation originates genetically, the angular deposits are bilaterally symmetrical and are located somewhat behind the equator. This is the typical appearance of retinitis pigmentosa. Relatively diffuse angular pigment deposits in one eye only (pepper and salt fundus) are characteristic of syphilis. A sharply localized single patch of angular pigment may result from contusion.

Doughnut distribution of pigment, in an irregular halo around a "white" center, results from the disruption of old chorioretinitis, which displaces the pigment to the periphery of the lesion (see Figs. 8-41 and 8-42). (An acute chorioretinitis is a "white" lesion due to leukocytic infiltration and edema—the melanin changes take days or weeks to develop.) Like a tattoo, melanin deposits tend to remain as a lifetime scar.

Disc distribution of pigment, in irregularly rounded blobs, is usually due to the developmental hyperpigmentation of a choroidal nevus (see Fig. 8-52). Choroidal nevi are not elevated, whereas neoplasms are. Actually, only a rare ocular melanoma is black; most are mottled gray, containing a vessel pattern visible by proximal illumination.

Diffuse scattering of focal hyperpigmentation mixed with depigmented areas is most commonly a degenerative change, although it may infrequently result from disseminated chorioretinitis.

SUMMARY

Ideally, this method of presentation has conveyed to the reader something of the exploring and questioning frame of mind that must characterize the successful ophthalmoscopist. Also, many of the more common ophthalmoscopic findings have been fitted into a logical diagnostic framework and have been matched with the appropriate questions that should run through the ophthalmoscopist's mind, almost subconsciously, as he tries to unravel the code whereby the fundus spells out the diagnosis of a multitude of eye, systemic, and central nervous system disorders. Good hunting!

chapter 9 Macular Disease

Because of the great functional importance of the macula, a detailed description of the abnormalities encountered in this region is included in this book. Being centrally located, this region can easily be observed even by the beginning ophthalmoscopist (provided the patient does not move his eyes, which commonly occurs because of the greater sensitivity of the macula to the examining light). Many of the conditions described here are rare; yet they are included to show that virtually every layer of the macular retina can be affected by disease. Another reason for inclusion of a few of these rare conditions is to convince the student of the fact that the ophthalmoscope is capable of diagnosing a great number of unusual systemic disorders. The examples cited are only representative and by no means include all rare diseases with characteristic eye findings.

The manner of presentation of these macular disorders follows the diagrammatic pattern of interpretation explained in Chapter 8. These general principles of ophthalmoscopic interpretation are, of course, equally applicable to the macula as to any other part of the fundus. Please observe that the diagnosis of a given disorder does not rest solely on its *depth* within the fundus (as illustrated in the diagrams); the *area of its distribution* (as described in the text) is also an important diagnostic feature.

The macular area is subject to the same diseases as most other parts of the fundus; however, the appearance of these diseases is somewhat modified by the regional anatomy.

An extremely important diagnostic point is that recognition of the depth of a lesion within the fundus is an excellent guide to its etiology. This is because the various layers suffer from their own unique disorders, as outlined in this chapter.

SURFACE-WRINKLING RETINOPATHY

Beginning on the inner surface of the retina and progressing backward, we encounter first a change due to contraction of a delicate membrane adherent to the inner surface on the retina (Fig. 9-1). Formation of this membrane is most often secondary to vasoocclusive retinal disease or intraocular inflammation, but it may also occur as an apparently spontaneous degenerative change of the vitreoretinal interface. The condition occurs primarily in the aged eye—60 years or older.

The membrane contraction produces delicate striations that may be either parallel or stellate in distribution, depending on the way in which the membrane happens to contract.

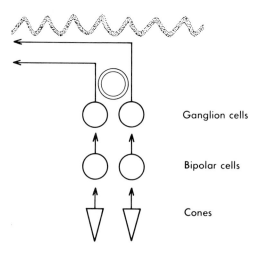

Ganglion cells

Bipolar cells

Cones

Fig. 9-1. Surface-wrinkling retinopathy.

These striations are best appreciated by observing the reflections of the ophthalmoscope light from their surface. Moving the ophthalmoscope slightly from side to side changes the pattern of surface reflections and aids in their study.

Distortion of the macula with associated visual distortion is variable, depending on the thickness of the membrane and the amount of contraction. Tortuosity of the underlying retinal vessels occurs if contraction is marked, but it is usually absent. The membrane does not itself cause pigmentary changes, intraretinal hemorrhages, or exudates.

The area involved by such a patch of preretinal contraction is rarely greater than several disc diameters across. The lesion may occur at any portion of the retinal surface, not only at the macula.

In most cases the retinal distortion produced by such a membrane is permanent. Infrequently, the membrane spontaneously separates from the retina, and vision returns to normal. No surgical or medical treatment is effective.

RETINAL EDEMA

Edema of the full thickness of the retina. Edema affecting the entire thickness of the retina (Fig. 9-2) cannot be due to disease of either the central retinal artery or the choriocapillaris alone, for each of these circulations independently nourishes half the thickness of the retina. The most likely cause of such retinal edema is ocular contusion. Full-thickness retinal edema after contusion is such a characteristic disorder that it has its own name—Berlin's edema.

Contusion edema may affect any part of the retina. Direct blows to the anterior portion of the eye may cause edema of the immediately underlying retina. Hydraulic shock waves may be transmitted to cause edema of the posterior retina. Edema affecting the macula is

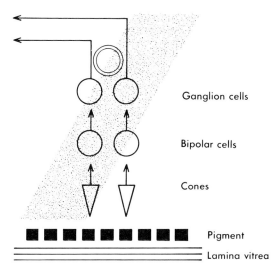

Ganglion cells

Bipolar cells

Cones

Pigment

Lamina vitrea

Fig. 9-2. Retinal edema—full thickness.

more often seen, undoubtedly because the accompanying central visual loss leads the patient to seek medical attention.

Full-thickness retinal edema appears as a dense gray discoloration that completely conceals the underlying pigment and vessel pattern of the choroid. The retinal vessels, being superficially located, are not concealed. A distinctive point is that the fovea also appears gray, although less densely so than the much thicker surrounding macula. In the fovea, only outer retinal layers exist. Entirely nourished by the choriocapillaris, these outer layers remain transparent in occlusion of the retinal artery but are affected by contusion edema.

The area of the retina involved by contusion edema is unpredictably variable, depending on the distribution of the injury. Its borders are sometimes surprisingly well defined. An important distinction is that contusion edema is not confined to the nutritive area of a retinal arteriole, whereas arteriolar branch occlusion is always so confined.

Contusion edema is responsible for the loss of vision that may last for several days after a blow to the eye. Unless structural damage to the fundus occurs (which may be recognized by pigment disruption), vision will return to normal spontaneously. Disappearance of edema is probably not enhanced by any medical management. Nevertheless, careful ophthalmoscopic examination of the ora serrata by a specialist is appropriate after severe ocular contusion, because an inconspicuous tear of the peripheral retina may coexist. Insidious, late retinal detachment will result if such a tear is not detected and sealed.

Edema of the inner half of the retina. Edema of the inner half of the retina (ophthalmoscopically recognizable as a gray discoloration obscuring the choroidal markings and as a cause of enhanced surface reflections) results from occlusion of retinal arterioles

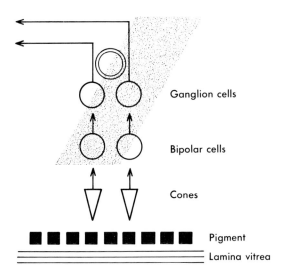

Ganglion cells

Bipolar cells

Cones

Pigment

Lamina vitrea

Fig. 9-3. Retinal edema—inner half.

and subsequent infarction of the inner retina (Fig. 9-3). The extent of the affected area is always related to the distribution of the occluded arteriole. The fovea, composed of outer retinal structure only, is not nourished by retinal arterioles and remains transparent despite occlusion of the entire central retinal artery. Because the posterior retina is much thicker than the peripheral retina, the gray appearance of infarcted retina is most prominent surrounding the macula but may become imperceptible equatorially. Within a few weeks the dead cells are absorbed, and the gray discoloration disappears.

Infarction of the retina causes immediate death of the retina, with irreversible blindness of the affected portion. Visual loss occurs within a minute. Comparable symptoms due to arteriolar spasm may be transitory.

Embolism, the usual cause of retinal arteriolar occlusion or spasm, is almost always due to occlusive disease of the internal carotid artery. Fragments of intimal debris break off and are carried to the brain or to the eye. Because of the development of techniques for successful carotid endarterectomy, diagnosis of carotid occlusive disease is of great significance in preventing cerebrovascular occlusions. Certain diagnosis of an embolus is easily possible by recognizing the whitish fragment within a retinal arteriole. The embolus will be located at the arteriolar bifurcation immediately proximal (on the disc side) to the area of gray retinal discoloration.

Edema of the ganglion cell layer. Selective death of the ganglion cell layer of the retina and of comparable cells within the brain occurs as a genetically transmitted, fatal degenerative disorder of infants—Tay-Sachs disease. In this rare disorder, the previously normal infant weakens and becomes listless and emaciated for no obvious reason. The

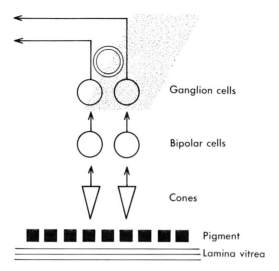

Fig. 9-4. Retinal edema—ganglion cell layer.

characteristic ophthalmoscopic findings are easily observed and are usually the first clue to the nature of the problem (Fig. 9-4).

As would be expected, the appearance is a gray discoloration concealing the pigmentary and choroidal vascular details but not the retinal vessels. The gray density is most marked surrounding the macula, fades away into the periphery (where there are fewer ganglion cells), and does not involve the fovea (where no ganglion cells are present). Both eyes are involved.

The involved area bears no relationship to the distribution of retinal vessels. Because pigmented structures are not involved, no pigment abnormalities occur. No hemorrhages or exudates occur.

Tay-Sachs disease is an excellent example of the value of careful ophthalmoscopy in the evaluation of an obscure generalized or cerebral disorder, whether occurring in adults or in children.

MACULAR CYSTS

Cystic degeneration affects the molecular layers of the retina between the layers of cell nuclei (Fig. 9-5). The far periphery is most susceptible to cystic degeneration, which is present in all eyes, even in childhood. Secondary to injury or inflammation, but most often due to aging, cysts may occur in the macula. The most characteristic appearance is a perfectly circular, uniform thinning in the exact center of the fovea. As would be expected, the edges of a cyst are as sharply defined as those of a soap bubble. Through the transparent center of the cyst, the underlying pigment and vessel markings are seen with

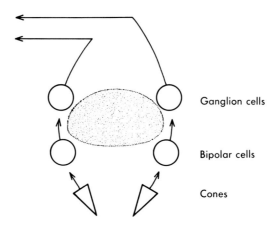

Fig. 9-5. Cystic degeneration.

unusual clarity. A macular cyst may be tiny or may reach a size half as large as the disc, rarely larger. Much smaller satellite cysts may occur, encircling the central cyst.

Visual acuity cannot be predicted from the size of the cyst, but depends on the integrity of the cones, which may or may not be damaged early. When a cyst ruptures and pigment disturbance becomes visible, cone integrity is damaged and a central scotoma results. The observer must remember that a fine granularity of the pigment layer is a normal finding at the macula and should not be misinterpreted as a pathologic irregularity.

Through-and-through rupture of a macular cyst to form a retinal hole, leading to retinal detachment, is extremely rare.

MACULAR EXUDATES

Lipoid infiltrates within the retina in the macular region conform to the anatomy of Henle's nerve fiber layer, a radially oriented communication between the foveal cones and their surrounding parafoveal bipolar cells (Fig. 9-6). The pattern of Henle's fibers causes exudates in this layer to assume a radial (star or fan) shape (see Fig. 8-48). This appearance is so characteristic as to permit easy ophthalmoscopic diagnosis.

Star- or fan-shaped figures in the macula usually indicate the presence of systemic diseases affecting the arterioles—for example, malignant hypertension (see Plate 23), hypertension secondary to renal disease, and pheochromocytoma. Infrequently, star-shaped figures result from nearby foci of acute chorioretinitis. Inspection of the adjacent fundus permits differential diagnosis.

The marked visual loss resulting from these macular infiltrates is, fortunately, reversible if the hypertension is medically controlled. This is a good example of a serious medical condition first presenting an eye complaint.

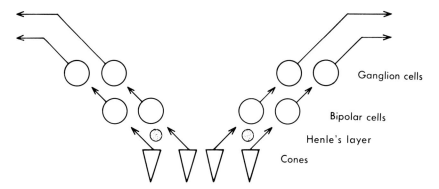

Fig. 9-6. Macular exudates.

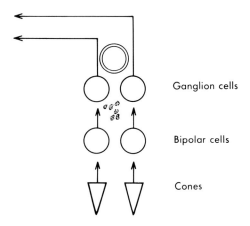

Fig. 9-7. Paramacular microaneurysms.

PARAMACULAR MICROANEURYSMS

Diabetic retinopathy characteristically affects the posterior portion of the fundus. The presence of scattered small microaneurysms (Fig. 9-7) about the macula is almost pathognomonic of diabetes. Small hemorrhages commonly occur, and in advanced diabetic retinopathy, neovascularization develops on the retinal surface.

Diabetic retinopathy is the leading cause of new blindness in the United States and is highly significant because of its frequency and disabling nature and because it is a readily observed finding that not only is diagnostic of diabetes but also is of great prognostic value. Only a few years of life expectancy remain after diabetic retinopathy limits sight.

Retinal microaneurysms sometimes occur overlying areas of choroidal inflammation or degeneration. The presence of such choroidal lesions is so conspicuous as to cause no diagnostic confusion. Diabetic retinopathy does not cause ophthalmoscopically recognizable choroidal changes.

MACULAR DEGENERATION

Selective abiotrophy of the macular cones is a genetically transmitted tendency that causes gradual development of a central scotoma. In its early stages only the cones are involved, and ophthalmoscopic changes are therefore almost imperceptible (Fig. 9-8). With progression of the degeneration, the underlying retinal pigment becomes mottled by irregular proliferation and rarefaction. More extensive changes such as hemorrhages and exudates are not encountered in this core abiotrophy type of degeneration.

Although every ophthalmologist is acutely aware of the frequency of visual loss due to senile macular degeneration, the disease is scarcely mentioned in statistics on blindness. This paradox is readily explained by the fact that the peripheral retina is never involved by macular degenerative processes. Deterioration of the various components of the macula is common enough as a cause of loss of central visual acuity in elderly persons that every physician should be familiar with its characteristics.

The ophthalmoscopic appearance of senile macular degeneration is subject to great individual variation and may closely simulate chorioretinitis, hemorrhage, or even neoplasm. Such gross discrepancies may exist between the ophthalmoscopic picture and the degree of functional loss that it is never safe to predict visual acuity on the basis of fundus

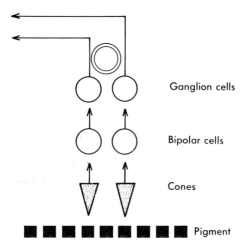

Fig. 9-8. Senile macular degeneration.

findings. Macular changes may include the following appearances or combinations thereof:

1. Absent foveal light reflex
2. Discrete punctate pigmentation
3. Ill-defined grayish discoloration (see Plate 19)
4. Irregularly rounded atrophic spots through which the larger choroidal vessels are visible
5. Hemorrhages, sometimes of a crescent shape (choroidal hemorrhage produces dark, elevated masses; this type of macular degeneration may be mistaken for a melanoma)
6. Gray subretinal proliferations (see Plate 20), usually rather discrete, and often arranged in a roughly circular pattern
7. Macular elevation, yellowish gray or slate colored
8. Macular cysts or holes

Despite any known therapy, all forms of senile macular degeneration are slowly progressive. Clearing of hemorrhages may result in transitory visual improvement. The physician should never fail to reassure the patient that senile macular degeneration does not involve the peripheral retina and therefore never causes blindness. Until he is told this fact, the elderly patient who has had his central vision gradually fade to the point where he cannot read or recognize his friends is convinced that in a short time he will become totally blind.

Genetic predisposition is the most important etiologic factor in all forms of senile macular degeneration.

RETINAL DETACHMENT

Separation of the rods and cones from the underlying pigment epithelium by intervening fluid (Fig. 9-9) may occur as a localized macular change secondary to inflammation or

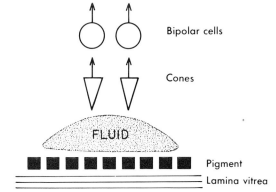

Fig. 9-9. Serous retinal detachment.

to disciform degeneration of the macula. The presence of such fluid beneath the retina is recognized by a glistening irregularity in the retinal appearance when the retina is viewed by retroillumination. Also, the layer of fluid obscures the underlying pigmentary and vascular markings. When macular serous detachment is secondary to inflammation or degeneration, conspicuous pigmentary changes are always present and are much more readily recognized than is the detachment itself.

Progressive retinal detachments originate from through-and-through retinal holes, which are almost always located in the far periphery. If the detachment extends to involve the macula, the patient recognizes that his field defect progresses to involve his central vision. The diagnosis of a relatively low retinal detachment is commonly missed, for there are no conspicuous ophthalmoscopic findings. Finding the peripheral hole is beyond the capability of the casual user of the ophthalmoscope. Only the faint translucency of the thin layer of subretinal fluid betrays its presence. The diagnosis of such a case is most easily and reliably made through the typical history of a gradually progressive field defect.

The prompt recognition of a retinal detachment caused by a hole is of great practical importance, because this condition can be cured by surgical closure of the hole. Ideally, the detachment should be detected and corrected before the macula is affected at all. If progressive detachment has already involved the macula, the sooner the macula can be restored to its normal position, the better will be its function. Retinal detachments occur more commonly in myopic eyes and in eyes that have suffered injury; however, most cases are a result of spontaneous degeneration of the peripheral retina with age.

CENTRAL SEROUS CHOROIDOPATHY

A special type of macular retinal detachment is characterized by the presence of tiny focal leaks through the lamina vitrea (Fig. 9-10). These leaks are readily visible after intravenous injection of fluorescein, which stains such areas of abnormal permeability within the eye. Unaided ophthalmoscopy detects the presence of submacular fluid, because it blurs deeper structural markings and reveals small nodular inflammatory deposits on the posterior surface of the detached retina. The involved area is always circular or

Fig. 9-10. Central serous choroidopathy.

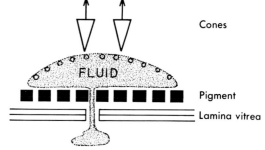

oval, is very sharply circumscribed, and in the active stage is outlined by a well-defined linear reflection from the fluid edge.

Central serous choroidopathy cases moderate blurring of central acuity but not an absolute scotoma. Most cases spontaneously resolve within a few months. The cause is probably a minor local inflammation, but the course is not shortened by antibiotic or corticosteroid therapy.

SUBRETINAL EXUDATES

Whitish deposits beneath the retina in the macular area are distinguished from intra-retinal exudates because they are not arranged in the typical star or fan pattern, but are scattered in a haphazard manner. An exception is the ring of subretinal exudates surrounding the central mass of disciform degeneration of the macula. (This condition is discussed subsequently.)

Irregularly distributed subretinal exudates (Fig. 9-11) located in the macular region in the absence of any other recognizable local disease are of unique diagnostic significance. They indicate the presence of a peripheral vascular abnormality with pathologically increased permeability. Because of absorption by the dense bed of macular choroidal capillaries, lipoid debris leaking into the subretinal space from these peripheral lesions migrates posteriorly and selectively accumulates beneath the macula.

Von Hippel–Lindau disease is an inherited angiomatosis of the retina and the cerebellum; it is also associated with renal tumors. Early diagnosis of this condition is impossible except by the typical ophthalmoscopic findings of greatly dilated vessels in one sector of the retina. These dilated vessels lead to the angiomatous tumor, which is a rounded, slightly elevated, sharply circumscribed, mottled reddish mass. If detected in its early stages, the retinal angioma can be surgically destroyed, so that further retinal damage is prevented. If the angioma is neglected, the continuing subretinal exudation causes extensive and irreparable retinal detachment.

Similarly, early detection of the cerebellar or renal faults may be important to the patient's general health.

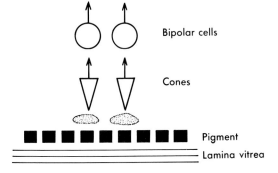

Fig. 9-11. Subretinal exudates.

Another condition characterized by peripheral vascular leakage resulting in subretinal exudates at the macula is Coats' disease. Coats' disease, a peripheral telangiectasis of unknown etiology, is a cause of monocular loss of vision in children. Recognition of the macular exudates should lead to a search of the periphery for the characteristic dilated blood vessels. These vessels can be destroyed surgical'y, which results in arrest of the disease.

DISCIFORM DEGENERATION

Accumulation of connective tissue, new blood vessels, hemorrhage, lipoid debris, and pigment may result from rupture of the lamina vitrea beneath the macula (Fig. 9-12). This degenerative change is ordinarily bilateral, but many years may elapse before the second eye is affected.

The involved macula shows a conspicuous dark elevation that may be mistaken for a malignant melanoma. In this location disciform degeneration is statistically far more common than a melanoma, and enucleation of the eye may be a tragic error. Often a partial ring of whitish subretinal exudates (circinate retinopathy) encircles disciform degeneration. Such a ring is of great diagnostic value, for it virtually excludes melanoma. Hemorrhage is characteristic of disciform degeneration but is uncommon in a small melanoma. Blood vessels are present in both types of disease.

Because large drusen (hyaline deposits in the lamina vitrea) predispose the patient to disciform degeneration, the presence of drusen in the opposite macula favors the diagnosis of disciform degeneration rather than melanoma.

Systemic disorders of elastic tissue predispose the patient to breaks in the lamina vitrea and to the resultant disciform degeneration. These disorders include pseudoxanthoma elasticum, Paget's disease, and senile elastosis. Large breaks in the lamina vitrea appear as irregular cracks in the posterior fundus, somewhat resembling blood vessels—hence the name, angioid streak. For some reason, angioid streaks also may occur in sickle cell anemia.

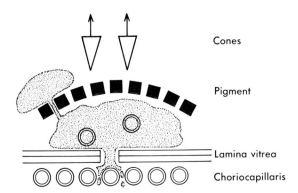

Fig. 9-12. Disciform macular degeneration.

PIGMENT EPITHELIUM

The pigment epithelium (Fig. 9-13) is selectively affected by vitelliform degeneration of the macula and by fundus flavimaculatus. The affected pigment is a light yellowish color.

Vitelliform degeneration is a dominant, very rare condition that produces a prominent yellow-orange disc almost the size of the optic nerve, in the center of the macula. This disc looks almost exactly like an egg yolk. Although the egg yolk appearance is present from early childhood, vision is normal for at least several decades. Gradually, a disturbance of the pigment appears in the macula, and the "egg" looks as though it has been fried. With the pigmentary change, central vision fails.

Ophthalmoscopy is important in young members of an affected family, for it can detect in childhood those individuals who will lose reading vision in early adult life. Such knowledge is helpful in the choice of a career.

Fundus flavimaculatus is characterized by the random distribution of irregular light-colored spots throughout the fundus. These spots are usually much smaller than the disc—they are perhaps a tenth as large. They may be numerous. Usually no visual symptoms or systemic disorders are associated. The condition is so rare as to be of little practical importance.

The main significance of fundus flavimaculatus is that it somewhat resembles and may be mistaken for exudates—small, readily observed, light-colored fundus changes that indicate serious nutritional disorder due to either systemic or local disease. It may be associated with juvenile macular degeneration (of Stargardt).

Rupture of the pigment epithelium. An appropriately severe ocular contusion may cause a tear of the retinal pigment epithelium, the lamina vitrea, and the choriocapillaris (Fig. 9-14). Depending on the severity of the blow and the strength of the individual eye, various combinations of damage to these structures (and other parts of the eye, including even rupture of the entire eye) may occur. Surprisingly, the delicate retina is relatively resistant to such rupture, because it is more elastic than the pigment layer.

The ophthalmoscopic picture, as would be expected, shows a conspicuous defect in the pigment epithelium and choriocapillaris, through which the white color of the sclera is obvious. The deeper large choroidal vessels are more than normally apparent as they cross the defect. The overlying retinal vessels are intact.

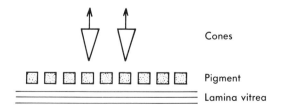

Fig. 9-13. Pigment epithelial degeneration.

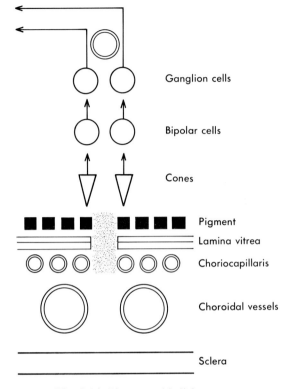

Ganglion cells

Bipolar cells

Cones

Pigment

Lamina vitrea

Choriocapillaris

Choroidal vessels

Sclera

Fig. 9-14. Pigment epithelial rupture.

Pigment epithelium–choriocapillaris ruptures are characteristically linear or curvilinear, may reach 3 or 4 DD or more in length, are usually narrow (perhaps ¼ DD wide), tend to occur in the posterior portion of the fundus, and are usually oriented concentric (not radial) to the disc. If they disrupt the macula (which is not anatomically more likely than adjacent areas to suffer rupture), permanent corresponding visual loss occurs. Hence, the presence or absence of pigment disruption at the macula is of great prognostic significance in ocular contusion, and evaluation of a patient with ocular contusion requires inspection of the macula.

An acute rupture of pigment-choriocapillaris causes localized subretinal and choroidal hemorrhage, as well as edema of the overlying retina. The extent of these acute changes is highly variable in the individual case and will determine whether the pigment rupture is concealed or visible. If subretinal hemorrhage (originating from choroidal vessels) is present after injury, the ophthalmoscopist may infer that rupture of the pigment epithelium must be present to have permitted the entry of blood into this space.

The outcome of a rupture of the macula is determined by the severity of the injury rather than by subsequent skill in medical management.

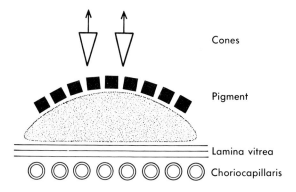

Fig. 9-15. Pigment epithelial detachment.

Detachment of the pigment epithelium. Fluid may (uncommonly) accumulate between the pigment epithelium and the lamina vitrea (Fig. 9-15). Being deep to the pigment epithelium, such fluid will appear relatively dark to the ophthalmoscopist, even though it may be serous fluid. Evaluation of the lesion by proximal illumination rather than direct illumination (shine the ophthalmoscope light adjacent to the lesion rather than directly on it, as in Figs. 8-56 and 8-57) will usually permit detection of a translucent glow if the lesion contains serous fluid. Blood or malignant melanoma (or any opaque lesion) will absorb the proximal illumination so that translucency is not observed. Obviously, there is an important clinical distinction between a slightly raised dark appearance caused by a malignant melanoma and a comparable lesion due to serous fluid beneath the pigment epithelium.

Pigment epithelial detachment occurs in degenerative (disciform degeneration of the macula) or inflammatory (presumed histoplasmic chorioretinitis) changes and is particularly likely to affect the macula. The conditions causing pigment epithelial detachment are relatively destructive and usually cause permanent impairment of sight in the affected area of the retina.

DRUSEN

Formation of hyaline nodules on the lamina vitrea (drusen) is a common change occurring with age. Inconspicuous small drusen are scattered about the fundus of almost every old eye. When such a nodule becomes large enough to displace the overlying retinal pigment epithelium (Fig. 9-16), it becomes visible as a discrete pale rounded spot. Drusen are haphazardly distributed and do *not* form patterns such as circles, stars, or fans. This absence of pattern formation reliably distinguishes drusen from intraretinal hard exudates, which are localized nutritional changes conforming to the anatomy of the retina. Because drusen are common, distinguishing them from possibly serious disease changes (hard exudates) is important.

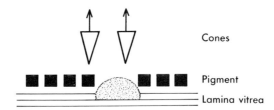

Fig. 9-16. Drusen.

Although drusen affect all parts of the retina, selective concentration sometimes occurs in the macula or in other areas of the fundus (for example, a cluster may occur in the nasal equatorial area). The distribution of drusen is genetically determined; hence, bilateral symmetry is the usual rule. This is not to say that the exact number or arrangement of macular drusen will be bilaterally identical, but that a patient with prominent macular drusen on one side will almost always have some drusen at the other macula.

Drusen, even if numerous, do not significantly affect vision. Sometimes, however, associated changes such as weakness of the lamina vitrea or choriocapillaris deficiency will destroy the macular cones, with a resultant central scotoma.

ANGIOID STREAKS

The lamina vitrea is actually composed of two layers, an inner cuticular layer deposited as a secretion from the retinal pigment epithelium and an outer elastic layer. The elastic layer is affected by systemic diseases of elastic tissue. Recognizable abnormalities of the lamina vitrea occur in pseudoxanthoma elasticum, Paget's disease, senile elastosis, and sickle cell anemia, and as solitary ocular disorders.

A spontaneous rupture of the lamina vitrea (Fig. 9-17) is the classic fundus manifestation of these diseases. Such a rupture is termed an angioid streak because it somewhat resembles a choroidal vessel. The narrow channel of the rupture is irregularly variable in width, a significant distinction from the uniform caliber of a blood vessel. Being deep to the intact pigment epithelium, angioid streaks are relatively indistinct to direct illumination and are best appreciated by proximal illumination.

Angioid streaks do not directly cause changes of the overlying retina, but progressive thinning of the lamina vitrea may permit growth of choroidal vessels across this normal barrier, especially at the macula. Should this vascular ingrowth occur, subretinal and subpigmentary hemorrhages result and cause the form of macular deterioration called disciform degeneration (see Fig. 9-12).

The significance of angioid streaks, therefore, is that they anticipate disabling visual loss, they identify a group of rare systemic diseases, and they aid in accurate differential diagnosis (for example, the distinction between melanoma and disciform degeneration in a patient with pseudoxanthoma elasticum).

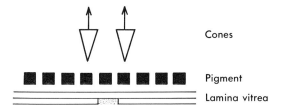

Fig. 9-17. Angioid streak.

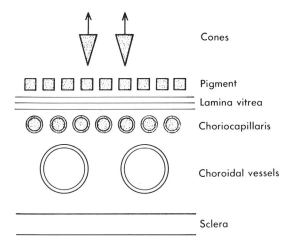

Fig. 9-18. Choriocapillaris atrophy.

CHORIOCAPILLARIS ATROPHY

Focal atrophy of the choriocapillaris is a common change occurring with age that may affect any portion of the fundus. Because the choriocapillaris nourishes the retinal pigment layer and the rod and cone layer of the retina, failure of the choriocapillaris always causes simultaneous disappearance of these two retinal layers (Fig. 9-18). The ophthalmoscopist recognizes this defect because of the abnormal visibility of the sclera and large choroidal vessels seen through the gap in the choriocapillaris and retinal pigment. Overlying retinal vessels, if any, are undisturbed.

Focal choriocapillaris atrophy causes discrete rounded or oval areas that commonly increase in size to a magnitude as large as 1 or more DD in the far periphery, although they are usually smaller in the macula. The edges of such defects are usually surprisingly sharply defined, indicating the abrupt edge of living tissue. Little, if any, debris or scar tissue remains within the atrophic area—even the pigment granules disperse.

Focal lesions due to inflammatory chorioretinitis are distinguished from nutritional

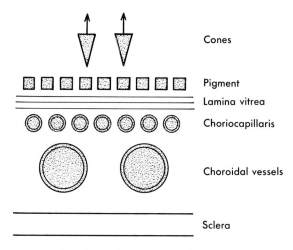

Fig. 9-19. Choroidal vessel atrophy.

atrophy by their characteristic hyperpigmentation adjacent to the lesion and irregularly dispersed within the lesion. Gross hyperpigmentation almost never accompanies nutritional atrophy at the macula.

Choriocapillaris atrophy of the macula is a characteristic type of senile macular degeneration, typically tending to affect both eyes. It is not uncommon in eyes suffering from severe arteriosclerosis but is absolutely not exclusively related to ocular or systemic arteriosclerosis.

LARGE VESSEL CHOROIDAL ATROPHY

Not only the choriocapillaris but also the large choroidal vessels are subject to focal atrophy. Degenerative myopia, arteriosclerosis, and genetic predisposition are among the causes. The appearance (Fig. 9-19) is similar to that of focal choriocapillaris atrophy (see Fig. 9-18), except that the involved area may be many disc diameters across and all or most of the large choroidal vessels are absent, leaving the sclera uninterruptedly visible. Choroideremia and gyrate atrophy are examples of such diseases.

MELANOMA

Although malignant melanomas can and do occur in any portion of the choroid, including the posterior pole of the eye, the diagnosis of macular melanoma must always be viewed with suspicion. This statistical generalization is based on the fact that melanoma is a rare disease in comparison with simulating disorders such as disciform degeneration of the macula and macular choroiditis. All three of these lesions are dark, elevated, and sight destroying. Melanoma, however, requires enucleation of the eye, whereas in macular degeneration or inflammation the peripheral vision and the eye itself are saved.

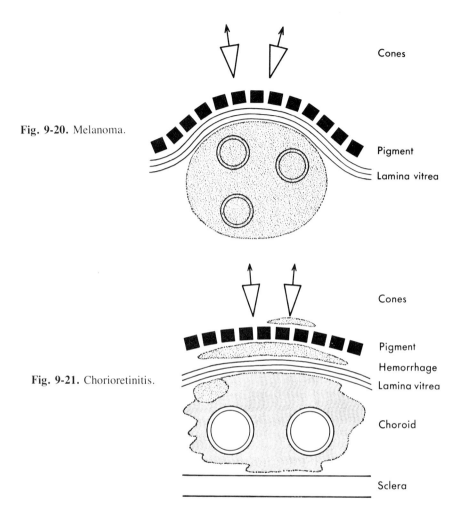

Fig. 9-20. Melanoma.

Cones

Pigment

Lamina vitrea

Fig. 9-21. Chorioretinitis.

Cones

Pigment

Hemorrhage

Lamina vitrea

Choroid

Sclera

The differential diagnosis of these lesions is of such significance that it must be entrusted to an experienced ophthalmologist. His conclusion that melanoma (Fig. 9-20) exists will be based on recognition of an elevated fleshy rounded mass containing visible nutrient vessels and located deep to the retina. Such a mass is typically associated with some overlying atrophy of the retina and usually causes some serous leakage, manifested as a gravity-dependent shifting retinal detachment. It is rarely associated with hemorrhage and exudate of the amount characteristic of degenerative or inflammatory masses of comparable size.

CHORIORETINITIS

Inflammation of the choroid and retina may be due to a large variety of microorganisms. Histoplasmosis and toxoplasmosis are currently believed to be among the more common causes of chorioretinitis. Basically, the condition may be considered to be an acute abscess of the choroid with subsequent scarring. In the acute stage, leukocytic infiltration causes a pale discoloration of the affected area. Edema is always present, overlying and surrounding the lesion, and is recognized by a faint gray discoloration of the retina, along with enhanced reflections surrounding its periphery. Bleeding from damaged vessels is common and leads to choroidal hemorrhages and, if the lamina vitrea is disrupted, to hemorrhage beneath the retinal pigment layer or subretinal hemorrhage (Fig. 9-21).

The scar remaining in old, inactive chorioretinitis is always surrounded by a conspicuous increase in retinal pigment, appearing as a more or less complete, dark ring of irregular width. The central portion of the scar is a variable mixture of focal pigment proliferation alternating with total pigment destruction. Extensive white areas exist within such a scar and may represent patches of scar tissue or transparent gaps through which the underlying white sclera is visible. Hemorrhages, leukocytes, and edema are no longer present when the scar is in the inactive stage.

EXTERNAL PRESSURE

Orbital neoplasms, if they are located immediately behind the eye, may indent it slightly, causing a typical appearance of diagnostic value (Fig. 9-22). This appearance is not so much a gross elevation (the intraocular pressure and the free mobility of the eye resist gross indentation) but a delicate parallel striation of the fundus. The mechanism of this change is a redundancy of tissue. Flattening of the surface of a sphere (Fig. 9-22) decreases the area of the flattened portion. Since the eye tissues are not perfectly elastic, they do not shrink to the new smaller area but are distorted into tiny folds. Although this folding affects all layers, it is most conspicuous on the inner surface of the retina, which is a sufficiently smooth and discrete interface so that conspicuous reflections originate from its surface.

A study of these reflections (move the ophthalmoscope light back and forth) will reveal the underlying corrugated contour. A distinction between the similar appearance of

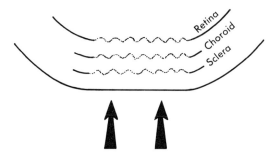

Fig. 9-22. External ocular pressure.

full-thickness folding of external pressure and the inner wrinkling of surface-wrinkling retinopathy (see Fig. 9-1) is made on the basis of the delicate white membrane of surface-wrinkling retinopathy and the greater irregularity of the folds produced by its shrinkage.

Orbital neoplasms are suspected on the basis of exophthalmos. Definitive diagnosis requires demonstration of the mass through palpation, x-ray examination (technically difficult, since most orbital neoplasms are radiolucent and do not erode bone), CT scan, or ophthalmoscopic recognition of the typical indentation of the fundus. The most common cause of unilateral exophthalmos is not neoplasm but thyroid disease.

SUMMARY

This chapter has presented, in superficial detail, representative examples of the disorders that affect the macula, arranged in an anatomic classification. The diagnostic criteria for judgment of the anatomic depth of such lesions are given in Chapter 8. Ideally, the description of these diseases has led to a better understanding of the concept that each layer of the fundus is peculiarly susceptible to its own diseases, which may reflect comparable disorders of similar tissues elsewhere in the body.

Ophthalmoscopic diagnosis is based on knowledge of the depth of a fundus lesion, its horizontal extent and distribution, and its components (for example, pigment, hemorrhage). In addition, the physician must know the nature of tissue responses to disease (for example, neoplasm, inflammation). The responses of the eye tissues to disease are, of course, entirely comparable to those of any other part of the body and hence are more familiar to the physician than he ordinarily realizes.

chapter 10 A Method of Learning Ophthalmoscopy

Let me be honest with you. I know that ophthalmoscopy is by far the most important clinical skill I can transmit to you. I have tried my best to describe ophthalmoscopy and have devoted a major portion of this Synopsis to that task. Unfortunately, reading and rereading all of this will not make you a good ophthalmoscopist. Reading about playing tennis or the piano will not enable you to do that, either.

Every year since 1954 I have taught ophthalmoscopy to Ohio State University medical students. We have evolved a system that will teach the entire class ophthalmoscopy in only 3 hours. This method will work for small or large groups. The general principle is to divide ophthalmoscopy into a sequential series of simple steps. Each step is so simple that anyone can perform it. Immediately after the step is described, all students perform it. As more sequential steps are progressively presented, each student repeats in order all the preceding steps, terminating with the newly presented step. This method develops the proper habit patterns that make use of the ophthalmoscope almost automatic.

Since enough patients are not available for a group of students, they must examine each other's eyes. The real key to the success of this method of teaching is an orderly rotation that permits each student to examine the eyes of half of the group. The opportunity of seeing many different eyes provides experience in technique and demonstrates a number of normal variations.

You can, as an individual, proceed through these steps in the examination of a friend or a patient. Alternatively, you can arrange a class exercise under the guidance of an ophthalmologist, as at Ohio State. The experience of having your own eye examined helps you understand the importance of gentleness and not too bright a light.

In a class setting, the students are arranged in two seated rows, with each student paired with one from the opposite row. In one row, all right eyes are dilated (tropicamide 0.5%, a very short acting cycloplegic). In the other row, all left eyes are dilated. This permits a right-eye–dilated student to use his undilated left eye to examine the dilated left eyes of that half of the class. One row remains stationary; the other row moves in the same direction a distance of one student at whatever interval a new partner is needed. In an auditorium, alternate rows can be right or left eye dilated. To allow examining room in an auditorium, every other seat must be left vacant.

188

Your instructor will have his own convictions as to the smaller details to be presented and will not agree exactly with the following outline. As a reader, you may consider the material "too detailed." However, successful teaching and learning do not "just happen," but require careful and detailed preparation.

Step 1. Hold the ophthalmoscope properly, with your forefinger positioned to spin the lens wheel. You must turn the lens wheel during ophthalmoscopy. Start with the small round white light and a zero lens (unless you have a marked refractive error, do not wear your glasses during ophthalmoscopy, but dial your own refractive error into the ophthalmoscope).

Step 2. Position the ophthalmoscope aperture in front of your eye, bracing it there by resting the top of the ophthalmoscope against your brow. Turn your head and look around the room through the aperture, making sure you do not lose alignment through the aperture. Do this with both eyes. You will use your right hand and right eye to examine the patient's right eye, and your left hand and left eye to examine the patient's left eye.

Additional stability is achieved by bracing your hand against your cheek.

Step 3. The ophthalmoscope handle should be displaced temporally about 20 degrees. This results in better matching of examiner-patient facial contours. Again hold the ophthalmoscope properly braced against your brow and tilted.

Step 4. Although at first you may have closed the other eye to be sure you are seeing through the aperture, you must keep both eyes open and *not accommodate* during the examination. With the properly held and braced ophthalmoscope, and with both eyes open, look around the room at the distant walls and objects.

During a real eye examination, knowledge that the object under view is only 2 inches away will cause automatic accommodation and convergence. However, the optics of the ophthalmoscope do not require any accommodation. You should pretend that you are looking through the patient's head, at the distant wall, just as during this practice session you are looking about without a patient.

> *The purpose of steps 1 through 4 is to familiarize the student with the way one looks through the ophthalmoscope.*

Step 5. While looking through the ophthalmoscope aperture and with its top against your brow, rotate the ophthalmoscope *slightly* on its long axis by pronation and supination of your hand. This moves the light from side to side. Direct the light on the palm of your other hand, held about 1 foot away from the ophthalmoscope.

Step 6. Consider the ophthalmoscope to be articulated on your brow, just as the top of the humerus is articulated to the shoulder, permitting free ball-and-socket rotation as well as joint displacement. Again look at your palm and move the light from top to bottom by vertically swinging the ophthalmoscope handle nearer and farther from your face, the "ball joint" of rotation being at your brow.

Step 7. Now look at your palm again and direct the light in a circle around your palm.

This is achieved by combining steps 5 (long-axis rotation) and 6 (vertical swing from brow).

Step 8. You *must* be able to change the direction of the light freely and easily. Again look at the palm of your opened hand. This time guide the light around the outside contour of your hand, tracing the outline of your thumb, fingers, and palm. Note that this requires a combination of four motions: horizontal (step 5), vertical (step 6), slight displacement of the point of ophthalmoscope-brow contact (as movement of the scapula displaces the shoulder joint), and some turning of your head. Continue to trace the outline of your hand with the light until you can do this freely and easily without losing your view through the aperture.

> *The purpose of steps 5 through 8 is to enable the student to change the direction of the light as the ophthalmoscope is in use.*

Step 9. Position the patient, comfortably seated, with his face tilted upward (for easy access by the examiner), looking at a designated spot perhaps 10 to 20 degrees up and temporal. Position the ophthalmoscope in front of the patient's eye almost exactly the same as in front of the examiner's eye except that the ophthalmoscope is reversed to direct the light toward the eye and it does not touch the patient's forehead. The ophthalmoscope should be as close as possible to the patient without bumping into the eye. Its handle should be directed 20 degrees temporally, as described in step 3.

Since you wish first to examine the disc, the ophthalmoscope light should be aimed at the disc. The disc is 15 degrees nasal to the macula. The visual axis (direction in which the eye is looking) extends from the macula out through the center of the pupil. The "disc-examining axis" enters the center of the pupil and strikes the disc. Therefore, in order to see the disc as soon as you look in, position the ophthalmoscope on an axis exactly 15 degrees temporal to the patient's visual axis. (It is situated 15 degrees lateral to his straight-ahead gaze.)

Position the ophthalmoscope before the patient's eye with light beam orientation on the disc-examining axis. Note that the patient does not like an excessively bright light.

Step 10. You know how the ophthalmoscope should be positioned with respect to your head (steps 2 and 3) and also with respect to the patient's head (step 9). Now combine these two positions. Place the ophthalmoscope properly before the patient's eye. Stand beside the patient and bend over with your head tilted so that your own position corresponds properly to your side of the ophthalmoscope. Never mind looking inside the eye—all we want is your proper position with respect to the patient.

If you are using auditorium seats, you cannot stand beside the "patient." The "patient" must turn in the seat so that his side faces you.

> *The purpose of steps 9 and 10 is to enable the student to position the patient, the ophthalmoscope, and himself in correct alignment.*

Step 11. Look at Plate 1 on the red reflex. You are to look at the patient's eye from a

1-foot distance and see the red reflex. If you cannot see it, either you are not looking through the ophthalmoscope aperture or the light is not directed on the dilated pupil. (The room is darkened, and the ophthalmoscope lens is set at zero.)

For teaching purposes, row 1 is designated as examiners; row 2 as patients. As soon as the examiner observes the red reflex, the "patient" takes his turn as examiner. With subsequent steps, the examiner-designated row alternates, thereby preventing repeated unfair time usage by the first examiner.

Step 12. All the students in row 1 move a distance of one student, thereby matching everyone with a new partner. Again find the red reflex at a distance of 1 foot. Now use the red reflex as a guide to approach the eye until your forehead touches the patient's. If you lose sight of the red reflex, back away to 1 foot, find the reflex, and approach again. Do not look for fundus details in this step.

> *The purpose of steps 11 and 12 is to show the student the red reflex, which is inherently useful in study of the clarity of the media and which is a guide for alignment as the ophthalmoscope approaches the eye.*

Step 13. Row 1 moves again, now and before each subsequent step. Look at Plate 14 as an example of what might be seen on first view if you miss the disc. Be aware that fundus photographs show a larger area than is visible at one time with the ophthalmoscope.

Now repeat everything again—correct ophthalmoscope positioning, red reflex, approach the eye. This time you are to adjust the lens wheel to the clearest focus. Do this as you would focus a microscope back and forth to the best view.

It does not matter whether you are looking at the disc, a vessel branch, or some pigmented structure. Achieving a clear focus is the proper action now. Remember to keep both eyes open and pretend you are looking through the patient's head into the far distance.

Unless you or the patient, or both, are myopic, the lens you select need not be minus (red). The strength of the red lens selected will indicate the amount of unnecessary accommodation you are exerting; if it is more than 2 or 3 diopters, you should again practice looking at the distant wall with both eyes open.

> *Focusing detail is an important aspect of ophthalmoscopy. Discovery of an out-of-focus area that requires plus focusing (black) identifies elevated abnormalities (always serious).*

Step 14. Look at Plate 14. Which direction is the disc? Retinal vessels branch at acute angles that always point toward the disc. This step is to locate the disc.

Find a vessel, any vessel you happen to focus on. Follow it either way to a branch; then go in the correct direction toward the disc. Do this just as you followed the outline of your hand (step 8). If you happen to find the disc first, follow any vessel out to a bifurcation and verify that the angle points to the disc.

Step 15. With a new partner, again find the disc. (At this stage, at least 90% of the students will have been able to find the disc. Since the subsequent steps also involve the disc, the remaining few students must continue to try to follow vessels correctly with each new partner.)

Step 16. Again find the disc. Remember that the purpose of this serial sequence is to learn by practice the habit of doing each step again and again in proper order. Note that you are doing this very quickly already. The instructor can reinforce this process by repeating the steps verbally. The ''patients'' can listen and think as they hold their eyes still.

This time consider its *size*. Compare it to the diameter of the small round ophthalmoscope light, which is a constantly available standard for measurement. If you think the disc is unusually large, you are probably misinterpreting some type of adjacent abnormality as being part of the disc.

Step 17. Again find the disc. Consider its *shape*. Round or vertically oval shapes are acceptable. A horizontally oval shape means misinterpretation of adjacent disease as being part of the disc.

Step 18. Again find the disc. Consider its *color*. Is the color uniform? Is it paler centrally and temporally?

Step 19. Again find the disc. Note its size, shape, and color as before. What is the ratio of the horizontal width of the physiologic cup as compared with the total horizontal width of the disc (C/D ratio)? (The great importance of the C/D ratio is explained in Chapter 15.)

Step 20. Again find the disc. Consider its *margins*. Are they equally distinct on both the nasal and the temporal sides? Are pigment (black) or scleral (white) rims present (common normal variants)?

> *Steps 14 through 20 require you to locate the disc and think of it in terms of size, shape, color, and margins. These are the features whereby you determine normalcy or disease. The C/D ratio is a special subdivision of color.*
> *This should have taken about 1¹/₂ hours, and it is time for a 15-minute break.*

Step 21. Look at Fig. 5-26, illustrating the pupil as the center of rotation of the ophthalmoscope light beam. To see into the periphery, your head and the ophthalmoscope must move in the opposite direction as the part of the fundus being observed; for example, you move down to see the upper fundus.

Find the disc and the blood vessels leaving its upper temporal edge. Follow these vessels as far out into the periphery as you can. Note the relative *size* of the arterioles and veins and the progressive decrease in size occurring at each vessel bifurcation.

Step 22. Repeat with the lower temporal vessels. Note their shape (gently curving).

Step 23. Repeat with the lower nasal vessels. Note the relative color of the arterioles and veins, and the width of the arteriolar light reflex.

Step 24. Repeat with the upper nasal vessels. Note the vessel margins, especially at arteriovenous crossings (the location of the "nicking" of veins, partially concealed by arteriosclerotic arterioles).

Steps 21 through 24 afford practice in scanning various parts of the fundus in a clockwise routine (see Fig. 8-15). Also, it reinforces the concept of describing details in terms of size, shape, color, and margins.

Step 25. Look at Plate 6. The macula is the dark spot larger than the disc, located 2 DD to its right side. The pinpoint central light reflection (fovea) does not show in this photograph, but it is usually conspicuous in a healthy young eye.

Request the patient to look directly at the ophthalmoscope light. You will now be looking exactly at the fovea.

Step 26. Resume the standard approach. Find the disc, then move 2 DD temporal to it. This is again the macula.

Steps 25 and 26 show how little detail is present in the macula as compared with the disc.

Step 27. You can see farther into the periphery if the patient looks in the same direction (he looks up as you are examining the superior fundus). Try this.

Step 28. Now examine the inferior fundus as he looks down. You cannot see in unless you lift the eyelid by pushing the brow up with your thumb.

Any lesion found in the periphery should also be described in terms of size, shape, color, and margins (also elevation).

Step 29. Dial a +10 (black) lens. Look through it at your hand 10 cm away. Note the magnified image. Now lock at the patient's iris, 10 cm away. This will convey some idea as to how you would be able to look at an elevated lesion such as a retinal detachment.

GENERAL COMMENTS

Do not try to do this learning technique in less than 3 hours. The instructor must *not* just talk and show pictures as in the usual lecture. You are learning a psychomotor skill, not cognitive facts, and *you* must actually *do it!*

chapter 11 Medical Ophthalmology

What can I leave out? The Synopsis is already too big. Be aware that I am deliberately omitting almost all of the information usually classified as medical ophthalmology and neuroophthalmology. Excellent presentations of this material are readily obtainable in larger textbooks such as Adler's textbook by Scheie and Albert and that by Newell (see recommended reading, p. 209). Furthermore, medicine and neurology are well represented in the medical curriculum and need not be duplicated here.

The general knowledge physicians possess about physiology and disease is easily applied to the eye and orbital area. Virtually all tissues exist here and respond to disease just as would be expected elsewhere. Bone and blood, muscles, nerves, fat, connective tissue, secretory glands, and skin are all present. Only endoderm is absent. Except for diseases unique to the digestive and reproductive tracts, practically all other human disorders have eye manifestations. Often such eye signs are of great diagnostic help.

DIABETES MELLITUS

Diabetes mellitus is an enormously important and expensive disease affecting 2% of the population. Its all pervasive blood vessel damage causes ischemic necrosis of the legs, nerves, kidneys, heart, eyes—everything. Your general knowledge of the way in which other tissues and organs are damaged by diabetes permits you to predict what will happen to the eye. Directly correlated with the duration and severity of diabetes, vascular disease develops, causing ischemia within the eye. The very high metabolic rate of the retina results in its selective damage. In fact, diabetic retinopathy is the most common cause of new blindness in the United States, being responsible for 15% of such tragedy.

Any of the wide variety of retinal changes associated with diabetes may be present in other diseases; therefore, none are pathognomonic of diabetes. Nevertheless, an experienced ophthalmoscopist can confidently diagnose diabetes on the basis of proper distribution of certain characteristic features of the disease.

Retinopathy does not appear until diabetes has been present for a number of years; therefore, a large group of patients with early diabetes will not have retinal changes. Recognizable changes first appear in the posterior pole of the eye, are often concentrated about the macula, and usually extend only out to the midperiphery except in severe cases. The distribution is fairly uniform unless disease of a vascular branch accelerates the damage in its tributary region. Bilaterality is the rule, but more often than not the severity of involvement differs in the two eyes.

Ophthalmoscopic findings

Components of diabetic retinopathy include microaneurysms, neovascularization, newly formed connective tissue, hemorrhages, hard exudates, cotton-wool exudates, arteriolar changes, venous changes, and lipemia retinalis.

Microaneurysms. These small rounded or oval red dots are sharply outlined, although they may cluster so closely that they almost seem to coalesce (see Plate 21). Rarely will a microaneurysm exceed the diameter of an artery at the disc, and most of them are much smaller.

Microaneurysms vary in size and occasionally reach 100 μ in diameter. Those who do not fully appreciate the magnifying potential of the 60-diopter refractive power of the eye often express disbelief in the visibility of such a tiny structure. A simple calculation reveals that the 1.5 mm optic disc is 1,500 μ in diameter. The large arterioles at the disc margin have a diameter about one fifteenth that of the disc and therefore are 100 μ in size. The resolving power of the observer's eye permits recognition of details one tenth the size of a large retinal arteriole, indicating that the fine pigment granules often seen ophthalmoscopically in the fundus are single pigment cells. Unquestionably, therefore, microaneurysms are large enough to visualize easily with the ophthalmoscope.

Neovascularization. At first, an exceptionally fine capillary network is detected, resembling a hemorrhage thinly spread on the retinal surface. As these vessels grow, they remain readily recognizable as pathologic by their extreme tortuosity. Less commonly, vessels and accompanying supporting tissue proliferate into the vitreous (see Plate 22). These new vessels are continuous with the main retinal vasculature.

Does neovascularization precede hemorrhage, or do new vessels grow into and organize preexisting hemorrhages? Clinical experience indicates the former, since it is common to find early neovascularization without hemorrhage. Conversely, the majority of intraocular hemorrhages, excluding those associated with diabetes or venous occlusion, do not result in neovascularization. Finally, recurrent hemorrhages are most likely to occur when neovascularization is already present. Contracture of newly formed connective tissue causes rupture of vessels and the consequent hemorrhage.

Newly formed connective tissue. Newly formed connective tissue is the meshwork that, in varying amounts, always accompanies diabetic neovascularization. Ophthalmoscopically invisible at first, it eventually forms an irregular, glistening sheen, simulating the appearance of wrinkled cellophane on the inner retinal surface, or it may extend throughout the vitreous cavity in strands or sheets.

Cross sections of the retina readily demonstrate such a fibrovascular membrane. If the fibrous membrane tears and the fibrovascular sheet subsequently retracts, discrete sharp edges are easily recognized. These defects may be banana shaped, just as are some tears in Descemet's membrane. A large semicircular tear may retract, leaving a folded straight edge like a taut bowstring. In more extensive tears, the fibrovascular sheet may retract into a grayish clump that protrudes slightly anterior to the retina. Recognition of this sheet and its retraction clarifies the appearance and behavior of retinitis proliferans. For example, why do we see ruler-straight bands of proliferating tissue? Such linear primary growth seems almost impossible, but the ability of the membrane to retract into a taut "bowstring" fold easily explains such configuration. How do vessels, preexisting and newly formed, assume such bizarre convolutions? Such patterns form easily when contiguous adherent fibrous tissue contracts. Why do repeated small and large hemorrhages occur? Rupture of small vessels crossing a tear in the membrane explains many of them. Intravitreal bleeding more often occurs from tears of the abnormal fibrovascular membrane than from the underlying retina.

In advanced stages of proliferating retinitis the entire retina is subject to traction detachment due to contraction of glial strands throughout the vitreous and on the retinal surface.

Hemorrhages. Many types of hemorrhage accompany diabetic retinopathy. Scattered small intraretinal hemorrhages differ from microaneurysms in that they have indistinct margins. Irregular patches composed of multiple small hemorrhages tend to exist in the neighborhood of microaneurysms or neovascularization and probably originate from rupture of vessels or by diapedesis through the weakened walls of diseased vessels. Contractures of connective tissue sometimes cause superficial retinal hemorrhages that are due to consequent tearing of associated vessels. Vitreous hemorrhages represent forward extension of similar but more extensive hemorrhagic tendencies.

Hard exudates. As a result of many chronic retinal diseases, localized lipoid infiltrates appear within the deeper retinal layers. These deposits are called edema residues or "hard" exudates. Ophthalmoscopially, they appear as discrete, sharply outlined, light gray areas (see Plate 21). Retinal exudates are etiologically nonspecific. The presence of exudates is an easily observed sign of retinal disease but does not in itself indicate the nature of the disease.

Hard exudates may mimic benign drusen in appearance, but with experience it is usually easy for the examiner to differentiate the two conditions. The hard exudates have discrete borders, although adjacent exudates may be confluent. Because of their relatively superficial location as compared with drusen, the whitish surfaces of hard exudates are seen in clear detail. Drusen never form circular or radial patterns, in contrast to exudates, which are frequently distributed in such a manner. Macular exudates, unlike drusen, cause serious reduction in vision.

Cotton-wool exudates. Cotton-wool ("soft") exudates are larger and fuzzier in appearance and usually somewhat grayer than the hard exudates. They represent tiny infarctions of the inner retinal layers. Cotton-wool exudates appear in the large variety of systemic diseases that affect small arterioles and are just as nonspecific as hard exudates.

Arteriolar changes. Arteriolar changes may be sclerotic or hypertensive. Widening of the light reflex, arteriovenous crossing changes, and coppery discoloration of arterioles are well-known features that identify arteriolar sclerosis. Hypertensive disease betrays its presence by premature sclerotic change, focal or general attenuation of arteriolar caliber, and, rarely, papilledema. These arteriolar changes occur only when secondary vascular disease develops as a complications of diabetes.

Venous changes. Venous changes include slight fullness of the veins, not infrequently a hyperemic appearance of the disc, and, rarely, a peculiar beadlike dilatation of a venous segment.

Lipemia retinalis. The rare but characteristic picture of lipemia retinalis appears during diabetic coma when the serum lipids exceed 3.5% (see Fig. 7-2). Both arteries and veins become cream colored because of the high fat content.

Ophthalmoscopic diagnosis

Retinal microaneurysms, neovascularization, or both, located posteriorly and preferably bilaterally, are pathognomonic of diabetes *in the absence of* indications of venous occlusive phenomena (distributed in the tributary area of the involved vein) or chronic inflammatory or degenerative disease. One swallow does not make a summer, and neither do one or two microaneurysms make diabetic retinopathy. Isolated microaneurysms are found in other diseases, including hypertension, glaucoma, inflammation, and venous occlusion.

Characteristic of diabetic retinal changes, but representing nonspecific degenerative changes, are such findings as exudates, hemorrhages, arteriosclerotic or hypertensive vascular changes, and newly formed connective tissue.

Other findings

Neovascular glaucoma. As the disease advances, neovascularization and new connective tissue proliferate on the surface of the iris and occlude the trabecular meshwork. Spontaneous anterior chamber hemorrhage may occur, accounting for the term ''hemorrhagic glaucoma.'' However, the glaucoma is not caused by the hemorrhage but by the proliferating tissue in the anterior chamber angle. Neovascular glaucoma is a rapidly progressive and devasting problem.

Lens changes. Osmotic changes in the lens increase its dioptric strength during periods of hyperglycemia, resulting in myopic refractive changes. Conversely, hypoglycemia causes hyperopia.

Rapidly developing cataract is a rare consequence of severe diabetic coma. Diabetic patients tend to require surgery for senile cataracts at a younger age than nondiabetics.

Neurologic changes. Transient paralyses of the extraocular muscles, as well as optic neuropathy, may be caused by diabetes. Sparing of the pupil innervation in association with oculomotor paralysis is characteristic of a diabetic etiology.

Management of diabetic eye problems

Very careful control of hyperglycemia may be helpful in preventing ocular vascular damage; it is of no benefit when retinopathy or neovascular glaucoma has already developed.

Laser treatment may be beneficial but is far from being a panacea. The theory is that some type of metabolic response to retinal ischemia is the mechanism whereby the eye is destroyed. Logically, therefore, elimination of the ischemic retina should be helpful. The procedure is termed panretinal ablation and consists of applying several thousand retinal burns of 50 to 100 μ diameter, scattered throughout the retina except in the macula. These burns are applied in several outpatient sessions. The flashes of laser light are painless and require no anesthetic.

Laser treatment is advised whenever neovascularization appears, preferably before the development of recognizable proliferation of connective tissue. Collagen shrinks with heat, and laser treatment of advanced retinitis proliferans may precipitate a retinal detachment.

Obviously, several thousand retinal burns are not without disadvantages. Marked loss of dark adaptation occurs and is a significant handicap at night. Some constriction of the visual field results, although this is less than would be expected. The slow progress of retinopathy often continues, requiring retreatment after several months. Hemorrhages, cataract, and retinal detachment can result. In general, however, at least partially useful vision may be preserved longer with laser therapy than without it. Panretinal ablation may eliminate iris neovascularization also.

Referral of a diabetic patient to an ophthalmologist for evaluation and possible laser therapy is advised whenever the patient develops symptoms referable to the eyes or if fundus changes are recognized.

HYPERTENSION

Lesser degrees of increased blood pressure exhibit minimal ophthalmoscopic changes or nothing at all. However, typical retinal changes accurately reflect the severity of advanced hypertension and permit positive diagnosis through ophthalmoscopy.

Ophthalmoscopic findings

Components of hypertensive retinopathy include arteriolar attenuation, arteriolar sclerosis, hemorrhages, exudates, and vascular occlusions.

Arteriolar attenuation. Narrowing of arteriolar caliber may be either in focal segments or throughout the arteriolar tree (see Plate 23). Whether the attenuation is focal or generalized has no practical significance. Focal narrowing is easier to recognize because it is obvious that a thin segment should not exist between two areas of normal caliber. Focal attenuations may be few in number, and the whole arteriolar tree must be scanned in orderly sequence to detect such changes. Apparent narrowing of an arteriole may normally be seen overlying the disc because the vessel is partially hidden in connective tissue; therefore, if the only visible arteriolar attenuations overlie the disc, they do not justify the diagnosis of hypertension.

Obviously, vessel branches are naturally narrower than the parent vessel, and arterioles grow smaller as they branch toward the periphery. Less apparent to the beginner is the fact that the caliber of the arterioles near the disc depends on the number of branches formed from the central retinal artery. If many arterioles cross the disc margin, their caliber will be smaller than if only several branchings have occurred. Comparisons of arteriolar with venous calibers are meaningless unless this matter of the number of branches is taken into consideration. In general, arteriole-vein ratios are valid only when vessels that supply an equal amount of tributary retinal area are compared. Specifically, a tiny arteriolar branch leading to part of the macula cannot be compared with a huge vein draining the entire lower retina.

The custom is to estimate the degree of general attenuation of arterioles by comparison with venous caliber, and the supposed normal ratio is for an arteriole to be about two thirds to three fourths the size of its corresponding vein. However, the preceding remarks concerning the variable branching of arterioles and veins indicate that sound judgment is necessary to reach a diagnosis of generalized attenuation. Even the yardstick of venous diameter may be misleading if venous congestion and dilatation exist. My most valid criterion is my own experience as to the apparent size of normal arterioles in relation to the disc size. The difficulty of making accurate arteriole measurements in terms of veins could be compared to the problem a pediatrician would face if he measured the height of children in terms of dog lengths—and used different dogs!

Nevertheless, with experience you will be able to state definitely that arteriolar constriction exists, and this constriction will be the main criterion on which the diagnosis of hypertensive retinopathy is based. In preparation for making this judgment, you should carefully observe the arteriolar caliber in all your normal patients.

The degree of constriction and the severity of hypertension are directly related. In fact, the crucial distinction between grade II hypertensive retinopathy (usually "benign") and grade III ("malignant") is the presence of unequivocal arteriolar constriction. With increasing severity of hypertension, the arterioles usually become progressively narrower.

Arteriolar sclerosis. Although sclerotic changes in the arteriolar walls are not necessarily related to hypertension, they do occur with greater frequency in hypertensive patients. Perhaps the simplest concept is that sclerotic changes occur with age but may be prematurely accelerated through adverse circumstances that increase vessel wear and tear. Hypertension is one of the outstanding causes of premature arteriolar sclerosis. In fact, if excessive retinal arteriolar sclerosis is observed in a young person, a tentative diagnosis of hypertension is justified. Grade I hypertensive retinopathy is the condition in which more sclerotic changes exist than would normally be expected for the patient's age. Grade II hypertensive retinopathy represents yet more advanced sclerosis. It should be clearly understood that the ophthalmoscopist is *not* justified in diagnosing grade I hypertensive retinopathy on the basis of the fundus picture alone. He must know from the patient's history that hypertension exists, and by making a diagnosis of grade I, he indicates that minimal vascular damage is observable. Grade II changes in a younger person are severe enough to suggest a tentative guess at the diagnosis of hypertension.

Emphasis is laid on the age of the patient because many older patients develop arteriolar sclerosis without having blood pressure elevations. Even severe arteriosclerotic changes in the retina of an older person do not warrant any estimate as to the presence of hypertension.

Criteria used to diagnose arteriolar sclerosis are discussed later in this chapter.

Hemorrhages. "Typical" hypertensive hemorrhages are described as being linear or flame shaped. This orientation is due to their position in the nerve fiber layer of the retina. Radiating out from the disc, the nerve fibers force hemorrhage at this level into a radial, linear pattern. Although commonly occurring in hypertension, linear hemorrhages are seen in association with many other diseases, including subarachnoid hemorrhage, papilledema, blood dyscrasia, and trauma. The typical linear hemorrhage of the nerve fiber layer is much smaller than the disc, somewhat comparable in size to a segment of a small retinal vessel. Many such tiny hemorrhages may become almost confluent to produce the appearance of a large hemorrhage. Such nerve fiber layer hemorrhages in occlusion of the retinal vein (a complication of hypertensive or arteriosclerotic disease, usually) typically extend across large areas of the fundus.

Microaneurysms and smaller rounded hemorrhages occur if venous occlusions complicate the hypertensive retinopathy. Infrequently, massive vitreous hemorrhages may occur.

Although none of these hemorrhages are diagnostic of hypertensive retinopathy, they are easily observed, definite signs of retinal disorder and are therefore most helpful in calling the ophthalmoscopist's attention to the presence of disease. Almost always there will be numerous hemorrhages and exudates present in grade III hypertensive retinopathy, although the really significant feature of grade III is marked arteriolar attenuation.

Exudates. Exudates are grayish discolorations of the retina occurring in definite patches. "Hard" exudates have more discrete borders and a smoother surface. They represent degenerative lipoid deposits within the retina, and they usually require considerable time to develop. "Soft" exudates appear as fluffy clouds with indistinct edematous edges and surfaces. They represent minute superficial retinal infarctions surrounding a tiny occluded arteriolar capillary and may appear fairly rapidly. Soft exudates may gradually disappear completely or leave a small irregular scar. Both types of exudates are commonly present in grade III hypertensive retinopathy—and also in many other diseases. Since they occur in many conditions, exudates are treacherous criteria on which to base an etiologic diagnosis, and you are well advised not to attempt to do so. Exudates about the macula frequently arrange themselves to form radial or circular patterns (see Plate 23), in contrast to the similar-appearing benign hyaline deposits known as drusen, which never form patterns.

Vascular occlusions. Hypertensive retinopathy, especially of the more severe grades, is often complicated by occlusions of branches of the central retinal artery and vein. The typical pictures of these occlusions are described in Chapter 8. Involvement of macular vessels will result in serious visual impairment.

Ophthalmoscopic diagnosis

A practical classification of hypertensive retinopathy is as follows:

Grade I	More arteriolar sclerosis than expected in a young person
Grade II	More pronounced sclerosis than in grade I
Grade III	Definite arteriolar attenuation, either focal or general; usually also hemorrhages and exudates
Grade IV	Grade III changes plus papilledema

Grade I is simply an estimate of minimal vascular damage occurring in persons with known hypertension. Grade II is only a tentative diagnosis, which might be inaccurate. Grades I and II occur in "benign" hypertension. Grade III carries a much graver significance, occurs in "malignant" hypertension, and may be positively identified through the presence of arteriolar attenuation. Exudates and hemorrhages alone do not permit etiologic diagnosis but serve admirably to call attention to the presence and severity of disease. Papilledema indicates that the severity has progressed to hypertensive encephalopathy. Whether or not arteriolar sclerosis is present in grade III hypertensive retinopathy depends on the duration of the disease.

Actually, it is more precise to specify the changes present within an individual eye than to state simply a rough numerical catchall classification of hypertension (or any other disease, for that matter).

Hypertensive retinopathy occurs regardless of the cause of the systemic hypertension. Except for differences related to the duration of hypertension, there are no ophthalmoscopic differences between "renal" hypertension, "malignant" hypertension, toxemia of pregnancy, or any other cause of marked elevation of blood pressure. Retinopathy seems to be related to diastolic levels. A high systolic pressure in aortic insufficiency will not cause hypertensive retinopathy.

Because of the importance of arteriolar attenuation in hypertensive retinopathy, several other causes of attenuation unrelated to hypertension require mention. Occlusion of the central retinal artery often results in severe attenuation of the arteriolar branches. These persons are blind and show optic atrophy. Pigmentary degeneration of the retina characteristically shows marked arteriolar narrowing. These patients are night-blind and have constricted visual fields. Pigment deposits may be scanty but occur in the midperiphery as linear or chicken-track black streaks, often deposited around vessels.

Summary

Retinal arteriolar attenuation is the classic sign of severe hypertension and is usually accompanied by hemorrhages and exudates. Milder, chronic hypertension in a younger person is recognizable through premature arteriolar sclerosis.

ARTERIOLAR SCLEROSIS

Degenerative changes manifest themselves slightly differently in vessels of dissimilar caliber. Almost the entire visible retinal arterial tree is really composed of arterioles. (An arteriole has a discontinuous muscular layer. This discontinuity appears after the first branching of the main trunks of the central retinal artery.) Ophthalmoscopic estimations of retinal sclerotic change are therefore almost entirely descriptions of arteriolar sclerosis. Arteriolar sclerosis is a process that tends to be distributed fairly uniformly throughout the body in vessels of this caliber, whether in the retina, kidney, or brain. The severity of arteriolar sclerosis may be more marked in some organs than in others, however, and localized complete occlusions (as of a branch of the central retinal artery) may cause a great deal more damage than has occurred elsewhere. In general, it is safe to assume that the presence of considerable retinal arteriolar sclerosis means that arteriolar sclerosis is widespread throughout the body. Unless modified by local disease, the severity of arteriolar sclerosis is almost always similar in the two eyes. In itself, arteriolar sclerosis does not significantly affect vision, even when it is of grade IV severity. Blindness, total or partial, may result from arteriolar occlusions of vessels supplying the retina or visual pathways. Such occlusions occur predominantly in individuals with considerable sclerotic disease.

An obvious ophthalmoscopic criterion of arteriolar sclerosis is widening and discoloration of the arteriolar light reflex. This reflection of light runs along the central portion of an arteriole. Normally, the width of the light reflex is about one fourth to one third that of the arteriolar diameter. The width of this reflex may normally be quite variable, even along the course of the same vessel. Widening of the light reflex is one of the earliest signs of arteriolar sclerosis and is due to loss of transparency of the vessel walls. A subtle color change accompanies sclerotic degeneration of the vessel, and the light reflex is noted to become gradually more yellowish orange, then coppery, and finally gray as the walls become so opaque as to conceal completely the underlying blood.

Thickening and opacification of arteriolar walls cause varying amounts of distortion of retinal veins at sites of arteriovenous crossings. At crossings the arteriole and vein share a common adventitial coat of fibrous tissue that binds them together in a figure-eight configuration. Thickening of the arteriole within this fibrous band causes displacement or compression of the vein, which results in the appearance of "nicking" of the vein, a common characteristic of arteriolar sclerosis. Severe sclerotic changes impede venous flow, resulting in dilatation of the distal venous segment. Eventually the venous branch may become completely occluded at the site of an arteriovenous crossing. When attempting to make a diagnosis of arteriolar sclerosis, the ophthalmoscopist should carefully seek out and study the arteriovenous crossings.

A useful classification of the severity of retinal arteriolar sclerosis is as follows:

Grade I	Recognizable widening and discoloration of the arteriolar light reflex
Grade II	More marked light reflex change and definite arteriovenous crossing changes
Grade III	Arterioles resembling a copper wire
Grade IV	Arterioles resembling a silver wire

BLOOD DYSCRASIA

Considerable similarity exists in the fundus appearances of the various blood dyscrasias. Although it is impossible to differentiate reliably between leukemia, aplastic anemia, and thrombocytopenic purpura with the use of the ophthalmoscope, it should be possible to identify the fundus picture as that of blood dyscrasia. Typical fundus appearances are present only during severe stages of the disease. During remission, all retinal evidence of blood dyscrasias may completely disappear.

Diffuse hemorrhages are the most characteristic finding in blood dyscrasia. They may be quite large, usually are irregularly oval in shape, and in their most typical form contain a gray central portion. Flame-shaped and small rounded hemorrhages may also occur but are less characteristic. The presence of retinal hemorrhages is correlated with the degree of anemia and platelet reduction. The retina is a better place than the skin to look for petechial hemorrhages because it is completely transparent and because the optical system of the eye produces a 15× magnification. A hemorrhage only 1.5 mm in diameter is as large as the optic disc.

Venous dilatation and tortuosity are sometimes prominent. Especially in the leukemias there may appear gray linear streaks paralleling the retinal vessels. These are due to perivascular collections of cells.

Polycythemia causes a characteristic enormous dilatation of both retinal arterioles and veins, imparts a dusky and cyanotic color to the retina, and produces a crowding of dilated vessels about the disc, somewhat simulating papilledema.

EXOPHTHALMOS

Exophthalmos refers to forward protrusion of the eyeball from the orbit and is measured in terms of the anteroposterior distance between the lateral orbital rim and the corneal apex. This measurement will not normally be in excess of 18 mm except in a few blacks. Normally the difference between the two eyes does not exceed 2.5 mm. Measurement to this degree of accuracy requires use of an exophthalmometer.

The main causes of exophthalmos are systemic disorders, tumors, inflammation, trauma, and congenital anomalies.

Probably the most common of all causes of exophthalmos is thyroid disease. The logical assumption that such a systemic disorder would always cause bilateral exophthalmos is erroneous. Very, very often thyroid exophthalmos is considerably more marked on one side. Indeed, the most common cause of unilateral exophthalmos is *not* orbital tumor but thyroid disorder.

An attempt has been made by some clinicians to divide these cases into thyrotoxic and thyrotropic types. Since all gradations exist as a continuous spectrum between these two extremes, it is difficult to insist that they are separate entities. Nevertheless, prognostic and therapeutic characteristics of the two types differ enough to warrant such clinical classification.

The *thyrotropic* type of exophthalmos (Fig. 11-1) is characterized by orbital infiltra-

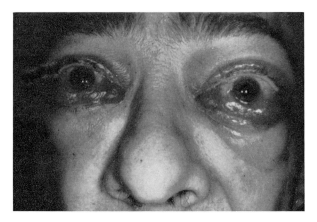

Fig. 11-1. This person with thyrotropic exophthalmos shows pronounced proptosis, chemosis, conjunctival edema and venous engorgement, corneal scarring, resistance to compressibility of the orbit, and limitation of extraocular movement.

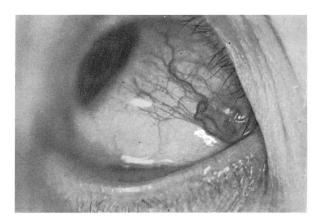

Fig. 11-2. Venous engorgement in the region of the rectus muscles is one of the earliest definite signs of the thyrotropic or malignant nature of exophthalmos. It occurs here because of the preexisting large vessels and because of the muscle involvement by thyrotropic infiltration. This vascular engorgement is an important clinical sign because it strongly contraindicates surgical thyroidectomy (which will cause a predictable exacerbation of exophthalmos in these patients).

tion with inflammatory cells, fat, and edema fluid, causing more marked exophthalmos; is firm and resists compression of the eye backward into the orbit; shows considerable venous engorgement, seen earliest as tortuous and dilated veins overlying the rectus muscle (Fig. 11-2); is associated with considerable edema of the lids and conjunctiva; commonly causes extraocular muscle paresis with diplopia; may result in serious exposure keratopathy or nutritional damage to the optic nerves; is associated with minimal lid retraction; and commonly is severe with normal or even low thyroid function. The thyro-

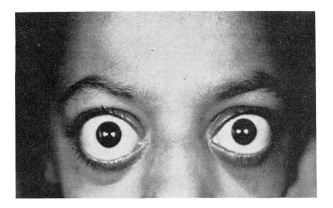

Fig. 11-3. Despite a tremendous lid retraction, this patient with thyrotoxic disease has perfectly white eyes and no ocular disability. Compare with Fig. 11-1.

tropic type is obviously much more serious and requires careful medical attention that should include the use of lubricants to prevent corneal irritation. Thyroidectomy makes thyrotropic exophthalmos *worse!*

The *thyrotoxic* type (Fig. 11-3) of exophthalmos seems to be more functional. Lid retraction is conspicuous and causes the exophthalmos to appear much worse than it actually is. Lid lag is commonly seen. The eyes can usually be compressed backward into the orbits quite easily. Since orbital pressure is normal, venous congestion and conjunctival edema are not conspicuous, and the eyes are often quite white. Extraocular muscle paralyses are uncommon. Serious ocular sequelae are not anticipated. Systemic evidence of thyrotoxicosis is ordinarily marked.

Lid lag refers to the failure of the upper lid to follow smoothly the downwardly rotating eye. The sign is demonstrated by having the patient look high up at the examiner's finger and then follow it downward slowly. Move the finger downward so slowly that a period of 5 seconds is required to traverse the distance from upward to downward gaze. Instruct the patient to hold his head steady and to move only his eyes. The normal downward following movement of both eye and upper lid is smoothly coordinated, with no grossly recognizable interruptions of lid movement. If lid lag is present, the lid descent lags behind, or fails to follow equally, the descent of the eye. Rather than being smooth, the lid descent occurs in a number of jerky, stepwise movements.

Lid retraction is due to an increased sympathetic tone of the smooth muscle, which elevates the upper lid and causes a characteristic pulling backward into the orbit of the upper tarsus. Conspicuous exposure of the sclera above the cornea is the most obvious feature of lid retraction. Testing for lid lag exaggerates the appearance of lid retraction and aids its recognition. Lid retraction and lid lag are almost pathognomonic of thyroid dysfunction. Their presence virtually excludes tumor as a cause of exophthalmos. Cirrho-

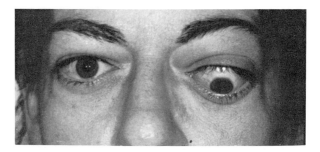

Fig. 11-4. Within 1 year after thyroidectomy this patient developed pronounced unilateral proptosis and paralysis of upward gaze. Obviously, investigation of thyroid status is an essential part of the evaluation of a patient with unilateral exophthalmos without a demonstrable tumor mass.

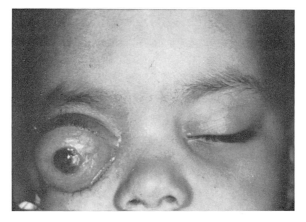

Fig. 11-5. Unilateral exophthalmos due to optic nerve glioma in von Recklinghausen's neurofibromatosis.

sis of the liver is a rare cause of lid retraction, presumably because of failure to metabolize circulating sympathomimetic substances.

Exophthalmos may also be caused by Paget's disease, Hand-Schüller-Christian disease, scurvy, and other systemic conditions.

Tumor-induced exophthalmos is ordinarily unilateral. Because of the previously mentioned tendency of thyroid disease to cause unilateral exophthalmos (Fig. 11-4), surgical exploration of the orbit should not be undertaken unless a definite mass is palpable or demonstrable by CT scan or x-ray examination. Orbital neoplasms may be metastatic from any source (adrenal neuroblastoma commonly spreads to the orbit), may invade from adjacent structures (as, for example, in sinus carcinoma, intracranial meningioma, and ocular melanoma), or may be primary in the orbit (as in hemangioma, dermoid, lipoma, lacrimal gland tumor, granulomatous pseudotumor, lymphoma, and neurofibroma [Fig. 11-5]). The medical workup of such an entity obviously should include a careful general physical examination; an eye, ear, nose, and throat evaluation (Fig. 11-6); x-ray films of

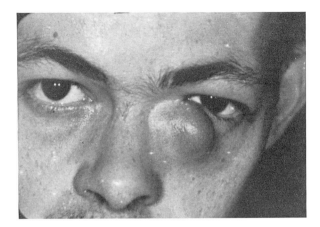

Fig. 11-6. This mucocele of the maxillary sinus closely resembles dacryocystitis. Mucoceles usually appear within the orbit and must be differentiated from orbital neoplasms.

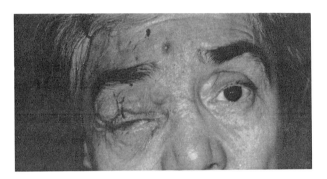

Fig. 11-7. After an auto accident 8 years previously, this 60-year-old patient developed an intracranial bruit, slight exophthalmos, marked venous engorgement around the right eye, and reduced vision. Note on the forehead the dark spots that are engorged venous loops. These findings are typical of a carotid cavernous fistula. Carotid ligation is not without danger in an elderly patient but may be seriously considered in a younger person or if there is progressive impairment of vision.

the orbit and adjacent structures; and thyroid studies (unless a discrete tumor is demonstrable).

Orbital cellulitis characteristically causes definite exophthalmos, marked conjunctival redness and edema, and extraocular muscle paralysis. A common cause is extension of an ethmoidal sinusitis through the lamina papyracea into the orbit. Penetrating trauma may introduce infection into the orbit. Rarely, organisms are metastatic. Posterior extension may cause cavernous sinus thrombosis and death.

Orbital contusion may result in considerable hemorrhage and edema of the retrobulbar spaces. Protection of the cornea is most important if it protrudes between the lids. A carotid cavernous arteriovenous fistula may be caused by trauma (Fig. 11-7). Such a fistula produces a characteristic pulsating exophthalmos, with engorged surface and retinal veins, and bruit audible through a stethoscope placed on the closed lids or against the temple.

Congenital shallowness of the bony orbit as seen in the various craniostenoses (oxycephaly, and so on) may produce severe exophthalmos, sometimes leading to blindness.

OTHER DISEASES

A great variety of other systemic diseases produce more or less characteristic eye disorders. Perhaps the greatest importance of these changes is that they provide readily observable evidence that systemic disease really does exist and thus encourage the physician to seek further for the diagnosis. Many of these diseases manifest themselves through vague and diffuse complaints, and it is easy to misdiagnose the patient's condition as neurosis. Careful fundus examination will help avoid such diagnostic errors.

A brief and incomplete listing will serve to emphasize the great variety of diseases that have eye findings.

Syphilis may cause disseminated chorioretinitis, primary or secondary optic atrophy, and corneal scarring.

Tuberculosis may cause severe chorioretinitis. In the miliary form of tuberculosis, multiple miliary nodules appear in the fundus.

Sarcoid may produce nodular deposits throughout the uveal tract (uveoparotid syndrome).

Toxoplasmosis may cause chorioretinitis. Especially characteristic is the bilateral macular lesion of congenital toxoplasmosis.

Cysticercus and other parasites are sometimes observed within the vitreous.

Sickle cell disease may cause retinal vessel occlusions with associated retinal hemorrhages and characteristic fan-shaped neovascularization.

Collagen diseases may cause perivascular sheathing and exudates. Periarteritis nodosa and disseminated lupus are especially likely to cause such a picture. Temporal arteritis is often associated with occlusion of the central retinal artery.

Lead poisoning and *chronic vitamin A intoxication* may produce papilledema.

Quinine poisoning causes severe arteriolar constriction.

Metastatic neoplasms appear as broad elevations of the choroid.

Phakomatoses (tuberous sclerosis, Sturge-Weber disease, von Recklinghausen's neurofibromatosis [see Fig. 11-5], and von Hippel–Lindau disease) each have a characteristic intraocular tumor, the presence of which will establish such a diagnosis. Please recognize how difficult it would be to diagnose von Hippel–Lindau disease (see Fig. 7-1), for instance, by any means other than ophthalmoscopy.

Cerebromacular degenerations such as Tay-Sachs juvenile amaurotic idiocy produce typical diffuse edema of the retina with conspicuous macular changes.

Hereditary afflictions such as the Laurence-Moon-Biedl syndrome show typical bone-corpuscle–like pigmentation of the midperipheral retina.

Albinism displays varying degrees of lack of ocular pigment.

Central nervous system tumor, hemorrhage, infection, or injury may result in obvious papilledema or optic atrophy.

Subacute bacterial endocarditis is a classic cause of infectious emboli to the retina, often producing characteristic white-centered hemorrhages.

Carotid artery ulcerations are the most common source of retinal emboli.

German measles during the first trimester of pregnancy causes a variety of developmental aberrations, depending on the time of infection. One of these defects, a pigmentary mottling of the macula, is so characteristic as to be pathognomonic of rubella infection at about the third month of pregnancy.

Demyelinating diseases, such as multiple sclerosis, may produce optic neuritis or optic atrophy.

This listing of diseases causing eye findings could be continued indefinitely.

SUMMARY

It is evident that many systemic disorders manifest themselves in the eye. Ophthalmoscopic examination is a rapid screening method that will detect the presence of such disorders and will often permit making a specific diagnosis. The capability of making such diagnoses will amply reward the student for the time he invests developing skill in the use of the ophthalmoscope. Only through *constant use* can one develop a high degree of proficiency in use of the ophthalmoscope.

Do not be awed by the problems of ophthalmoscopic diagnosis. Nothing more than recognition of a fundus abnormality will alert you to the need for further evaluation of the patient.

RECOMMENDED READING

Newell, F.W.: Ophthalmology: principles and concepts, ed. 5, St. Louis, 1982, The C.V. Mosby Co.

Scheie, H.G., and Albert, D.M.: Adler's textbook of ophthalmology, ed. 9, Philadelphia, 1977, W.B. Saunders Co.

chapter 12   Neuroophthalmology

Ophthalmoscopic examination, especially of the disc, is absolutely essential in the evaluation of every patient with headache. You cannot do an acceptable neurologic examination without looking at the eye.

Half the cranial nerves (II to VII, parasympathetic, and sympathetic) contribute to ocular function. Paralyses of these nerves are easily recognized and highly significant (Fig. 12-1). Details of the examination of the extraocular muscles and of the pupil and corneal reflexes are given in Chapters 5 and 16. Accurate interpretation of the meaning of various combinations of defective nerves requires a working knowledge of neuroanatomy and neuropathology that may be obtained from appropriate textbooks. Papilledema, optic atrophy, and perimetry are discussed in this chapter.

PAPILLEDEMA

Because papilledema is a readily observed sign of serious disease, the ability to recognize papilledema and to differentiate it from other disc abnormalities should be one

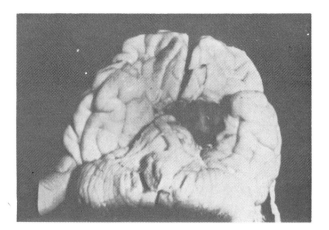

Fig. 12-1. This aneurysm arising from the circle of Willis caused death. Extraocular muscle paralyses are commonly seen in aneurysms and may permit early diagnosis and surgical cure of these serious vascular anomalies. The symptom of diplopia requires careful evaluation because of the grave significance of extraocular muscle paralysis.

of the skills of every physician. Indistinctness and elevation of the optic disc may be caused by conditions such as the following: papilledema, optic neuritis, central retinal vein occlusion, retinitis proliferans, degenerative changes, and physiologic variants.

Papilledema. Papilledema is actual edema of the optic nerve (see Plate 24) due to anterior transmission of increased intracranial pressure via the meningeal spaces surrounding the optic nerve. This pressure partially blocks the tiny veins that drain the optic nerve and causes their characteristic dilatation. These veins of the optic nerve and disc are entirely independent of the central retinal vein (which is itself also partially blocked by the elevated intracranial pressure surrounding the optic nerve). The cause of papilledema, therefore, may be anything that elevates intracranial pressure, including brain tumors (especially those causing internal hydrocephalus), subdural hematoma, and brain abscess, for example.

In view of the serious nature of such causes, papilledema demands prompt neurologic, medical, and ophthalmologic evaluation of the patient. Diagnostic procedures include confirmation of the diagnosis by an ophthalmologist, visual field studies, skull x-ray films, CT scans, and electroencephalography.

Diagnostic characteristics of papilledema may readily be remembered by considering the sequelae of increased venous pressure, which develop as follows.

1. Dilatation, tortuosity, and nodularity of the fine capillaries of the disc result in a hyperemic disc and are the earliest definite signs of papilledema.
2. Dilatation and tortuosity of the central retinal vein follow, with loss of the spontaneous (in 80% of normal persons) venous pulsation. In fully developed papil-

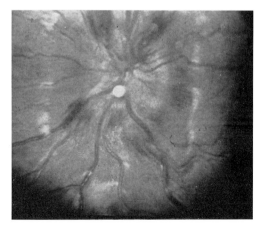

Fig. 12-2. Papilledema is easily recognized through dilatation of the disc capillaries and veins, blurring of the disc margins, and radial hemorrhages near the disc. Note the circular light reflections around the disc, which indicate the extent to which edema has infiltrated the surrounding retina. The changes of true papilledema are confined to the immediate neighborhood of the disc and do not extend far out into the retina as do the hemorrhages of vascular disease.

ledema, it becomes impossible to collapse the veins by digital pressure on the globe.

3. Leakage of fluid from the dilated vessels results in edematous elevation of the disc itself and also of the nearby retina. The disc margins become blurred and indistinct. The physiologic cup disappears. Extension of edema into the retina may be recognized by a circular reflection arising from the peripheral edge of the elevated tissue (Fig. 12-2).

4. More severe vascular stasis results in bleeding from the tiny disc capillaries. Such hemorrhage enters the nerve fiber layer, causing a radial, linear orientation of the blood, resembling small splinters of hemorrhage. Originating from the disc vessels, the blood must overlie the disc margins or be situated very near the disc (rarely more than 1 DD away). Multiple small linear hemorrhages may become confluent to form flame-shaped patterns extending from the disc.

Inasmuch as hemorrhages cannot be a normal variant, recognition of even a single small streak of blood is certain evidence of pathologic change. Consciously seek hemorrhages near the disc when you are considering the possible diagnosis of papilledema.

5. Prolonged leakage of lipoidal debris results in formation of the small white dots called hard exudates. These pattern-forming spots will be confined to the area near the disc, perhaps extending to involve the macula with a ''star'' pattern. They signify long duration of the papilledema.

6. The typical field defect, enlargement of the blind spot, is produced by edematous displacement of the rods and cones from the disc. If the etiologic lesion affects the visual pathways, it may be localized by visual fields. No subjective visual symptoms occur until the later stages, when there may be transient blurring of vision. At this point arteriolar attenuation may be ophthalmoscopically detectable. Transient blurring and arteriolar attenuation are the early indications of impending optic atrophy and blindness. Cranial decompression is urgent if sight is to be preserved. Pallor appears as optic atrophy progresses. If decompression or definitive brain surgery is done, many weeks may be required for clearing of the papilledema.

Be aware that many different conditions cause disc appearances that more or less closely resemble papilledema. Because of the tremendous significance of this differential diagnosis, consultation with an ophthalmologist will often be appropriate. Brief descriptions of conditions often confused with papilledema follow. You will recognize that these various optic nerve diseases can result in blindness or signify the presence of serious general disease. Proper management requires prompt and accurate diagnosis.

Optic neuritis. Optic neuritis is due to inflammatory blocking of venous outflow and hence may present *exactly the same ophthalmoscopic picture as papilledema*. Visual loss is usually of fairly abrupt onset (within a day or two), with a central scotoma—in contrast to the absence of visual symptoms in early papilledema. Involvement of peripheral portions of the optic nerve may cause sector losses of the peripheral visual field, called nerve fiber bundle defects. Because of irritation of the meningeal sheath of the optic nerve, movement of the eye is often painful. Unilaterality is more common in optic neuritis than in papilledema.

Demyelinating diseases are by far the most common cause of optic neuritis. They include multiple sclerosis, postinfectious encephalomyelitis, and the rarer demyelinating syndromes. Local inflammations such as juxtapapillary chorioretinitis, orbital cellulitis, meningitis, and, rarely, sphenoid sinusitis may cause optic neuritis. Diseases such as pernicious anemia and vitamin deficiency are infrequent causes. Poisons such as thallium (depilatory), lead (a special hazard to infants who chew painted articles), and methyl alcohol (beverage adulterant) may affect the optic nerve. Leber's optic neuritis is a rare, sex-linked, dominant affliction of young males.

The prognosis is relatively good, since the most common cause, multiple sclerosis, is characterized by spontaneous remissions. Most persons with optic neuritis regain useful vision over a period of several weeks to a month. Older patients are less likely to improve. Treatment of optic neuritis (with corticosteroids and vasodilators) does not greatly alter its course or the final outcome.

Retrobulbar neuritis has the same cause (usually demyelinating diseases) and symptoms as optic neuritis. However, retrobulbar neuritis attacks the posterior portion of the optic nerve and therefore causes *no* ophthalmoscopically visible edema or other early defect of the optic disc. The symptoms and prognosis of retrobulbar neuritis are identical to those of optic neuritis.

Both optic neuritis (affecting the disc) and retrobulbar neuritis (affecting the nerve more posteriorly) cause optic atrophy. The severity of disc pallor correlates with the amount of nerve fiber damage and the degree of visual loss.

Specific infections. Edema of the optic disc is produced by a focal toxoplasmosis lesion within the optic nerve or in the nearby retina. The *toxoplasma* organism grows selectively in central nervous system tissue (such as the retina). Massive leukocytic infiltration of the nerve, retina, and vitreous is typical of this infection. Dense, heavily pigmented scars remain in the fundus following healing of toxoplasmic retinochoroiditis.

Histoplasmosis selectively involves the choroid, often encircling the optic nerve. A ring of mottled peripapillary choroidal atrophy is very typical of this condition but causes little visual loss unless subretinal neovascular hemorrhages occur. The disc itself is not involved, but the immediately adjacent choroid is. The vitreous is not affected.

Direct spirochetal invasion of the optic nerve and meninges by *Treponema pallidum* was formerly a common cause of optic neuritis and atrophy. Because of penicillin therapy, syphilitic optic nerve disease is now uncommon.

Pyogenic sinus and orbital infections can invade the optic nerve.

Ischemic optic neuritis. Arteriolar insufficiency of the optic nerve and disc causes a pale (nonhyperemic) swelling of the disc. The involved disc has blurred margins comparable to those of papilledema. Radial hemorrhages near the disc or overlying it are common. Pale gray patches (soft exudates) near the disc represent microinfarctions of the nerve fiber layer and are very characteristic of ischemic disease.

Note that papilledema is a congestive disorder with a hyperemic appearance, whereas ischemic optic neuritis is a disorder of arteriolar insufficiency with a pale appearance.

Severe hypertensive disease (grade IV severity) is the most common cause of ischemic optic neuritis. Fortunately, control of the hypertension will usually arrest further progression of visual loss. Diabetes and collagen diseases are other causes.

Giant cell arteritis (temporal arteritis) causes an ischemic optic neuritis with a far worse prognosis. Blindness may occur within only a few days or even within hours and is usually irreversible. The second eye is often affected also. High-dosage, prolonged corticosteroid therapy may prevent progression of the damage or involvement of the second eye. Infarcted nerve fibers will not recover; hence, immediate recognition and treatment are necessary. Although loss of vision within hours or days may be an isolated symptom, pain in the temple or jaw is common. An elevated sedimentation rate is an important laboratory confirmation of the diagnosis.

Hypoxia due to chronic pulmonary disease, anemia, or other causes may result in disc swelling very similar to that of ischemic optic neuritis.

Central retinal vein occlusion. Characteristically, central retinal vein occlusion produces marked edema and hemorrhage of the disc area *and* also of most of the retina. Recognition of the peripheral retinal involvement rules out the diagnosis of papilledema. The retinal veins are engorged, tortuous, and without spontaneous pulsation. The disc is never markedly elevated as in severe papilledema. If originally present, the physiologic depression remains visible in central venous occlusion, whereas it fills with edematous tissue in papilledema. Occlusion of a branch of the central retinal vein produces hemorrhages and edema only in the involved quadrant.

Retinitis proliferans. Retinitis proliferans is an extension of vascular and connective tissue over the retina and disc, often extending far into the vitreous (see Plate 22). Diabetes, tuberculosis, and trauma are the more common causes. Although these membranes often overlie and obscure the disc, they are present elsewhere over the retina and have an irregular contour readily differentiated from papilledema. The visual defect is usually extensive and depends on the distribution of retinitis proliferans.

Degenerative changes. *Circumpapillary chorioretinal atrophy* consists of degeneration and disappearance of the choroidal and retinal elements immediately adjacent to the disc. The result is a crescentic or annular area of grayish white sclera about the disc—a rather confusing picture simulating a giant disc. The involved area is not elevated or edematous. Hemorrhages are not present. This type of atrophy may be a result of inherited chorioretinal defect, degenerative myopia, trauma, and so on. Visual fields show enlarged blind spots.

Hyaline deposits within the nerve may cause elevations closely resembling papilledema but without hemorrhage or retinal edema. If superficial, these hyaline bodies may be recognized as having a characteristic translucent appearance typically more conspicuous when viewed by proximal illumination. Nerve fiber bundle field defects may result. Tuberous sclerosis is one cause for hyaline deposits of the optic nerve. The term ''drusen of the disc'' has been applied to these lesions, which are entirely different from the common drusen of the lamina vitrea.

Physiologic variants. The physiologic variants discussed here, being extremely common, are often misdiagnosed as papilledema, especially when the patient has a history of head trauma or neurologic difficulty. All are perfectly normal.

Pseudoneuritis refers to a hyperemic, somewhat elevated disc, with considerable physiologic blurring of the disc margins. It is usually associated with hyperopia, is ordinarily symmetrical in the two eyes, and *never* produces hemorrhages or retinal edema. Spontaneous venous pulsation is present or is readily elicited by pressure on the globe.

High central branching describes the appearance of vessels that appear to arch forward into the vitreous before bending posteriorly to the retina. Extreme cases are termed ''epipapillary vascular loop.''

A *glial veil* is a translucent membrane overlying the disc, resembling a piece of cellophane with curled edges. It represents persistent embryonic tissue.

Myelinated nerve fibers are glistening whitish plaques usually in apposition to the disc (see Plate 14). They commonly have characteristic fine feathery edges representing the irregular extent of myelination of each individual nerve fiber.

The *myopic disc* often has a prominent temporal crescent of sclera and may have a nasal ''supertraction'' crescent of retina encroaching over the disc margins.

Physiologic blurring refers to the normal irregularity of pigment and tissue at the disc margins, which are usually less sharp nasally than temporally.

Summary. An important guide to the presence of intracranial disease, papilledema closely resembles optic neuritis. Both may be confused with some types of intraocular inflammation, vascular disease, or degenerative changes and in some respects are simulated by physiologic variants in the structure of the optic disc.

OPTIC ATROPHY

Optic atrophy is the dreaded sequel to inadequately treated papilledema, optic neuritis, or other lesions of the anterior visual pathways. Older writers divided optic atrophy into primary and secondary types, which have no significance as to etiology but merely indicate whether or not the disc was involved by the causative process. For the diagnosis of either type of optic atrophy, the disc must be grayish white and the fine capillaries overlying the disc must be reduced in number. (The normal infant disc has this appearance, which may unnecessarily alarm the examiner.) Vision is often uncorrectably decreased, and visual field defects are demonstrable by perimetry.

The pallor of optic atrophy must extend from center to edge of the disc. Only a sector or the entire disc area may be involved. Do not confuse this pallor with a central pale area (physiologic depression) or a pale area adjacent to the disc (sclera, exposed by developmental or acquired absence of overlying pigment and vessels), in both of which the normally pink disc peripheral rim is intact.

Primary optic atrophy. The appearance of primary optic atrophy results from a causative lesion behind the entry of vessels into the nerve (1 cm behind the globe), a location that does not produce engorgement of the disc. The disc is free of gliosis and has a prominent physiologic cup and lamina cribrosa, and no perivascular sheathing is present. Some classic causes are syphilis, skull fracture with transection of the optic nerve, and pituitary tumor.

Secondary optic atrophy. In secondary optic atrophy, the damage is located at the disc, leaving characteristic visible features as follows:

1. Grayish glial deposits lie on and about the disc and neighboring vessels, obscuring the physiologic cup and lamina cribrosa. Pigment and lipoid deposits are often arranged concentrically around the disc.
2. In glaucomatous atrophy, there is characteristic cupping extending to the disc margin, often with overhanging edges and vanishing vessels. Absence of the normal peripheral rim of disc tissue differentiates this cupping from physiologic cupping.
3. Vascular atrophy after occlusion of the central retinal artery often may be diagnosed by the characteristic narrow arterioles. Quinine idiosyncrasy also produces marked vasoconstriction.
4. Consecutive atrophy is subsequent to obvious retinal disease such as retinitis pigmentosa, extensive chorioretinitis, trauma, and so on.

Therapy. Three points should be remembered in the treatment of optic atrophy:

1. Determine the cause! It may enable you to save the other eye or perhaps the patient's life.
2. Telescopic lenses are rarely helpful.
3. Good solid white canes help the advanced cases. Do not let your patients with papilledema or syphilis reach this stage!

PERIMETRY

Perimetry refers to visual field measurement. Characteristic defects of localizing value are produced by any damage of the visual pathways—which have an extensive distribution from the eye all the way to the posterior tip of the brain. Diagnosis depends not on the field alone but also on complete ophthalmologic study. The reason is that purely ocular lesions may produce field defects simulating those of neurologic disease.

The field extent may be roughly estimated by the confrontation method with a pencil or similar small object. The eye not being examined must be completely occluded. Emphasize the importance of looking steadily straight ahead and watch the patient's eye during examination to be sure it does not wander. The limits of the peripheral visual field usually extend 90 degrees temporally, 70 degrees inferiorly, 60 degrees nasally, and 50 degrees superiorly (see Fig. 5-21).

Much earlier defects may be demonstrated by the more delicate methods of quantitative and qualitative perimetry, which employ small test objects of different sizes and colors at varying measured distances under controlled illumination. Since angiograms and other neurosurgical diagnostic procedures are uncomfortable and do carry a slight risk, it would seem desirable to employ the safe and nontraumatic techniques of perimetry as a preliminary screening examination in patients with headaches and other minor neurologic complaints.

Perimetry is a highly subjective examination and is markedly variable with fatigue and reduced concentration. Testing should be repeated at a later date if it becomes evident that the results are inconstant. Some judgment should be used in referring patients for perimetry, since semiconscious, nauseated, or pain-racked individuals do not give reliable responses.

Perimetry is particularly useful under the following circumstances:

1. Visual loss unexplained by ocular findings and not correctable by refraction will almost invariably be found to be due to a field defect.
2. Perimetry is extremely valuable in following the progress of explained visual loss (chorioretinitis or retinitis pigmentosa). Proper management of glaucoma requires perimetry at least every 3 months. Perimetry informs you of the extent of retained visual function. It is of academic interest in almost all ophthalmoscopically visible disease.
3. Perimetry is part of the complete examination of any patient with suspected central nervous system disease. Unexplained headaches indicate careful perimetry. Visual field studies are part of the complete workup of a patient with a brain tumor.
4. Malingering and hysteria can be nicely demonstrated perimetrically. Unfortunately, organic brain disease, such as multiple sclerosis and frontal lobe neoplasm, may have a functional overlay and may closely simulate functional fields.

Importance of ophthalmoscopic examination in the interpretation of visual fields

The place of perimetry in neurologic diagnosis is secure. Nevertheless, it must be emphasized that no diagnosis can be made by perimetry alone. Supplementary information from the history, general and neurologic examination, and laboratory findings must support the diagnosis. Since field defects simulating almost any intracranial defect may be produced by purely ocular disease, no perimetric diagnosis is reliable without ophthalmologic examination.

Knowledge of the anatomic structure of the retina and choroid permits accurate prediction of the defect expected from a given ocular lesions. Conversely, the extent of involvement is evident from the field defect.

1. A choroidal lesion produces field defects only to the extent that the rods and cones are damaged.
2. Disease of the outer retinal layers, up to but not including the nerve fiber layer, causes field defects coextensive with the disease.

3. Damage to the nerve fiber layer results in visual loss not only in the area of damage but also in the entire distribution of the nerve fiber layers peripheral to the lesion.

4. An opaque lesion, whether cataract or retinal hemorrhage, causes visual reduction proportionate to the extent and density of the shadow cast on the neuroepithelium.

The multiplicity of causes of an *enlarged blind spot* may be chosen to illustrate the necessity for fundus examination. Lateral displacement of the rods and cones by the swollen disc is the well-recognized cause of an enlarged blind spot in papilledema. Similar displacement occurs in optic neuritis, a process so like papilledema that it cannot be distinguished ophthalmoscopically. (Differentiation is readily made through the central scotoma or sector defect of optic neuritis.) Far more common than papilledema as a cause of an enlarged blind spot is atrophy of the choroid and retina about the disc. On a genetically determined basis, this circumpapillary atrophy is frequently encountered as a normal aging process. The temporal crescent of myopic chorioretinal atrophy appears at an early age in degenerative myopia. Structural damage consequent to chorioretinitis may appear at any age.

Myelinated nerve fibers overlap disc margins and neuroepithelium, producing an enlarged blind spot and a blurred papilla, simulating inflammation or edema to the inexperienced observer. The feathery edges, characteristic gray-white color, and absence of vascular abnormality clearly differentiate myelination from papilledema.

As part of a general field depression, glaucoma may cause an increase in the size of the relative scotoma surrounding the blind spot, eventually creating a defect of absolute intensity. Localized pressure damage may cause Seidel's scotoma (an elliptic prolongation of the blind spot).

Even sharply delineated *quadrant* and *hemianopic defects* (which usually are caused by intracranial disease) may be produced by retinal disease. Occlusion of a branch of the central retinal artery or vein will affect only the involved retinal quadrant. Arteriolar occlusions are characterized by sharp-edged, absolutely blind, permanent defects that may have a straight horizontal boundary corresponding to the temporal raphe of retinal nerve fiber distribution. Vascular variations, such as the cilioretinal arteriole present in 20% of people, may cause sparing of the macula or centrocecal areas. Venous occlusions produce relative field defects. Branch venous occlusions have their highest incidence in the upper temporal quadrant, supposedly because of the greater number of arteriovenous crossings in this quadrant. (Branch vein occlusion almost always occurs at the arteriovenous junctions.)

Trauma to the nerve fiber layer produces absolute, sharp-edged defects of quadrant, sector, or arcuate distribution, corresponding to the extent of injury. Choroidal ruptures produce only small, localized field defects. Chorioretinitis adjacent to the disc is much more likely than peripheral chorioretinitis to involve the nerve fiber layer with the production of sector defects. Nerve fiber bundle defects, especially the arcuate Bjerrum's scotoma, extending around the macula from the disc to the temporal raphe, are classic findings in glaucoma. Extensive myelination of the nerve fibers may give a similar picture. Retinal detachments produce defects of any extent and location, usually beginning peripherally, that are absolutely blind only where high detachment is present. A relative defect occurs in areas of low detachment, and sometimes a sharp-edged defect occurs if a ballooning overhang is present. Choroidal detachments are similar in extent but produce much denser visual defects.

Although *central scotomas* may be caused by occipital pole lesions, posterior chiasm defects, or optic nerve involvement, by far the majority of such scotomas result from ophthalmoscopically visible macular disease. A common cause is macular degeneration, a slowly progressive hereditary affliction that is much more common in the elderly and is usually bilateral. More often seen in the younger age group is chorioretinitis, an inflammation usually involving only the outer retinal layers and therefore producing a defect coextensive with the lesion. Uncommonly, chorioretinitis will penetrate to the nerve fiber layer and will cause visual loss from the peripheral area supplied by these fibers.

Ocular contusion not infrequently causes a central scotoma, because the fovea is a particularly thin and easily injured part of the retina. Thermal trauma resulting from the viewing of a solar eclipse while unprotected by dark glasses produces a similar central scotoma. Retinal detachment involving the macula usually destroys the possibility of future foveal vision. Occlusions of the small arteriolar or venous branches supplying the macula result in irregular central scotomas. Hemorrhages and exudates such as those seen in diabetes and hypertension will, of course, cast shadows on the underlying rods and cones.

Adequate ophthalmoscopic examination will be greatly facilitated by mydriasis such as that obtainable by the use of 2½% phenylephrine hydrochloride, one drop in each eye, repeated in 5 minutes. Before mydriatics are used, the patient should be asked whether he has glaucoma. No other absolute contraindication to dilatation exists—from the ophthalmologic viewpoint. Fifteen to 20 minutes are required for mydriasis.

Because of the importance of pupil signs to the neurosurgeon, dilating drops should not be used in a patient suspected of having acute intracranial damage (for example, after head injury) or during the recovery period after brain surgery.

Summary. Pathologic changes limited to the eye commonly cause visual field changes exactly simulating those produced by lesions of the visual pathways. These field changes include an enlarged blind spot, quadrantanopia, hemianopia (altitudinal and lateral), and central scotoma. It therefore cannot be too strongly emphasized that ophthalmoscopic examination is indispensable in accurate interpretation of visual field abnormalities. Interpretation of a visual field defect cannot be made by a technician or nonmedical practitioner.

Simplified method of measuring visual fields

The previously described confrontation method will fail to detect early evidence of damage to the visual pathways and hence is unsatisfactory for clinical use (unless, of course, a large defect is clearly demonstrated with confrontation testing).

Quantitative measurement of the visual field is a much more accurate and certain method of detecting, evaluating, and following visual pathway damage. Measurement of the visual field should be included in the complete neurologic examination and in the evaluation of many eye complaints (for example, unexplained loss of visual acuity that is uncorrectable with glasses, possible malingering or hysteria, and ocular or head aching of undetermined cause). Although visual field testing is by habit relegated to the ophthalmologist, it is basically a simple test that is much easier to learn than percussion.

The patient is seated comfortably on a chair and positioned so that his eyes are exactly ⅓ meter from the perimeter. One eye at a time is examined, the other being completely occluded by an eyepad.

The patient is instructed to watch the fixation mark constantly and to report when he sees the test object appear or disappear in his side vision. The temptation to watch the object move or otherwise to stray from the fixation point is great, and almost all patients will require multiple reminders to look at the fixation mark. During field testing, the examiner must frequently observe the patient's eye to be certain it is not wandering from fixation. Accurate visual field study is impossible if the patient cannot fix reasonably well.

Study of the normal blind spot should be done first in order to show the patient what is wanted and to confirm that his fixation and responses are reliable. The blind spot will be found 15 degrees temporal to the fixation point. It is usually vertically oval. Since measurement of the blind spot is important per se and since the same approach is used in mapping out any other central field defect, proper technique will be described in detail.

The test object is shown to the patient, who must understand that his response is sought to the object—not to the wand, the examiner's hand, or other extraneous stimuli.

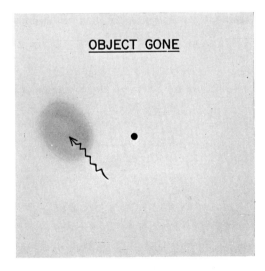

Fig. 12-3. Disappearance of the test object into the blind spot.

As the patient observes the fixation spot, the test object is moved temporally toward the blind spot. The patient is told that the object will normally disappear somewhere in this area and is requested to say "gone" when it disappears. If he does not respond as expected, the examiner must prompt him by asking, "Is it gone yet?" Normally, the patient will recognize without too much trouble the disappearance of the object, as shown in Fig. 12-3. Having found the area of the blind spot, the examiner must now map its exact dimensions. Holding the object within the blind area, he asks the patient, "Is it still gone?" If it is, the patient is instructed to say "back" when he sees the object return to sight.

In mapping any blind spot, whether normal or abnormal, the most accurate responses are obtained by moving the object from the blind to the seeing area. Seeing-to-blind movement encourages involuntary following of the object. The wand handle should point away from the direction of movement so that the object will pop suddenly into sight and not be preceded by the handle. Do not move too fast, lest delayed reaction time give an erroneous result. The most rapid and efficient measurement of any blind spot will be

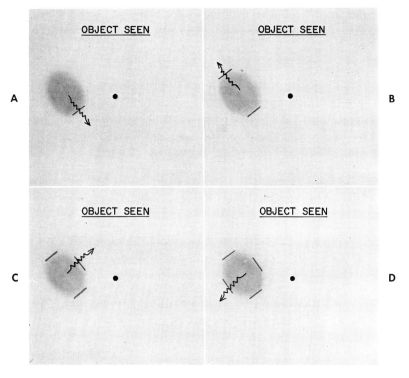

Fig. 12-4. **A,** The object again becomes visible when it emerges from the blind spot. **B,** Appearance of the object on the opposite side of the blind spot. **C,** Position of the third mark in mapping of a blind spot. **D,** Appearance of the object at the site of the fourth mark in mapping of a blind spot.

accomplished if the object is first moved from the blind region directly back to the area where it was last seen. As soon as the patient says "back," place a chalk mark there (Fig. 12-4, *A*). Now return the object to the blind area and move it in the opposite direction until the response "back" is again marked (Fig. 12-4, *B*). Now place the object exactly halfway between the first and second mark and move it perpendicular to an imaginary line connecting them until the patient again sees the object (Fig. 12-4, *C*). The fourth mark is found by moving the object opposite from the third mark (Fig. 12-4, *D*).

Bounded in this fashion by four marks (Fig. 12-5, *A*), the blind spot is reasonably accurately identified (although it is good practice to check four more points, one between each of the original four). Although insistence on a routine such as this may seem arbitrary, reference to Fig. 12-5, *B*, shows that four points recorded by movement of the object in repeated, almost parallel paths will provide much less information than do the recommended four points. Since pathologic blind spots are of unknown extent, if is particularly important to explore them with four initial movements 90 degrees apart, as described. Disregarding this recommendation will often throw a beginner into hopeless confusion when he finds a central field defect.

After identification of the normal blind spot (Fig. 12-6), the test object should be moved in concentric circles around the fixation mark (Fig. 12-7) in search of any field defect. During this procedure the patient is instructed to respond with "gone" if the object disappears and is occasionally prompted with the question, "Has it disappeared yet?"

Recording of any defects found in the visual field can be done by copying the position of the fixation point, the normal blind spot, and the defect in accurate proportions and relationships on an ordinary sheet of paper.

Although study of the visual field should be as objective as possible, it is true that the examiner is more likely to find that for which he looks. Hence, a brief review of the anatomy of the visual pathway (Fig. 12-8) is appropriate. Since nerves from both eyes

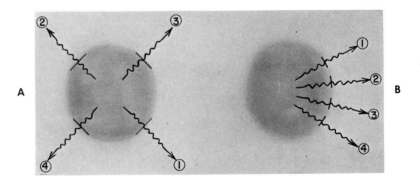

Fig. 12-5. A, The extent of a blind spot is fairly well established by four marks if they are located 90 degrees apart. **B,** Four marks immediately adjacent to each other provide much less information as to the extent of a blind spot.

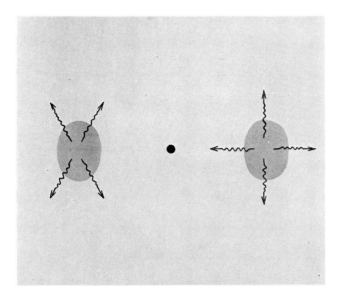

Fig. 12-6. The sinuous lines represent movements of the test object in mapping of the normal blind spot. Eight equally spaced meridians adequately measure the limits of the usual blind spot.

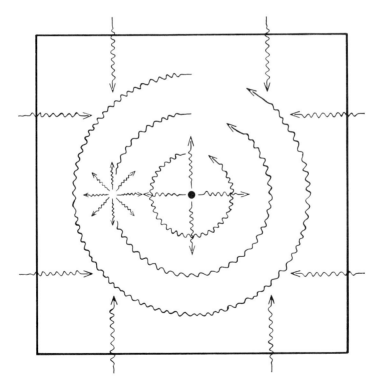

Fig. 12-7. Composite representation of the movements made in screening a normal central visual field. If some such methodical pattern is followed, the examiner will most likely detect any significant defect.

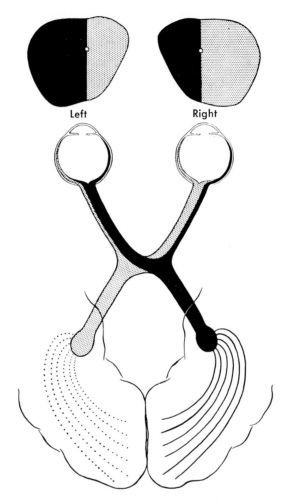

Left   Right

Fig. 12-8. Representation of the visual field in the optic pathways.

intermingle behind the chiasm, lesions posterior to the chiasm will impair the opposite half of the visual field of both eyes (homonymous hemianopia). Lesions at the chiasm may cause a wide variety of defects, usually involving both eyes. Midline chiasm damage (as from pituitary tumor) damages the crossing fibers from the nasal retina and classically causes bitemporal field loss. Naturally, damage to one optic nerve will affect only the field of the involved eye. A visual field defect indicates only the location of a lesion of the visual pathways, not the type (for example, vascular, neoplastic, or inflammatory) of lesion.

    The anatomy of the nerve fiber layer of the retina (Fig. 12-9) will determine the pattern of field defects caused by retinal disease. Macular defects cause a central blind spot.

Text continued on p. 228.

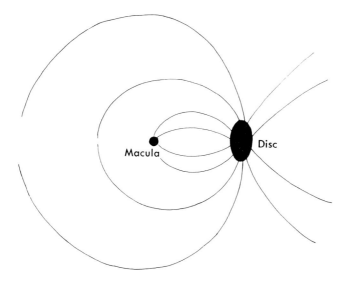

Fig. 12-9. Distribution of nerve fibers within the retina.

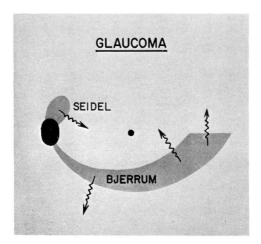

Fig. 12-10. Nerve fiber bundle defects are typical of glaucoma. These may be small (Seidel) or more extensive (Bjerrum). Enlargement of the blind spot and concentric constriction may also be found.

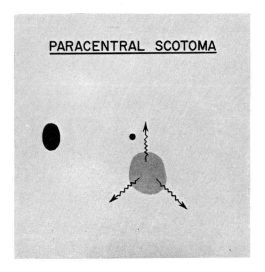

Fig. 12-11. Chorioretinitis near the fovea will cause a paracentral field defect. Repeated visual field measurements are the most accurate way of following the progress and response to treatment of such a lesion.

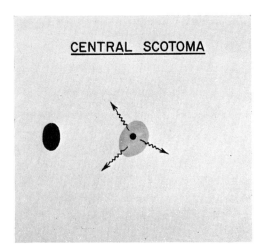

Fig. 12-12. A central defect of the visual field is commonly caused by macular degeneration, chorioretinitis involving the fovea, or ocular contusion. Such a lesion always reduces visual acuity.

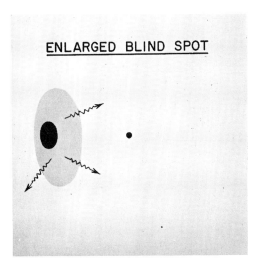

Fig. 12-13. Enlargement of the physiologic blind spot occurs in lesions such as papilledema, juxtapapillary chorioretinitis, or circumpapillary chorioretinal atrophy. The patient is unaware of this type of field loss.

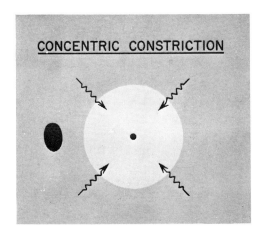

Fig. 12-14. Loss of the periphery of the visual field is characteristic of hysteria, malingering, glaucoma, retinitis pigmentosa, syphilitic optic neuritis, and some types of optic atrophy. A patient suffering from genuine (as opposed to hysterical) field constriction will readily bump into obstacles.

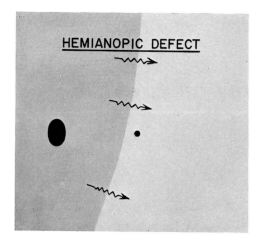

Fig. 12-15. Loss of half of the visual field of both eyes is caused by central nervous system damage to the visual pathways. Monocular extensive field loss may be due to optic nerve damage, retinal detachment, choroidal melanoma, or similar purely ocular diseases.

Edema of the optic disc enlarges the blind spot. Localized damage to a group of nerve fibers (as by injury, infection, or glaucoma) will cause a sector of blindness corresponding to the involved area of the retina.

Malingering and hysteria cause variable, bizarre, and nonphysiologic defects of the visual field. The most common functional defect is marked constriction, and the patient may claim to see nothing beyond 10 degrees from the fixation point. That he actually does see peripheral to this area is clear from his behavior, for he does not bump into chairs and so on, as does the diseased patient who actually cannot see peripherally.

Classic types of field defects and the direction of movement of the test object for most efficient examination are shown in Figs. 12-10 to 12-15.

chapter 13 Diagnosis and
Management
of Eye
Injury

You must realize that in many cases of serious eye injury, useful vision may be salvaged through prompt care (Fig. 13-1). In contrast, rough handling and poor management may irretrievably destroy the injured eye. Because of the thinness and delicacy of the eye structure, major damage may be caused by slight trauma that would be inconsequential elsewhere on the body. Specifically, a tiny laceration 1 mm deep represents a serious penetrating ocular injury, although on a finger it would require only a small bandage.

Do not forget the significance of future blindness when examining patients with injury about the eyes. What residual damage would most affect *your* life 1 year after an accident to the upper face? Certainly, blindness of one or both eyes would handicap the majority of us far more than would any other scars.

RECOGNITION OF INJURY

Failures to detect eye injury can be practically eliminated through attention to the history of injury, reduced vision, persistent discomfort, techniques of examination, objective signs, and finger tension estimation.

History of injury

A history of injury to the eye mandates careful examination. Most likely to be overlooked are the perforating injuries of small, high-speed particles such as those produced by the hammering or machining of metal or by the use of high explosives. Secondary fragments such as slivers of glass from broken spectacles should be searched for carefully whenever the patient's glasses have been shattered by the accident. Serious eye injuries from tiny, high-velocity fragments may be almost *painless*. A search for a possible intraocular foreign body by diagnostic x-ray examination is indicated when the eye injury is caused by speeding fragments.

Reduced vision

Reduced vision after injury will alert the physician to the probability of eye damage. Measurement of visual acuity with a Snellen type of chart should be routine in the

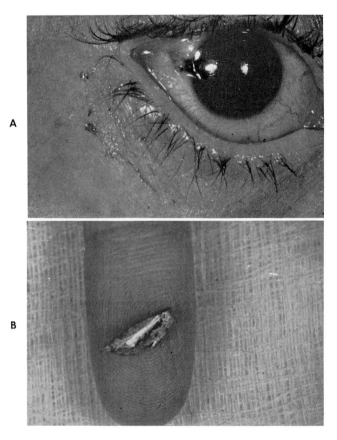

Fig. 13-1. A, A large penetrating wound of the limbus is easily recognized. This eye still contains the huge piece of metal shown in **B.** Pressure carelessly directed into the eye during examination could have destroyed it. Delay in recognition and in starting antibiotic therapy would probably have resulted in serious infection. Proper care restored 20/20 vision.

evaluation of a potentially injured eye. *The importance of visual acuity measurement cannot be overemphasized.*

Persistent discomfort

Persistent discomfort subsequent to eye trauma indicates at least some degree of injury. Adequate explanation for this discomfort should be found through physical examination techniques.

Remember that a recent penetrating wound may no longer hurt!

Techniques of examination

Simple techniques of examination include inspection, proper separation of the lids, and oblique, moving illumination.

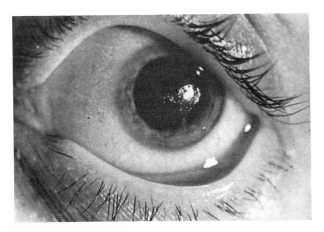

Fig. 13-2. Note the conspicuous reflections seen when a corneal abrasion is illuminated obliquely. Study of the cornea with an obliquely directed, moving, bright flashlight is the best way to locate irregularities of the corneal surface. Fluorescein staining is unnecessary if the lesion can be demonstrated in this fashion.

Inspection. Inspection is self-explanatory; however, do not overlook the value of comparing the two eyes for asymmetry due to injury (for example, fractured orbital rim).

Proper separation of the lids. During separation of the lids of an injured eye, *pressure should never be directed on the eyeball.* The upper lid is easily raised by pushing up on the brow against the frontal bone. The lower lid is safely depressed by pulling the cheek down with pressure against the maxillary rim of the orbit. With the examiner's thumb and forefinger resting against the lower and upper orbital margins, the lids may be safely spread without causing further damage to a lacerated eye. Erroneous pressure on the lids and underlying eyeball is not more effective in exposing the eye and is potentially destructive. *Until proved otherwise by adequate examination, all suspected eye injuries should be treated with as much caution as if they were known to be penetrating wounds.*

Oblique, moving illumination. Oblique, moving illumination is the secret of successful examination of transparent structures. A bright, well-focused pencil flashlight is most convenient. Defects of the cornea appear as grossly irregular reflections in the normally mirror-smooth surface (Fig. 13-2), provided that the light is directed from the proper oblique angle. Conspicuous shadows will be cast on the iris by almost invisible corneal lesions. Slow movement of the light will emphasize these moving shadows. Differentiation between corneal and lenticular opacities is easy through oblique illumination. Straight-ahead illumination is almost useless for detection of fine details, is much more uncomfortable for the patient, and is invariably used without success by the neophyte physician.

Objective signs

Objective signs suggesting eye injury are particularly important to the examining physician.

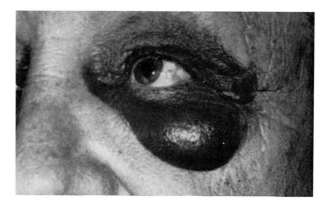

Fig. 13-3. Subcutaneous hemorrhage from a blow to the orbital margin dissects freely beneath the thin lid skin and is not usually associated with ocular damage. However, a similar picture may be produced by direct trauma on the lid or eyeball. Ophthalmoscopic examination is necessary to rule out intraocular injury.

Lid abrasions, ecchymoses, lacerations, and paralyses. The frequency with which we see uncomplicated black eyes engenders a false sense of security (Fig. 13-3). Trauma sufficient to cause lid hemorrhage may also cause intraocular bleeding or other damage to the underlying eye. The eyelids are thin, and a laceration that is only a little deeper will involve the eyeball. Repair of a lacerated eyeball has a high priority over suturing a torn lid! (Fig. 13-4). *Do not fail to examine the eye completely before concluding that only external damage is present.*

Conjunctival hemorrhages and lacerations. Conjunctival hemorrhages and lacerations (Fig. 13-5) are unimportant in themselves but may conceal a penetrating scleral wound (Fig. 13-6). Although the sclera is a relatively inert tissue, its surface vessels bleed freely when cut. The common and harmless spontaneous subconjunctival hemorrhages (Fig. 13-7) must be differentiated by the history and examination from those appearing when a small, sharp fragment strikes the eye.

Superficial corneal abrasions and foreign bodies. Superficial corneal abrasions and foreign bodies are extremely common (Figs. 13-8 and 13-9). Oblique, moving illumination is the best technique for detection. Look carefully for irregular reflections or shadows, which may be extremely tiny. Fluorescein will stain corneal epithelial defects a bright green, permitting easy diagnosis. Administer the fluorescein by touching the end of a sterile fluorescein paper strip to the moist lower conjunctival sac (see Fig. 5-9). Allow it to remain until a visible amount of stain has dissolved into the tears. Irrigate the excess out with a generous amount of normal saline solution. Do not undertake this manipulation until you have ruled out penetrating injuries. Stain will be retained only by damaged surfaces. Use of a magnifying loupe is helpful in detecting tiny defects.

Do *not* subject an eye with a known penetrating injury to the manipulation of staining.

Text continued on p. 237.

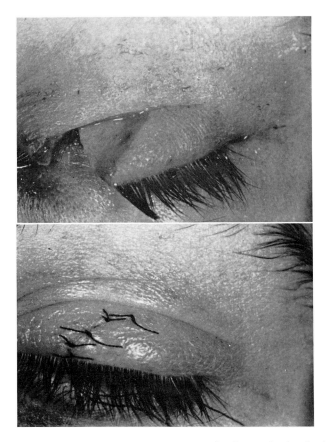

Fig. 13-4. The most important step in care of this lid laceration is examination for injury of the eye itself. If the eye is uninjured, the lid should be sutured in three separate layers, which are clearly visible here. The deepest layer is the tarsal plate; the surface layer is skin. Between them lies the layer of the orbicularis muscle. The lid margin must be very accurately approximated. No sutures should protrude deep to the lid, where they might injure the cornea. The final result from such an injury should be perfect except for an almost imperceptible scar. Poor apposition and careless suturing would leave conspicuous, unsightly defects.

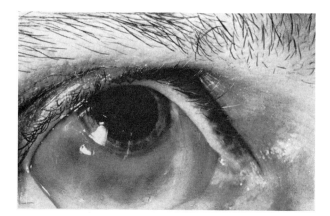

Fig. 13-5. Dilatation of the pupil is advisable when traumatic subconjunctival hemorrhage exists. Thorough ophthalmoscopic examination is impossible through a small pupil and is necessary to detect possible intraocular damage. Phenylephrine, 2½%, is a good mydriatic for this purpose.

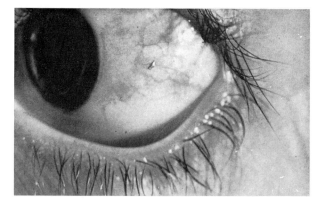

Fig. 13-6. The end of a metal splinter is protruding from the sclera. A considerably longer portion of the splinter lies within the eye. Had a more massive subconjunctival hemorrhage occurred, the penetrating wound could have been completely concealed from external detection. The internal projection of metal was easily seen with the ophthalmoscope.

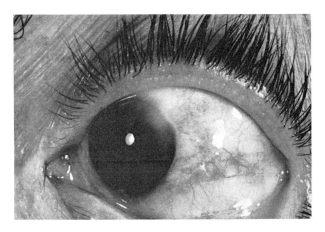

Fig. 13-7. Absorbing subconjunctival hemorrhage assumes a peculiar, mottled appearance. Gravity may cause progressive downward migration of blood, which does not mean that fresh bleeding has occurred. One or two weeks are required for clearing of a subconjunctival hemorrhage.

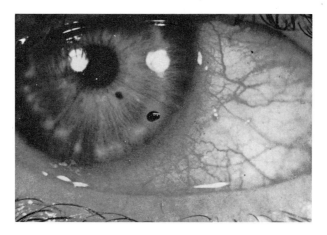

Fig. 13-8. Superficially imbedded metal particles produce a discoloration of the surrounding cornea known as a "rust ring." Marked redness and pain may be caused by an extremely tiny corneal foreign body barely visible by oblique, moving illumination. Irrigation or swabbing with cotton will not successfully remove such imbedded particles and usually succeeds only in damaging the surrounding epithelium.

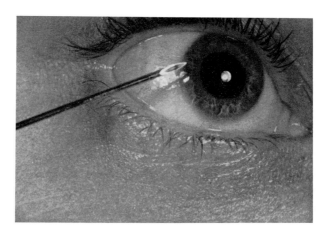

Fig. 13-9. Use of a No. 20 hypodermic needle is advised for removal of superficially imbedded particles because it is readily available, is sterile, is easily manipulated, and permits discrete removal of the foreign particle without damage to surrounding epithelium. Topical anesthesia, as with proparacaine, is adequate for this procedure. Topical antibiotics are useful in preventing infection until the wound heals.

To avoid infection, only fresh sterile drops (tetracaine, fluorescein, antibiotics, mydriatics, and so on) should be instilled on an injured eye.

The *corneal epithelium,* although only five cell layers thick, is an extremely effective barrier against infection. The intact epithelium is impenetrable to all the common pyogenic bacteria, but it is susceptible to the granulomatous infections (such as tuberculosis), to gonococci, and to some viruses. Because the unprotected deeper cornea is more susceptible to infection, topical antibiotics are recommended until any epithelial breaks have healed. The disappearance of pain usually signifies epithelial healing. Regeneration of the epithelial surface occurs by mitosis and by a sliding migration of adjacent cells. It is not unusual for these mechanisms to reepithelialize as much as one third of the entire cornea within 1 day. The epithelium heals without any scar.

Bowman's membrane is the extremely tough layer immediately below the epithelium. Because of its strength, the great majority of minor corneal abrasions and foreign bodies do not damage more than the epithelium and therefore do not leave scars. Injury of Bowman's membrane or of the deeper corneal stroma will leave a permanent scar.

Penetrating injuries of the cornea or sclera. Because of the dangerous nature of penetrating injuries of the cornea or sclera and the great importance of prompt therapy, recognition of this type of injury is vital. Many such injuries are not obvious at first glance. Their identification is aided by the following features:

1. A faint gray ring of edema usually surrounds corneal perforations.
2. Uveal tissue exposed through a scleral laceration is a conspicuous black or brown-black color.
3. Protruding transparent jelly certainly represents loss of vitreous or lens.
4. Collapse of the anterior chamber (so that the iris and cornea are in contact) indicates a leaking penetrating wound. Such a collapsed chamber is demonstrable through oblique illumination, which emphasizes the forward displacement of the iris (see Fig. 15-3).
5. Displacement of the pupil suggests prolapse of the iris through a wound on the side toward which displacement has occurred. Tearing of the iris from its base on the ciliary body also will result in pupil displacement.
6. Localized iris defects such as notches or holes (Fig. 13-10) almost certainly indicate penetrating trauma. Occasionally a small round hole within the iris is the only grossly visible sign of serious injury.
7. Intraocular bleeding may result from a penetrating injury or contusion. Blood within the eye is a readily observable sign in many persons with serious eye trauma.
8. Purulent material inside the eye (Fig. 13-11) means that the diagnosis of penetrating injury was made too late and that infection will probably destroy sight. Heroic amounts of antibiotics sometimes salvage partial vision. It is far more effective to begin prophylactic antibiotics within the first few hours after injury, before implanted bacteria have multiplied.

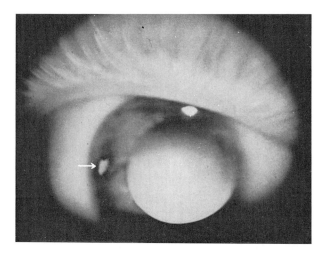

Fig. 13-10. The red reflex seen during ophthalmoscopy is transmitted conspicuously through a traumatic iris hole. With flashlight illumination such a hole is black (like the pupil) and somewhat resembles as iris nevus. A small iris defect is almost certain proof of penetrating injury. The peripheral iridectomy intentionally formed at the time of cataract surgery is a commonly seen example of such an appearance.

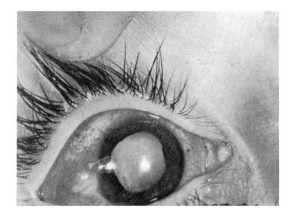

Fig. 13-11. This gray opacity of the vitreous appeared 3 days after a schoolmate had struck the patient's eye with a piece of chalk, inflicting an inconspicuous penetrating injury. Vitreous infection is already far advanced, and the eye was lost shortly afterward. Immediate recognition of the penetrating nature of the wound and vigorous use of prophylactic systemic antibiotics might have saved the eye with good vision.

Iris changes. Visible trembling of the iris with movement of the eye means dislocation or absence of the lens. (When in normal position, the lens supports the iris.) Apposition of the iris to the cornea (loss of the anterior chamber) indicates that aqueous has been lost through a penetrating wound. Distortion of the pupil occurs when the iris has prolapsed into a wound, when adhesions have developed between the iris and adjacent structures, or when iris innervation has been damaged. Paralytic dilatation of the pupil is not uncommon after severe contusions.

Lens changes. Cataract is one of the serious sequelae of eye injury and may follow a contusion as well as a penetrating injury. The presence of a cataract is indicated by grayish opacities immediately behind the pupil. Obviously, mydriasis aids diagnosis. Contusions may cause dislocation of the lens forward into the anterior chamber or backward into the vitreous. In the anterior chamber a dislocated lens is recognized as a smooth round or oval mass that is two thirds the diameter of the cornea. (Many physicians do not realize the lens is so large.) Diagnosis of posterior dislocation is best made by visualizing the lens with an ophthalmoscope.

Vitreous changes. Hemorrhage into the vitreous is confusing to the inexperienced ophthalmologist, for it obscures all details. The beginner is likely to attribute this finding to his own faulty technique with the ophthalmoscope, especially if the anterior part of the eye appears normal. Comparison of the red reflex of the normal eye with that of the injured eye is one of the most helpful methods of examination. The red reflex is the glowing appearance within the pupil, similar to the well-known luminous reflections from a cat's eye when a light strikes the pupil. The red reflex is easily seen in a dark room when the examiner sights through an ophthalmoscope with the lens set at zero and directs the light beam into the patient's eye from a distance of about 1 foot. Absence of the red reflex indicates opacities within the normally clear ocular contents. Hemorrhage, inflammation, cataract, and neoplasm are examples of disorders that may obscure the red reflex. A red reflex is readily seen through a perforating wound of the iris (provided that the ocular media remain transparent) and clearly differentiates such a wound from an iris freckle.

Fundus changes. Ophthalmoscopy is a necessary part of the evaluation of an injured eye and will permit recognition of such conditions as intraocular hemorrhage, edema, foreign bodies, or retinal tears. In blond fundi it is possible to see vortex veins in the far periphery. These veins appear as bright red areas several disc diameters across and are readily confused with hemorrhages unless the radiating red lines representing tributary choroidal veins are recognized as such. Choroidal hemorrhages underlie the retinal pigment layer and, depending on the pigment density, may appear slate gray and elevated, closely simulating a malignant melanoma.

Retinal edema after contusion is usually most pronounced surrounding the macula. Severe edema causes a gray discoloration of the retina, whereas lesser injury produces increased glistening reflections surrounding the macula. Since considerable variation exists in the normal macular pigmentation and in the physiologic retinal reflections, comparison of the injured eye wih the other normal eye is most helpful. (Normal variations are almost always symmetrical in the two eyes.)

The appearance of intraocular foreign bodies (see Plate 25) is striking, because the optical strength of the eye may produce up to 15× magnification. Magnification is greater the farther posteriorly the foreign body is located. Within days a considerable exudative reaction may surround and conceal such foreign bodies.

Traumatic retinal detachments usually lead to blindness if they remain untreated. Diagnosis is made by recognition of an elevated translucent area with an undulating surface. The detached portion is quite gray. Detachments almost always begin in the far periphery and cannot be recognized at an early optimal time without adequate dilatation of the pupil. Diagnosis of a fresh retinal detachment indicates emergency referral to an ophthalmologist. A history of progressive field loss is characteristic.

Use of 2½% phenylephrine or another mydriatic is strongly recommended to aid fundus examination in the majority of persons with serious eye injury. Few pupils are spontaneously large enough to permit adequate ophthalmoscopy of the peripheral fundus.

Orbital changes. Blunt contusions may cause a "blowout" of the orbit into the sinuses, ultimately producing enophthalmos (backward displacement of the eye), which is undesirable cosmetically. Plastic repair is best done within the first few weeks. Temporary exophthalmos results from orbital hemorrhage and may be accompanied by visual loss in many cases. Such visual loss is probably due to damage of the blood supply to the optic nerve and is not reparable surgically. Decompression of such an orbit is not feasible, because the hemorrhage will be found to have infiltrated diffusely throughout the orbital

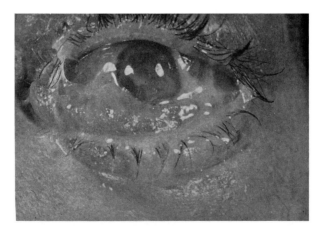

Fig. 13-12. Orbital cellulitis and endophthalmitis have destroyed this eye. Extension of infection from a sinus is the most common cause of orbital cellulitis. It is recognized by exophthalmos, paralysis of extraocular muscles, visual loss, pain, and systemic toxicity. Penetrating orbital trauma is another common cause.

fat and is inaccessible to surgical evacuation. Should x-ray examination show fracture of the optic canal, neurosurgical removal of bony fragments pressing on the nerve may restore vision. If the cornea is exposed, it must be protected by lubricant ointments.

Crepitus of the lids is readily perceived as a crackling sensation by the examining finger. Crepitus always means a fracture into a sinus. To avoid forcing more air into the orbit, the patient must be cautioned not to blow his nose. Prophylactic antibiotics minimize the possibility of orbital cellulitis (Fig. 13-12).

Reduced sensation in the distribution of the maxillary branch of the trigeminal nerve on the cheek is strongly suggestive of a blowout fracture of the orbital floor.

Finger tension estimation

Finger tension estimation should be done only if the preliminary survey discloses no evidence of a penetrating injury. In general, whenever it has been determined with certainty that an eye has suffered a penetrating injury, the examination should stop at that point and the patient should immediately be referred to an ophthalmologist. If, however, the eyeball seems uninjured in all respects, at this stage of the examination finger tension should be gently estimated. Excessive softness indicates a penetrating injury or rupture that may be located invisibly in the posterior half of the eye. Finger tension should *not* be estimated on an eye known to have sustained a penetrating injury.

Other tests

Further manipulations should now be considered safe if necessary. This would include fluorescein staining in a search for corneal abrasions as a possible cause for persistent pain. Eversion of the upper lid may disclose foreign particles lodged on the upper tarsal conjunctiva. Such inspection of the everted tarsal conjunctiva should certainly be done in all persons with unexplained persistent discomfort of sudden onset. Remember the importance of *oblique, moving, bright illumination.*

MANAGEMENT OF INJURY

Although the eventual outcome of an eye injury depends heavily on the severity of injury, blindness can often be prevented by prompt medical or surgical treatment. Methods of recognition have been stressed, because diagnosis is prerequisite to treatment. Management is discussed under the headings of birth injuries, burns, superficial abrasions and foreign bodies, contusions, penetrating injuries, and lid injuries.

Treatment

Birth injuries. Injury of an infant's eye may be of any type suffered by an adult and will have a similar appearance and prognosis (Fig. 13-13). It is interesting but of little practical significance that the process of normal birth produces transient small retinal hemorrhages in a considerable proportion of infants. A unique lesion is the corneal damage sustained from poorly applied obstetric forceps. Such pressure may cause a

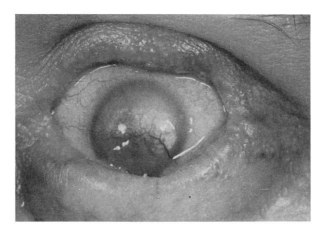

Fig. 13-13. Severe exposure damage of the cornea has produced this dense, white, vascularized scar. This was due to faulty development of the lids and inadequate protection of the cornea.

rupture of Descemet's membrane, which results in dense gray corneal edema. With regeneration of Descemet's endothelium, the cornea clears after weeks or months. A permanent corneal scar can always be seen with the slit-lamp microscope. Because of the unequal curvature of the torn cornea, marked astigmatism persists and will cause suppression amblyopia if proper glasses are not prescribed early. A child with such an injury should receive refractive correction before 1 year of age.

Chemical burns. Chemical burns of the eye are not uncommon and may originate from laboratories, industrial plants, or kitchens. A great variety of agents (acids, alkalies, cleaners, solvents, insecticides) may be encountered. Regardless of the type of chemical, emergency treatment is always the same. *Immediate, prolonged washing with plain water* will prevent permanent scarring more effectively than any other treatment. One should *not* search for a specific antidote such as baking soda or vinegar. Seconds are precious if the cornea is to be saved from a strong caustic. Water may be poured on the eye with a glass, squirted from a drinking fountain, and so on. The lids should be widely separated so that the water bathes the eye directly. Ordinarily, traces of irritant chemical will persist despite 10 minutes of irrigation, and therefore it is wise to continue washing for 15 or 20 minutes. First aid courses should include this information.

When the patient arrives at the physician's office, a repeated, thorough, prolonged irrigation is indicated. Tetracaine or proparacaine anesthesia of the cornea will make the patient more cooperative. Normal saline solution is better than water because it does not cause corneal edema. Particulate matter such as lye crystals must be identified and removed mechanically. The extent of epithelial damage is best assessed with fluorescein staining (Fig. 13-14). If more than one third of the corneal area is damaged or if gray discoloration indicates deep stromal damage, cycloplegia should be maintained with 1%

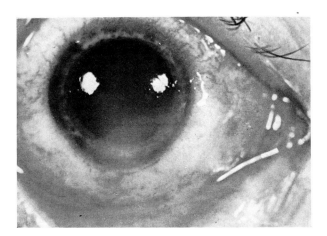

Fig. 13-14. This acetic anhydride burn of a chemist's eye has denuded the epithelium of the lower three fifths of the cornea as indicated by the extent of fluorescein staining. The lower conjunctival cul-de-sac has also been extensively burned. Immediate and prolonged washing with plain water is the most important step in care of such an eye injury. Note the irregularity of the corneal light reflections.

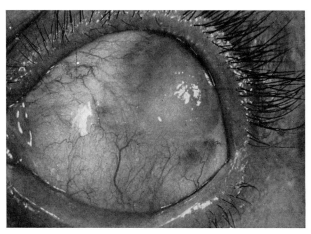

Fig. 13-15. A hot lye solution was thrown into this patient's eye with malicious intent. Dense, full-thickness scarring has resulted despite all therapy. Unfortunately, this type of injury responds poorly to corneal transplantation. Internal damage to the iris and lens further complicates such cases.

atropine twice daily. Topical antibiotics instilled every 2 hours will minimize the possibility of infection and should be used until the cornea no longer stains. If injury is severe enough that more than a few days will be required for healing, topical corticosteroids may minimize scarring (Fig. 13-15) and neovascularization. However, corticosteroids may cause rapid loss of the exposed corneal stroma, so dramatic that it is termed "melting." Corticosteroid use is potentially dangerous and requires frequent observation of the patient.

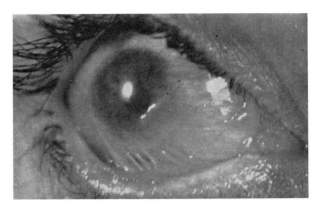

Fig. 13-16. After a chemical burn of the conjunctival cul-de-sac, the raw surfaces of the lid and eyeball were permitted to lie in apposition and healed together. Thick bands of scar tissue have fused together the lid and globe (symblepharon). Such fusion may interfere considerably with eye movements and with adequate lid closure. Some of this late difficulty is avoidable through frequent mechanical separation of the burned surfaces during the first few days after injury.

Denudation of apposing tarsal and bulbar surfaces will result in adhesions (Fig. 13-16) unless mechanical separation and ointment instillation are done every few hours. Pain is usually intense, requiring sedatives and narcotics. Topical anesthetics must *not* be used repeatedly, because they inhibit healing.

Ultraviolet burns. Sunlamps, welding arcs, germicidal lamps, or natural sunshine may cause ultraviolet damage to the corneal epithelium. Characteristically, these burns are relatively asymptomatic for some hours and then cause severe eye pain. Often this pain will awaken the patient from sleep. As observed with oblique light, the normally lustrous corneal surface will be dulled. Diffuse punctate fluorescein staining results. Photophobia, blepharospasm, and tearing are usually present. The conjunctiva is reddened. Discharge and crusting are absent. Diagnosis is most easily made from the history of a rather sudden, apparently spontaneous onset of pain accompanied by this clinical picture.

The pain of a severe ultraviolet burn usually disables the patient for a day or two. Topical proparacaine or tetracaine will relieve pain during the office examination. In general, topical anesthetics should never be prescribed for home use in treatment of corneal injury or disease, because they impair epithelial healing and predispose the cornea to additional unrecognized injury while it is anesthetized. Ice packs, analgesics such as aspirin or codeine, and sedatives should be prescribed for pain. Short-acting cycloplegics (2% homatropine or 1% cyclopentolate) will relieve pain due to associated iritis. Topical antibiotics should be used four times a day to prevent infection. The patient may be assured that the corneal epithelium will regenerate without scarring or visual loss.

Thermal burns. Usually the lid surface will have suffered most of the damage, the underlying cornea being protected. Gentle cleaning and thorough greasing with antibiotic

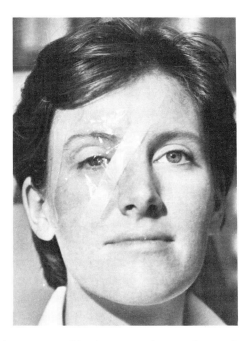

Fig. 13-17. Drying of the cornea resulting in exposure keratopathy may be prevented by an airtight covering with clear plastic wrap.

ointment is probably the best treatment for burned lids. Dressings need not be applied if the skin is kept covered with ointment. If the burn is so severe as to impair lid closure, the exposed cornea *must* constantly be kept covered with generous amounts of ointment (boric acid ointment is as inexpensive as any), or permanent corneal scarring will result. Covering the eye with plastic wrap may help protect the cornea (Fig. 13-17). Crusting and discharge should be removed by gentle mechanical swabbing or with the aid of warm, moist compresses.

Corneal burns are treated with antibiotic and cycloplegic (for associated iritis) drops. Rarely, a severe corneal burn may perforate. This serious emergency is recognized by collapse of the anterior chamber (the iris touches the cornea). If the peripheral cornea is strong enough to support a corneal transplant, such surgery may save the eye.

Superficial abrasions and foreign bodies. Superficial abrasions and foreign bodies of the conjunctiva are not dangerous. Without an anesthetic, foreign particles such as sand may be irrigated from the conjunctiva or picked out with clean moist cotton spindles. The natural resistance of the conjunctiva is high, and a single antibiotic instillation in the office is adequate prophylactic treatment.

Corneal injuries are much more serious, because resistance to infection is low, and even small scars may seriously impair vision if they are centrally located. Whenever the corneal epithelium is broken (and it is only five cell layers thick), a portal of entry for infection exists. Prophylactic use of topical antibiotics should be continued until the epithelium is healed. (Surprisingly large epithelial defects may heal within a day.) Healing is recognized through failure to stain with fluorescein or by complete disappearance of pain. Pain is much more marked with corneal foreign bodies than with conjunctival ones. Worth remembering is the practical point that all superficial ocular foreign bodies that continue to be painful will be found in one of two places, either on the cornea or on the tarsal surface of the upper lid that covers the cornea. These foreign bodies are usually vanishingly small and are completely overlooked by the physician who does not use *oblique, moving, bright illumination*. If left imbedded for several days, a corneal foreign body may cause severe keratitis and iritis, which will not heal until the particle is detected and removed. The possibility of multiple foreign bodies must be kept in mind. Examine the entire eye—do not stop when one foreign body is found.

Topical anesthesia is necessary for removal of an imbedded corneal foreign body. Proparacaine, 0.5%, repeated in 30 seconds, will give adequate anesthesia within a minute or two. Removal is best accomplished with a small, relatively sharp instrument such as an eye spud. *It must be sterile.* A No. 20 hypodermic needle is a satisfactory and easily obtainable substitute. With such a discrete tip, the average superficial particle is easily dislodged without damage to surrounding epithelium (see Fig. 13-9). It is wise to brace your hand against the patient's cheek and to have good illumination. The commonly employed cotton swabs are highly undesirable, because their use causes extensive damage to surrounding epithelium, thereby prolonging healing time. Furthermore, it is impossible to remove rust rings with a cotton swab.

Epithelial defects are always present after removal of a superficially imbedded corneal foreign body, and use of prophylactic topical antibiotics should therefore be routine (see Figs. 14-10 to 14-12). The best choice is a medication that is not used systemically, because bacteria are more likely to be susceptible to these less commonly used drugs. Bacitracin, neomycin, and polymyxin (often used in combination as Neosporin); nitrofurazone (Furacin); or sulfacetamide is effective and should be instilled every 2 hours while the patient is awake. Liquid vehicles are more desirable than ointments for this purpose. Recommendations concerning use of an eye patch vary among ophthalmologists. I routinely patch the eye after removal of a foreign body to prevent scuffing of the anesthetized eye by the patient himself (Fig. 13-18). After the first 30 minutes, when the anesthetic has worn off, I leave patching to the option of the patient, who determines whether the eye is more comfortable open or closed. Many ophthalmologists routinely patch such an eye for 24 hours, with firm pressure. Healing proceeds at the same rate whether the eye is patched or not. Patching encourages infection and should therefore never be used in the management of bacterial conjunctivitis or keratitis.

Do not prescribe topical anesthetics for home use in the injured eye. During anesthesia the mitotic and ameboid reparative activity of corneal epithelium is completely inhibited. Repeated instillation of anesthetics will cause breakdown of the epithelium of a healthy, undamaged cornea.

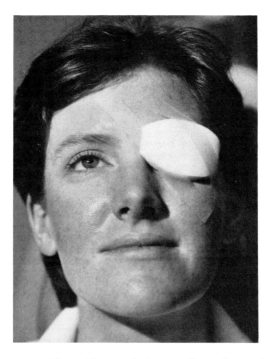

Fig. 13-18. To hold an eye pad in position, apply the tape diagonally, as shown. Beginners often apply a cross of tape, extending across the nose—an ineffective and uncomfortable position.

Corticosteroids are *not* indicated in the management of minor corneal abrasions. They are expensive and do not hasten healing. Neovascularization does not occur in these small wounds, and the extent of scarring depends on the amount of epithelial injury. Worst of all, steroids actually depress bodily defenses against bacteria, viruses, and fungi and may be responsible for the development of infection.

Use of atropine is *not* desirable for most minor corneal abrasions. Atropine produces prolonged cycloplegia (sometimes lasting 2 weeks), which is extremely annoying to anyone who must do close work. Traumatic iritis will develop only in neglected cases, in unusually extensive abrasions, or when a cotton applicator has been used unskillfully and has damaged a considerable area surrounding a foreign body. Such iritis is recognized by undue redness of the eye, particularly marked in a ring surrounding the cornea (limbal flush); by excessive and persistent pain; and by photophobia. Traumatic iritis responds well to cycloplegia (provided the cause is removed) such as is obtained with 2% homatropine or 1% cyclopentolate three times daily. Usually only a day or two of treatment is necessary. The duration of homatropine cycloplegia is usually not more than 2 days.

Conjunctival variants. *Conjunctival concretions* or *cysts* are small (1 to 2 mm) rounded, yellow-white, slightly elevated nodules seen frequently in the lower cul-de-sac

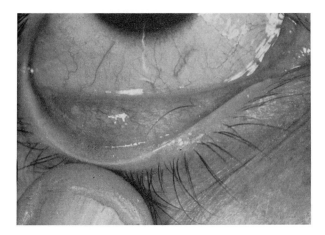

Fig. 13-19. The lower tarsal conjunctiva is normally redder and more vascular than the bulbar conjunctiva. The small white area in the lateral conjunctiva is a lipoid deposit, is commonly seen, and is not responsible for any symptoms. Note the loose eyelash lying on the tarsal conjunctiva. Removal of such a lash is easily accomplished with a cotton swab and does not require anesthesia.

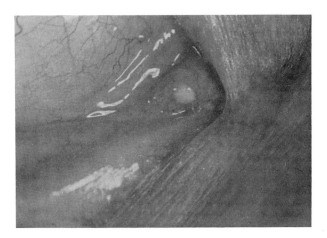

Fig. 13-20. A large sebaceous cyst is seen in the caruncle. This is asymptomatic.

(Figs. 13-19 and 13-20). They are asymptomatic and should not confuse the physician seeking an explanation for a foreign body sensation. *Lymphatic cysts* are similar in position and appearance, except that they are perfectly transparent (Fig. 13-21). These cysts are also asymptomatic.

Conjunctival pigmentation becomes gradually more pronounced with age, especially in dark-skinned persons. An increase in extent of a given pigmented area is a matter of

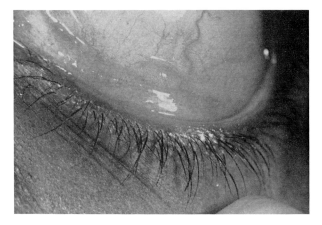

Fig. 13-21. An unusually large lymphatic cyst is just above the center. It is smoothly rounded and filled with transparent fluid.

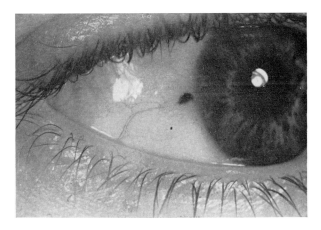

Fig. 13-22. Conjunctival pigmentation as dense as this in a white person occasions some concern as to malignancy. The surrounding pinkish vascular discoloration led to prophylactic excision of this nevus, which was found to be benign histologically.

some concern in a white patient's eye (Fig. 13-22). Elevation (Fig. 13-23) or very black color indicates excision of the lesion. This is easily done with the patient under local anesthesia, leaves no scar, and eliminates the fear of malignant transformation. *Intrascleral nerve loops* are localized pigment dots in scleral foramina (Fig. 13-24). Frequently these dots closely resemble a cinder or other foreign body, and futile attempts at removal may be made. Fortunately, these pigments dots are almost always situated in the upper

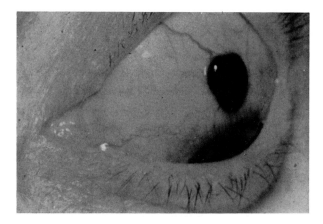

Fig. 13-23. Extraocular extension of a malignant melanoma of the choroid formed this elevated black mass. Enucleation is necessary to remove this growth.

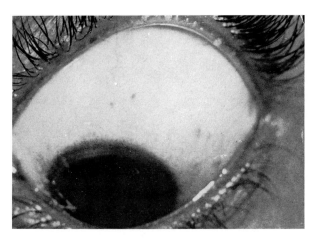

Fig. 13-24. The prominent pigment spots seen here in the upper sclera are uveal pigment that has spread through the foramina that transmit vessels and nerves through the sclera. They are ordinarily seen superiorly, about 0.5 cm above the limbus, and are more common in black patients. These common lesions are often mistaken for foreign bodies.

sclera, about 0.5 cm above the limbus. This area is always protectively covered by the upper lid, and I have never seen a genuine foreign body superficially imbedded in this location.

Hairs normally grow from the caruncle in the nasal cornea of the conjunctiva. These hairs do not cause eye irritation and should not be epilated in the treatment of a foreign body sensation.

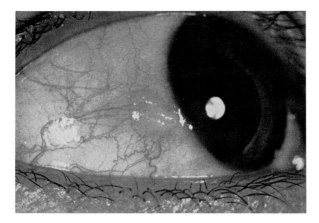

Fig. 13-25. A pinguecula is always situated in the horizontal meridian, nasally or temporally, is often bilateral, and is a slightly elevated gray mass. Usually there is no excess vascularization surrounding a pinguecula; this photograph was chosen for illustrative purposes because a minor inflammation exaggerated the appearance of the pinguecula.

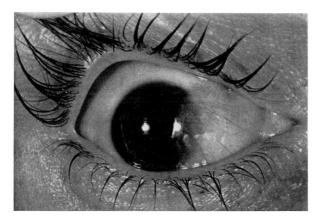

Fig. 13-26. A pterygium is a fleshy, vascular growth extending onto the cornea. A pterygium arises from environmental irritation of a pinguecula and may progress to involve much of the cornea. It should be excised before reaching the size shown here.

A *pinguecula* is a slightly elevated, irregular, gray elastic tissue deposit occurring in the conjunctiva within several millimeters of the limbus (Fig. 13-25). Pingueculae occur *only* in the horizontal meridian, nasally or temporally, an are ordinarily bilaterally symmetrical. They are asymptomatic and of no consequence but may cause the patient some alarm if he notices them one day in the mirror. If subjected to excessive irritation by ultraviolet radiation, a pinguecula may be stimulated to develop into a *pterygium* (Fig. 13-26), which is a flat, superficial vascular tissue mass encroaching on the cornea. If progressive, a pterygium should be excised before it extends very far on the cornea.

Contusions. Contusions (as caused by a golf ball or BB shot) of any magnitude carry a guarded prognosis. Intraocular hemorrhage, rupture of the globe, lens dislocation, macular edema and degeneration, retinal detachment, and similar serious complications may develop immediately or many months after the accident. It is probably wise to refer patients with obvious intraocular injury to an ophthalmologist for a decision as to whether surgical therapy is indicated or for optimal medical care. A good example of the complications that may be encountered is anterior chamber hemorrhage with secondary glaucoma. Within a few days this condition can cause blood staining of the cornea, a gray-brown discoloration that will obscure vision for years. Osmotic therapy or paracentesis may prevent this complication.

Penetrating injuries. Penetrating injuries are always emergency referral cases. Adequate instrumentation (including giant magnet and x-ray localization facilities), skill, and experience are required for definitive management. Proper shielding of the eye against injury is most important. Well-meaning friends and relatives may inflict serious additional injury through attempts to wipe away blood or tears. Almost instinctively the patient will

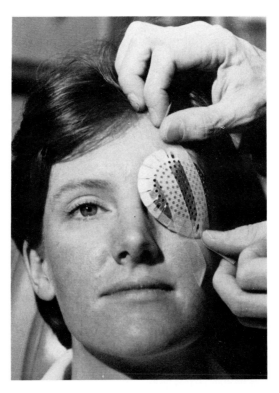

Fig. 13-27. Proper shielding of an injured eye. Assume that the patient and her well-meaning attendants and friends will further damage a lacerated eye *unless* you protect it and caution them.

press on a painful or weeping eye. *A metal or plastic shield should be firmly taped over the eye* (Figs. 13-27 and 13-28), and everyone concerned should be cautioned against putting pressure on the eye. I have had the unhappy experience of walking into the emergency room just in time to see a little girl squeezing vitreous out of an arrow wound in her own eye as the intern, nurse, and parents watched.

Since surgical repair will usually be performed with the patient under general anesthesia, the patient should be advised not to eat or drink. Systemic antibiotics (for example, chloramphenicol, 2 g) should be given. Tetanus prophylaxis and necessary analgesics are in order. Local medication should be limited to antibiotic drops.

Undue exertion must be avoided; however, the patient may ordinarily be transported sitting up in an automobile.

Lid injuries. Lid injuries are simply jigsaw puzzles. Accurate approximation of tissue fragments is time consuming but essential. Separate layer-by-layer closure of tarsus, orbicularis muscle, and skin will minimize scar retraction. Sacrifice of viable tissue through debridement is taboo. Lid margin wound edges require exact approximation. Delicate forceps and sutures should be used. The cornea must be adequately protected from exposure. *Never* repair a lid until you know that the underlying eyeball is *not* lacerated.

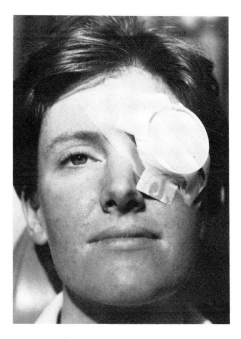

Fig. 13-28. If no metal shield is available, an effective substitute is easily fashioned from the bottom of a paper drinking cup.

Special attention must be paid to repair of a torn levator tendon, avulsed palpebral ligaments, and severed canaliculi. Lid tears or lacerations medial to the punctum will transect the lacrimal canaliculus. Primary repair of the canaliculus is relatively easy, requiring only threading of a polyethylene tube through the canaliculus and approximation of the cut ends. Failure to repair the canaliculus at the time of initial repair usually dooms the patient to permanent epiphora, because attempts at late repair are notoriously difficult and unsuccessful. Whenever the ends of the lids have been torn free from their orbital attachments, repair of the palpebral ligaments with deep sutures is essential. Skin suturing alone, although easy, tempting, and apparently adequate, will result in a loose lid that hangs away from the eye, and that will require further surgery.

Faults of lid structure or innervation may prevent proper corneal protection. Temporary protection against corneal exposure damage may be achieved by taping a piece of plastic wrap to form an airtight cover over the eye (see Fig. 13-17).

Prophylaxis

Prevention of eye injury is a legitimate medical concern. Rigid adherence to safety eyeglass rules eliminates eye injuries in most large industrial plants. Many eye injuries are sustained by individuals in small business or home workshops. Safety goggles are just as important in these small workshops as in large plants.

Children at play frequently suffer serious eye injury. Throwing missiles, waving pointed sticks, using BB guns or bows and arrows while unsupervised, experimenting with explosives, and having similar "fun" have cost many children the sight of an eye. Having seen many such tragedies, I vigorously condemn such activities, with complete disregard of the "spoilsport" complaints.

Finally, ordinary eyeglasses may be shatterproofed at little additional expense. This will prevent glass fragments in the eye should the lenses be broken during wear. Federal law now mandates the use of such break-resistant lenses.

SUMMARY

Recognition of even the tiniest eye injury can be important. Proper management of eye injuries will prevent many cases of blindness. Inquiries involving the interior of the eye should be referred to an ophthalmologist.

chapter 14 Diagnosis and Management of the Red Eye

Redness of the eye is a warning signal common to many diseases. Most frequently encountered are the relatively insignificant allergies and superficial conjunctival infections. Danger exists that the frequency with which minor conjunctival inflammations are encountered may engender a feeling of security in dealing with red eyes. Such an attitude will lead to regrettable delay in making an accurate diagnosis and instituting definitive therapy for the more serious eye diseases.

How can the physician be sure that he does not overlook the presence of one of the serious and potentially blinding causes of a red eye? It is actually easy to guard against such diagnostic errors. Although later in this chapter the more common diseases are discussed, it is unnecessary to learn the characteristics of a multitude of diseases in order to exclude the presence of major eye disease. Eight easily determined objective and subjective findings may be used as a checklist. Almost never will a really serious red eye fail to show the presence not only of one but usually of several of these criteria. Conversely, minor conjunctivitis does not present these findings.

FINDINGS IN A RED EYE SUGGESTING MAJOR DISEASE

Visual loss. Definite reduction in acuity occurring since the onset of redness should *always* be regarded with great suspicion. The patient will usually be aware of visual loss and should be specifically questioned on this point. Use of a visual acuity chart is an important part of the examination of a red eye. Minor allergic or bacterial conjunctivitis will *not* cause loss of vision.

Pain. Severe discomfort strongly suggests corneal damage or serious intraocular or orbital involvement. Although painful corneal abrasions usually heal without trouble, they represent a potential portal of entry for infection and cannot be disregarded.

Opacities. Fresh corneal infiltration or debris within the normally transparent eye structures is always serious (Fig. 14-1). Bright, obliquely directed, moving illumination, as from a small flashlight, is best for observation of anteriorly situated opacities. Opacities posteriorly situated in the lens or vitreous are best appreciated as dark shadows against the ophthalmoscopic red reflex.

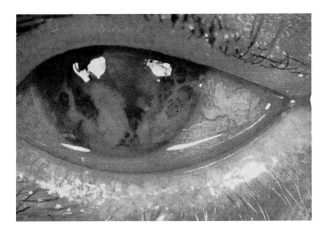

Fig. 14-1. Propelled by a glancing hammer blow, a nail perforated this eye and damaged the lens capsule, resulting in a fluffy traumatic cataract. This is a good example of the appearance of intraocular opaque debris, which should always be considered to indicate a serious cause of a red eye. Cataract surgery and fitting of a contact lens resulted in good vision.

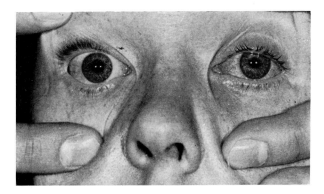

Fig. 14-2. One of the best diagnostic criteria in iritis is the smaller pupil in the affected eye. This is a case of traumatic iritis after general anesthesia, during which the left eye was not adequately protected against exposure keratopathy. Simply through the instillation of eye ointment, this patient could have been spared considerable discomfort. Note also the proper method of separating the eyelids by pressure over the orbital rims.

Irregularities of the pupil. Irregularities in the size and shape of the pupil result from intraocular inflammation or trauma. A smaller pupil on the side of a red eye is an excellent indicator of iritis (Fig. 14-2), whereas an enlarged pupil suggests acute glaucoma (unless it is due to mydriatic therapy).

Distribution of redness. A red halo immediately encircling the cornea (Fig. 14-3) (limbal flush) almost invariably indicates serious eye disease. Redness diffusely distributed throughout the conjunctival area may occur with either benign or serious causes of a red

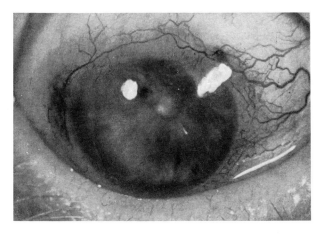

Fig. 14-3. Redness encircling the cornea is always an indication of serious eye disease. Shown here is a very poorly performed cataract extraction with retention of a large amount of lens cortex, displaced pupil, and iridocyclitis. Considerable variation exists in the technical skill and training of surgeons. Successful cataract extraction is a delicate operation.

eye and has no diagnostic significance. Engorgement of the deeper vessels is emphasized by some physicians as a sign of serious eye disease but is not readily differentiated from superficial hyperemia. Deep vessels are said to be straighter, bluish-red because of overlying tissue, and more difficult to blanch with topical epinephrine. Localized sectors of redness usually indicate episcleritis but may occur with focal infection or injury.

Alterations in pressure. Noticeable alterations in pressure of a red eye, either hard or soft as determined by finger tension estimation, indicate serious disease.

History. Redness in an eye known previously to have suffered from serious disease such as uveitis or glaucoma must be regarded as a recurrence until proved otherwise. The presence of bacterial conjunctivitis in other members of the family suggests the diagnosis of this simple, benign infection.

Failure to respond to therapy. Should diagnosis of a minor cause of the red eye have been made, failure to respond to adequate therapy within 2 or 3 days should cast doubt on the accuracy of the diagnosis. Sometimes this point has been misunderstood. I emphatically do *not* mean that you can wait 3 days to see whether a red eye will go away. During this time acute glaucoma could cause permanent blindness.

DIFFERENTIAL DIAGNOSIS

If, by means of the eight signals of major disease just discussed, a red eye is determined to have a serious cause, this cause should be diagnosed and the patient should receive specific treatment. Should the physician be unable to arrive at a diagnosis, urgent ophthalmologic consultation is in order.

A brief description of the more common causes of a red eye is in order at this point. Reference to Table 8 may be helpful.

Table 9. Differential diagnosis of the red eye

	Acute bacterial conjunctivitis	Acute iritis	Acute glaucoma	Corneal ulcer or trauma	Scleritis	Episcleritis
Only superficial vessels	Yes					
Superficial and deep vessels		Yes	Yes	Yes	Diffuse	Sector
Pupil	Not affected!	Small	Large	Small if secondary iritis	Small if secondary iritis	Not affected
Increased pressure		May have secondary glaucoma	Marked			
Opacity	Cornea uninvolved!	Iris and anterior chamber may be hazy	Steamy cornea	Corneal opacity, fluorescein staining	May encroach on cornea	
Ocular discharge	Yes			Yes		
Decreased vision	No!	Yes	Yes (rainbows)	Yes		
Severe pain			Yes (vomiting)	Yes		
History	Contagious	Often recurrent	Often hereditary	Often trauma	Often arthritis	
Therapy	Antibiotics	Atropine Cortisone	Pilocarpine Glycerol Surgery	Antibiotics	Systemic and topical cortisone	Topical cortisone
Prognosis	Self-limited, 3 to 5 days	*May be extremely serious without proper treatment*				Self-limited, 2 to 4 weeks

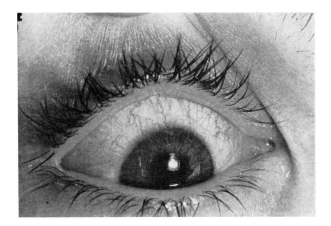

Fig. 14-4. In contrast to the limbal redness illustrated in Fig. 14-3 is the uniformly distributed redness of acute bacterial conjunctivitis. Such a conjunctivitis produces redness that is just as marked in the cul-de-sac as it is near the limbus. Superficial vessels become dilated and conspicuous and therefore seem more numerous. Absence in this picture of the characteristic crusting of the lids is due to cleaning of the lids by the patient before visiting the physician. Practically always the patient with bacterial conjunctivitis will report that the lids are ''sticky'' on awakening.

COMMON CAUSES OF A RED EYE

Acute bacterial conjunctivitis. Any of the common pyogenic bacteria may infect the conjunctival surface. Staphylococci are the most frequent offenders. This is the benign and self-limited disease known as ''pinkeye.'' Not only dilatation of surface vessels, but also multiple tiny petechiae, contribute to the redness. Distribution of the redness is throughout the conjunctiva and is not more marked near the cornea than in the periphery (Fig. 14-4). Invariably, some degree of discharge of crusting will be present on lid margins or corners of the eye. Usually this crusting will be quite conspicuous, especially in children. Mild cases such as usually are found in adults may be reported to show slight crusting only in the morning due to the night's accumulated secretions. This crusting of the lid margins is constant enough that its absence casts doubt on the diagnosis of bacterial conjunctivitis. Bear in mind that the patient may have cleaned his lids before seeing you. Usually both eyes are infected, either simultaneously or after a few days' incubation period. Above all, *remember* that pinkeye does *not* show the eight findings discussed previously as suggesting major eye disease!

Although acute bacterial conjunctivitis is self-limited and leaves no permanent scars, it is annoying, looks cosmetically bad, and may be quite contagious, especially among children. For these reasons treatment should be prescribed. Most appropriate are the antibacterial agents used for topical application only, such as neomycin, sulfacetamide, and gramicidin, or combinations that are commercially available. Corticosteroids reduce ocular resistance to bacteria; hence, their use is contraindicated in the presence of infec-

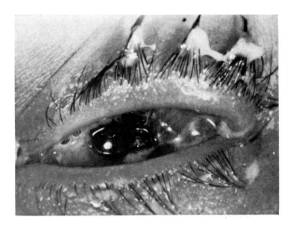

Fig. 14-5. Gonococcal conjunctivitis causes a copious amount of purulent secretion. This disease is very contagious. Permanent corneal scarring may result.

tious conjunctivitis. A liquid vehicle is preferable to an ointment. The patient should be instructed to instill one drop in the affected eye every 2 hours while awake. Warm, moist compresses (clean washcloth wrung out of hot tap water) help to remove crusts. An eye with a surface bacterial infection should *not* be bandaged, because covering the eye promotes bacterial growth. If this treatment does not cure the patient within 2 or 3 days, the possibility of misdiagnosis must be seriously considered (Fig. 14-5).

Obsolete drugs such as yellow oxide of mercury and boric acid are relatively ineffective.

Nasolacrimal duct impatency. The nasolacrimal duct, which is formed from a solid cord of epithelial cells and leads from the lacrimal sac to the nose, gradually develops a lumen and opens last at its lower end. This final opening usually occurs shortly after birth but may be delayed for several months. Since tears are not secreted during the first month, epiphora (pathologic tearing) is not noted early, despite failure of the duct to open. At about 1 month of age the affected infant (Fig. 14-6) is noted to have a "watery" eye, with frequent tearing down his cheek. Epiphora is naturally more pronounced when the child cries. Usually this symptom will spontaneously disappear before 3 months of age as the duct belatedly opens. If spontaneous cure does not occur by 3 months of age or if the lacrimal sac becomes infected, the child should be referred for probing of the nasolacrimal duct. Passage of a thin probe though the lacrimal drainage system and into the nose will break the imperforate septum and cure the child. This procedure may be done with a local anesthetic in the restrained infant but requires a 5-minute general anesthetic for a larger child. Infection of the blocked lacrimal sac is recognized by the accumulation of purulent discharge on the eyelids and canthi of the involved eye. Pressure over the sac will cause regurgitation of more purulent material, thereby confirming the diagnosis. Neglect of the infected stage of this disease will result in serious scarring of the duct, which will render probing impossible and necessitate performance of a major operation to create an artifi-

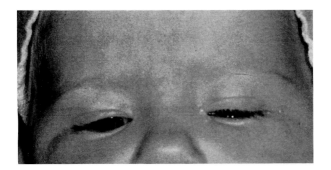

Fig. 14-6. Failure of the nasolacrimal duct to perforate into the nose results in epiphora, which appears at 3 to 4 weeks of age. Usually the lacrimal sac becomes infected, and purulent discharge accumulates on the lashes and corners of the eye. Despite all this discharge, the conjunctiva is usually perfectly white—a finding that differentiates this condition from conjunctivitis.

cial channel between the sac and the nose (dacryocystorhinostomy). When infection is recognized, topical antibiotics should be instilled and the child referred for probing.

Acute viral keratoconjunctivitis. Many types of acute viral conjunctivitis exist. Easiest to recognize are those associated with systemic febrile diseases such as rubella, rubeola, or the adenopharyngoconjunctival viruses. Indeed, the typical multiple small rounded follicles especially marked on the tarsal conjunctiva may be of help in diagnosing the systemic disease. No treatment is necessary in these patients unless a secondary bacterial infection should develop.

Not uncommon is herpes simplex keratoconjunctivitis. Particular stress is laid on identification of this disease because corticosteroid therapy may cause a considerable increase in severity of the infection and extent of the final scar. The possibility of viral infection is one of the major reasons for avoiding indiscriminate prescription of topical corticosteroids for eye inflammation. Herpes simplex characteristically produces a gradually progressive corneal lesion that is barely visible as a slight local haziness. Fluorescein staining makes the corneal ulceration more prominent and may permit identification of the pathognomonic zigzag shape of a dendritic ulcer. Most conspicuous, however, is the conjunctival redness that does not respond to antibiotic therapy. Untreated herpetic ulcers may continue for weeks and leave permanent scars. They should be referred as promptly as possible to an ophthalmologist for treatment of the involved cornea.

Superficial corneal infections due to herpes simplex respond to topical treatment with antiviral drugs such as idoxuridine, trifluorothymidine, and acyclovir. The antiviral medication must be instilled frequently, four to eight times daily, for several weeks. The older method of chemical cauterization of the corneal ulcers (using iodine or ether) is now rarely used. Although effective in eradicating the dendritic ulcer, cauterization can be very painful.

Occasional stubborn cases of conjunctivitis are encountered that do not seem to respond to any therapy and must be allowed to run their course of some weeks. It is presumed that these cases are of a viral origin, and careful study will sometimes result in isolation of many different kinds of viruses.

Allergic conjunctivitis. No diagnostic problem is presented by the reddened, itching, and weeping eyes associated with hay fever, allergic rhinitis, or asthma. Systemic antihistaminic or desensitization therapy may control the eye symptoms. Topical use of dilute sympathomimetic drugs, such as phenylephrine, 0.12%, is extremely effective in reducing the allergic response. Within 5 minutes the increased protein content of allergic tears will be reduced to normal by sympathomimetic drops. A comparable response to corticosteroid therapy requires 30 minutes or more. A variety of such sympathomimetic preparations are available as over-the-counter, nonprescription eyedrops.

In the past, corticosteroid drops were advised for treatment of ocular allergy. Although effective, corticosteroids may cause glaucoma and cataract. In addition, they cause immunologic incompetence, thereby rendering the eye vulnerable to infection. In short, prolonged use of corticosteroid drops for chronic conditions such as allergy is highly inadvisable.

Vernal conjunctivitis is a seasonal allergy affecting children and adolescents. Usually there are no systemic allergies coexisting. Itching is a prominent symptom and is accompanied by mild redness, weeping, and rubbing of the eyes. Crusting and discharge are not conspicuous in allergic conjunctivitis, in contrast to bacterial conjunctivitis. The most

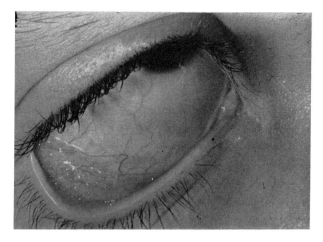

Fig. 14-7. Allergic conjunctivitis most often occurs in younger patients and characteristically itches. Confirmation of the diagnosis is made through recognition of the numerous small rounded follicles in the cul-de-sac. Glistening light reflections from the tops of these follicles are readily seen. Redness of the eye is often minimal.

characteristic objective finding is the presence of multiple tiny, somewhat flattened, semitransparent follicles (Fig. 14-7) that are most conspicuous on the upper border of the uper tarsal conjunctiva (Fig. 14-8). The upper lid must be everted to make the diagnosis in many persons. Therapy with topical sympathomimetic drugs such as 0.12% phenyl-ephrine is effective in relieving symptoms, but it does not cure the allergy, which often spontaneously disappears in adult life. Dosage is individual, the frequency of instillation being adjusted to the least amount necessary to relieve symptoms. More frequent use the first few days will cause the symptoms to disappear, after which instillation is tapered down to two to four times daily or however often is necessary. Desensitization and antihistaminics are not notably effective. Too many complications follow corticosteroid use to justify its prescription for minor allergies.

Episcleritis. Episcleritis is a peculiar localized hyperemia of the episcleral tissue (between the conjunctiva and the sclera). It is not uncommon. The cause is said to be bacterial hypersensitivity; however, other systemic manifestations are conspicuously absent. The affected eye has minimal irritation or may be almost asymptomatic. Distribution of redness is in a characteristic, somewhat pie-shaped sector (Fig. 14-9), which may be located in any meridian. The striking contrast between affected and adjacent perfectly normal white conjunctiva can never be seen in bacterial conjunctivitis, which spreads throughout the whole conjunctiva. Episcleritis is a benign process that does not damage the eye. Untreated, it may last for weeks, but with topical sympathomimetic drops it usually disappears in a few days. Prolonged maintenance therapy is unnecessary.

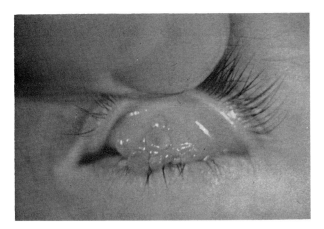

Fig. 14-8. Eversion of the upper lid is often most helpful in diagnosing allergic conjunctivitis. The largest lesions are usually on the superior part of the upper tarsal conjunctiva. Because of pressure from the cornea, these lesions assume a flattened, cobblestone-like appearance, which is well demonstrated in the unusually large allergic papillae of vernal conjunctivitis shown here.

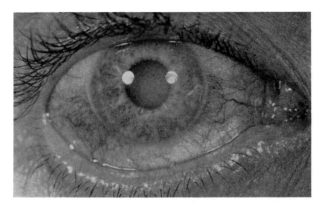

Fig. 14-9. A typical episcleritis is instantly recognizable because of the sharply limited sector distribution of redness. Whiteness of the immediately adjacent conjunctiva is unusual in other causes of a red eye.

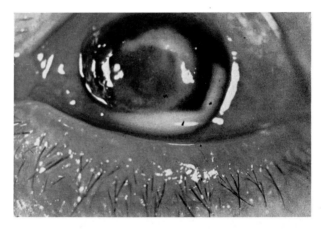

Fig. 14-10. A seemingly insignificant corneal foreign body was neglected in this eye. Bacterial infection ensued, resulting in rapid destruction of the central cornea. The inferior part of the anterior chamber is filled with leukocytes (hypopyon). Only 3 days elapsed between injury and this photograph.

A phlyctenule is similar to episcleritis except that a nodule is present in the center of the lesion.

Bacterial corneal ulcer. A variety of common bacteria (and also viruses and fungi) may gain entry to the cornea through an epithelial abrasion. Such an abrasion is the usual source of corneal infection, and for this reason routine use of topical antibiotics is advocated whenever significant corneal injury occurs. Depending on the virulence of the organism and patient resistance, there may develop a low-grade, self-limited, insignificant ulcer or a fulminating and destructive abscess that destroys the eye. *Pseudomonas* infec-

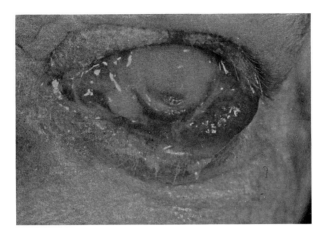

Fig. 14-11. Panophthalmitis refers to complete destruction of the eye by infection. It may often be prevented through prophylactic use of antibiotics in cases of corneal abrasion or a penetrating eye injury. Useful vision is never regained when intraocular infection reaches an advanced stage.

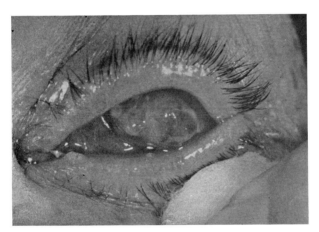

Fig. 14-12. Spontaneous rupture of the necrotic cornea represents the ultimate stage of destruction. Such loss of an eye can often be prevented through recognition of injury or infection and proper early care.

tions are among the worst. Bacterial corneal infections of any magnitude must be treated as emergencies, for only 24 hours delay may mean loss of the eye.

A dangerous corneal infection appears as a light gray infiltration surrounded by opalescent corneal edema (Fig. 14-10). Only the slightest crater is visible centrally. (After all, the whole cornea is less than 1 mm thick.) Pain is usually severe, and vision is definitely reduced. Angry, deep redness is present due to dilatation of both conjunctival and deeper vessels. Purulent discharge and crusting may be profuse. Some degree of iritis will always accompany severe corneal irritation of any type. Eventually, purulent discharge enters the eye, which shortly thereafter is converted to an abscess (Figs. 14-11 and 14-12).

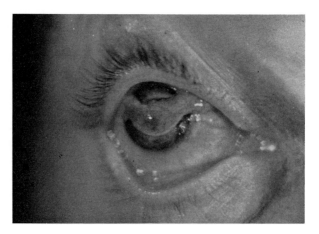

Fig. 14-13. A bridge flap of conjunctiva has been placed over a corneal ulcer in order to prevent its perforation. This procedure is only one of a variety of specialized techniques available for treatment of corneal disease. There should be no delay in seeking expert advice in the management of serious corneal infection.

Ophthalmologic consultation is important in the treatment of a severe corneal infection. Massive antibiotic therapy, both systemic and topical, should be started immediately. It is wise to take a culture and smear first (without causing delay in treatment) for a Gram stain, bacterial culture identification, and sensitivity studies. Should the infection not be controlled within the next 2 days, sensitivity studies may provide the clue to cure. Day and night, until the infection is controlled, appropriate topical antibiotics in an ointment vehicle should be instilled every 30 minutes. Warm, moist compresses should be used generously. Do not patch an infected eye. A very high dosage of systemic antibiotics selected for broad coverage of a variety of organisms should be started promptly. Atropine, 1%, three times daily, should be used for the accompanying iritis. Corticosteroids are *contraindicated,* for they reduce resistance and thereby enhance spread of the infection. Careful examination of the eye for injury is essential, and if any foreign bodies are present on or in the eye, they must be removed. Threatening perforation of the cornea may sometimes be helped by emergency surgery (Fig. 14-13). Delay has been fatal to many such eyes!

Acute glaucoma. A precipitous rise in pressure may occur in an eye predisposed to blockage of the outflow angle by the iris (see Fig. 15-6). This blockage occurs on a hereditary basis and is due to gradual forward displacement of the iris by the lens. Susceptible eyes often (not always) may be recognized by shallowness of the anterior chamber. The iris may seem to bulge forward until it almost touches the cornea. Sometimes the patient gives a history of preceding, less severe, similar attacks. Emotional upsets may precipitate an attack.

Acute glaucoma occurs within hours and is very obvious to the patient, who has extremely severe pain of the affected eye or the whole head. Vision becomes foggy, may pass through a stage where rainbow halos are seen around lights, and may be completely and permanently lost if proper treatment is delayed for several days. Most patients have reflex nausea and vomiting, which occasionally reaches such proportions that the dehydrated, pain-racked, semiconscious elderly patient is misdiagnosed as having a gastrointestinal disorder—a most regrettable error that may be avoided by a rapid look at the eyes of all such patients or by a good history. The pupil is always semidilated and does not react to light. Finger tension will be rock-hard. The cornea is steamy with edema.

A patient with acute glaucoma requires emergency referral.

Oral glycerol, 1 to 2 g/kg of body weight, is an effective agent in reducing intraocular pressure. If nausea precludes oral medication, a comparable dosage of intravenous mannitol will be even more effective. Pilocarpine, 1%, one drop every 5 minutes for three doses and then four times daily, will tend to open the occluded chamber angle. Pilocarpine should also be instilled in the other eye, because the predisposition to acute glaucoma is bilateral. A larger dose of pilocarpine is unlikely to be more effective and risks systemic toxicity. Timolol, 0.5%, one drop repeated in 10 minutes, will reduce the rate of aqueous formation and may be helpful.

Morphine will control pain and aid in producing miosis. Retrobulbar injections of lidocaine and hyaluronidase may be tried. As indicated above, the physician should never forget that both eyes are predisposed to this disease, and miotic therapy for the "good" eye is necessary also and should be started immediately after examination.

Should pressure be uncontrollable, emergency surgery becomes necessary and should be performed within 24 hours of the onset of the attack if at all possible. Even if the pressure is controlled medically, most patients should undergo surgery (see Fig. 15-7) within a few days.

A dramatic improvement in treatment of acute glaucoma resulted from the development of the ophthalmic laser. With this intense light flash, only milliseconds in duration, an effective iridectomy can be produced within minutes, requiring neither incision nor anesthetic.

Acute iritis. Inflammation of the iris is poorly understood except for the obvious cases due to injury or corneal irritation. The HLA-27 antigen is often present. A few patients are proved to have infection (tuberculosis, syphilitic, herpetic), but in many instances no cause is evident and an immunologic theory is proposed. Recurrences are frequent.

Before treatment, the affected pupil is characteristically smaller than the normal pupil (see Fig. 14-2). This sign is helpful. The normally clear iris markings become indistinct and fuzzy, which is appreciated better with oblique illumination. Sometimes, purulent exudate is recognizable in the lower part of the anterior chamber (hypopyon). Iritis is painful, and photophobia is usually marked. If the condition has been neglected for days or weeks, adhesions form between the pupil margins and the lens, and inflammatory membranes may permanently block the pupil (see Fig. 19-4). Interference to aqueous circulation may cause an acute secondary glaucoma. Destruction of ciliary processes may result in a shrunken, opaque, useless eye (see Fig. 19-5).

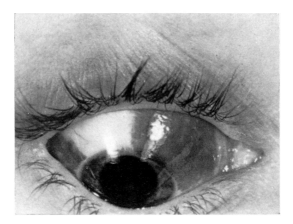

Fig. 14-14. Subconjunctival hemorrhages are more densely red than any other condition of the ocular surface. Initially the unaffected conjunctiva may be normally white, but with time, diffusion of hemoglobin may cause reddish or yellow discoloration of adjacent areas.

Less severe cases of iritis respond well to topical cycloplegics and corticosteroids. Minor traumatic iritis may require only several instillations of 2% homatropine. In more severe iritis with synechiae, the pupil should be dilated with frequent drops while the patient is in the office. Dilatation is maintained by 1% atropine and 10% phenylephrine, one drop of each three times a day. Topical corticosteroids every 2 hours during the day are desirable. Usually several weeks will elapse before the attack is cured. Some cases progress to serious damage despite topical and systemic care. Antibiotics are not helpful except in the few cases with a proved bacterial origin. A careful etiologic survey should be undertaken in difficult cases. I would recommend ophthalmologic consultation for any patient whose visual loss does not respond promptly to therapy or in whom obvious intraocular opacities can be seen.

Scleritis. Scleritis is similar to iritis except that the scleral coat is primarily involved. Movement of the eye is usually painful, and it is very red. Iritis usually accompanies scleritis. Treatment is similar to that for severe iritis.

Trauma. It is obvious that injury can cause ocular hyperemia and hemorrhage. This subject is discussed in a separate chapter (Chapter 13) but must be kept in mind in the differential diagnosis of the red eye (Fig. 14-14).

Defects of lid closure. Inadequate closure of the lids will result in drying, infection, and scarring of the cornea (see Fig. 5-4). This condition of exposure damage of the cornea, whether due to accident, serious disease such as meningitis, or surgical anesthesia, may occur in any unconscious patient. Bell's palsy, lid injury, or exophthalmos as in thyroid disease predisposes the patient to exposure damage of the cornea. Gray, opaque, irregular defects of the exposed cornea are evident, in addition to conjunctival redness, and may cause permanent loss of vision. This condition is easily preventable and

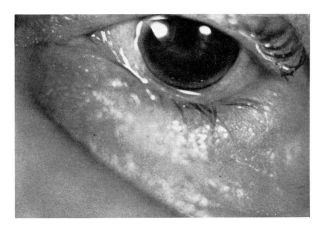

Fig. 14-15. Entropion, or turning inward of the lid margin, causes considerable redness and irritation of the eye through abrasion by the in-turned lashes. Occasionally a single aberrant lash causes a similar foreign body sensation and should be considered in the differential diagnosis of such symptoms.

should never occur—but does very often. Prevention consists of putting any type of eye ointment into the eye and closing the lids. Rarely, it is necessary to tape or suture the lids together. Care should be taken that any covering placed over the eye does *not* touch the cornea, or it may result in more damage than protection. Should exposure damage already have developed, the same measures should be taken and antibiotic ointment used to prevent infection.

In-turned lids (Fig. 14-15) or aberrant lashes may irritate the eye and cause considerable redness. Foreign body sensation is usually a prominent complaint in these patients. Treatment consists of removal of the offending lashes or surgical correction of the lid position.

Systemic causes. Redness of the eye may indicate systemic rather than purely local disease. Examples include the exophthalmic eye of thyroid disease (Fig. 14-16); conjunctivitis indicating that the eye was a portal of entry for tularemia (Fig. 14-17), syphilis (Fig. 14-18), gonorrhea (Fig. 14-19), or tuberculosis; the keratoconjunctivitis of acne rosacea; the extraocular muscle involvement of trichinosis; the chemotic eye occurring with primary or metastatic orbital tumor (Figs. 14-20 and 14-21); orbital cellulitis (see Fig. 13-12) secondary to ethmoid sinusitis or associated with cavernous sinus thrombosis; corneal breakdown (keratomalacia) caused by avitaminosis A (Fig. 14-22); iritis associated with brucellosis or toxoplasmosis; mucous membrane syndromes such as Stevens-Johnson disease (Fig. 14-23) or pemphigus; phlyctenular or intraocular disease associated with general tuberculous infection; the bleary red eye of chronic alcoholism; allergies to penicillin and other drugs (Fig. 14-24); and many types of viral infections. Discussion and treatment of these systemic diseases are not within the scope of this chapter; however, it is

Text continued on p. 274.

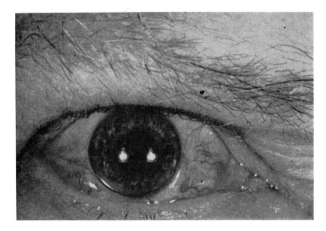

Fig. 14-16. Thyroid disease may be suggested by a reddened, staring eye with widened palpebral apertures or by retraction of the upper lid. Sometimes the eye symptoms are quite pronounced, although no other obvious manifestations of hyperthyroidism are present.

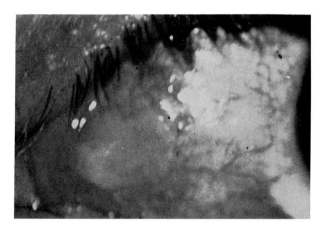

Fig. 14-17. The ''oculoglandular'' syndrome of preauricular adenopathy associated with a nodular, ulcerative conjunctivitis indicates infection caused by granuloma-producing organisms (such as tuberculosis, tularemia, lymphogranuloma venereum, or syphilis) or perhaps some types of viruses or fungi. Such an elevated, ulcerated nodule is therefore ordinarily indicative of systemic disease rather than simply a conjunctivitis.

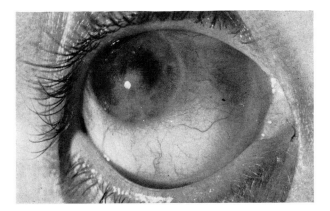

Fig. 14-18. Interstitial keratitis, a late manifestation of congenital syphilis, produces a typical vascularized corneal scar. The slit-lamp appearance is almost pathognomonic of a syphilitic origin. This photograph also shows the limbal redness of serious eye disease.

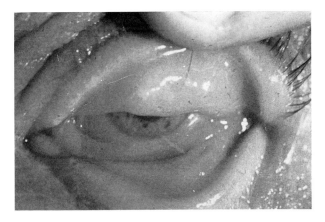

Fig. 14-19. An exceptionally severe and destructive conjunctivitis is caused by gonorrhea. The gonococcus is one of the few pyogenic bacteria capable of attacking an intact corneal epithelium. Without prompt antibiotic treatment, gonorrheal conjunctivitis ordinarily results in serious corneal scarring. This highly contagious disease may easily be transmitted to the eyes of physicians and nurses by unwashed fingers. Before antibiotics were discovered, the Credé method of 1% silver nitrate instillation into the eyes of newborn infants was developed to destroy gonococci acquired during delivery.

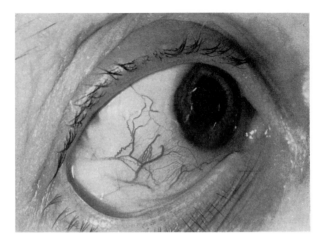

Fig. 14-20. Dilated large vessels in one sector of an otherwise white eye may signify increased blood flow to a malignant tumor. Within the inferior temporal anterior portion of this eye is a malignant melanoma.

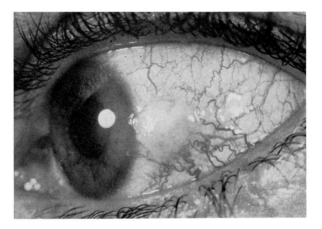

Fig. 14-21. Primary carcinoma of the conjunctiva causes a persistent redness of the involved area with obvious dilatation of surrounding vessels. Such carcinomas are slightly elevated, fleshy, translucent, pinkish lesions. At an early stage, local excision is successful, with retention of a perfectly normal eye. Prompt diagnosis is therefore of great value.

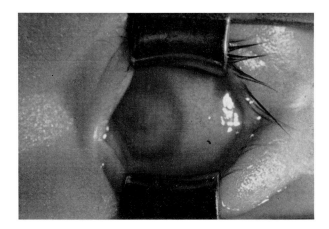

Fig. 14-22. Keratomalacia, the result of vitamin A deficiency, has destroyed the cornea of this 2-month-old child. Vitamin A therapy will reverse earlier stages of this process, recognizable through dryness of the conjunctiva and cornea and loss of corneal luster and transparency.

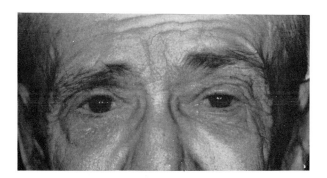

Fig. 14-23. Although this man was known to be allergic to sulfonamides, he was given sulfa therapy for a urinary tract infection. A severe exfoliative dermatitis ensued, as well as severe conjunctival involvement. A year afterward (at the time of this photograph) he still showed redness and irritation of the eyes and suffered severe ocular discomfort. Early treatment with topical corticosteroids sometimes seems to prevent prolonged eye disability.

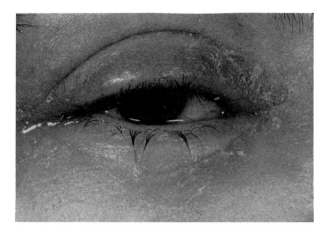

Fig. 14-24. This atropine sensitization shows the classic features of ocular drug allergy. The thin lid skin becomes edematous and thickened with surface maceration and crusting. Itching is pronounced. Surprisingly, redness and irritation are usually confined to the lids and do not extend to the adjacent parts of the face.

evident that appropriate ocular antibiotic, corticosteroid, lubricant, or other therapy will help many persons with red eyes.

Contact lenses. With great frequency, contact lens wearers will develop red eyes. Minimal redness and irritation is almost physiologic with the wearing of a contact lens and is often accepted without complaint just as swimmers accept the redness caused by chlorine in the pool water. However, the acute development of pain and redness in a contact lens wearer cannot be neglected. This may be due to problems in the lens itself (chipped edges, roughened surfaces due to deposited material, faulty fitting), accidents in lens manipulation (scratching the cornea with the edge of the lens or the inserting finger), the solutions used (preservative irritation, contamination with bacteria and fungi, allergy), or anoxic damage to the cornea (wearing the lens for too long a time period, too tight a fit, sleeping with an oxygen-impermeable lens on the cornea).

Most contact lens wearers have learned that the proper management for almost all these problems is to stop wearing the lens and consult the lens fitter. Problems may arise if the patient cannot see without the contact lens and therefore wears it despite redness and discomfort. Neither the patient nor the nonmedical fitter may be fully aware of the infrequent but serious infections that can arise from the combination of a corneal abrasion and microorganisms.

Your management of an acutely red and painful eye associated with contact lens wearing should be threefold. First, be sure that no other obvious cause of the condition is present. Contact lens wearers can get foreign bodies in the eye, suffer from acute glaucoma, or have any other red eye cause that would affect anyone else. Second, remove the contact lens, and leave it out until the redness has disappeared and the lens and solutions have been determined to be harmless. Third, never overlook the possibility of corneal infection, which can continue its devastating course even if the contact lens is removed. Proper and prompt antibiotic therapy is urgently necessary for corneal infection. Signs of such infection may include purulent discharge, ulceration or opacity of the cornea, reduced vision, small pupil (associated iritis), or hypopyon. Limbal redness, one of the eight danger signals, is commonly present from contact lens irritation and under such circumstances does not by itself necessarily indicate an imminent serious problem. Conversely, do not ignore contact lens irritation so severe as to cause limbal redness, and look carefully for any evidence of corneal damage. Actually, it is difficult to evaluate such a cornea adequately without a slit-lamp microscope.

SUMMARY

Many causes of a red eye have been described, together with their treatment. It is evident that accurate diagnosis is an absolute prerequisite to therapy. Specific, sight-saving treatments exist for many of these diseases. In some cases therapy must be started without delay. Confusion in diagnosis and treatment will destroy eyes; for example, erroneous treatment of acute glaucoma with atropine will lead to destruction of the eye. Delay in recognition of the serious causes of a red eye will also cause blindness and can be avoided by checking all red eyes against the eight-point list of *visual loss, pain, opacities, irregularities of the pupil, distribution of redness, alterations in pressure, history,* and *failure to respond to therapy*.

chapter 15   Glaucoma

Glaucoma designates eye disease characterized by increased intraocular pressure. It is of extreme importance because of its relatively high incidence, because glaucomatous visual loss is permanent, and because proper early therapy prevents visual damage. Adequate glaucoma supervision requires a specialist.

Glaucoma is present in about 2% of persons over 40 years of age, an incidence similar to that of diabetes. It is estimated that there are 800,000 cases of undiscovered glaucoma in the United States today, and 12% of all blindness is caused by glaucoma.

Glaucoma is due to obstruction of the trabecular and canal of Schlemm mechanism of outflow in the angle of the anterior chamber. Many causes and types of obstruction exist, but the most common is the genetic loss of trabecular permeability, resulting in open-angle glaucoma.

OPEN-ANGLE GLAUCOMA

By far the most common type of glaucoma is open-angle glaucoma. This disease has aptly been termed "the thief in the night," because without warning it gradually and irreversibly destroys vision. Both eyes are usually affected. It is usually painless or at most causes slight occasional aching of the eyes. Complete blindness can occur with *never any acute attack*. The elevated intraocular pressure causes slow nutritional damage, producing the characteristic arcuate scotomas that go unrecognized until they finally encroach on central vision. Advanced stages do not respond well to medical or surgical therapy and often progress to blindness, whereas early stages are usually controlled with medical therapy.

Diagnosis. Discovery of open-angle glaucoma is therefore *too late* when made by the patient's complaints. Early diagnosis and preservation of vision is possible only by routine screening examinations. Glaucoma should be especially strongly suspected under the following circumstances:

1. If the patient is over 40 years of age
2. If there is a family history of serious visual loss (glaucoma is hereditary)
3. If the corneal diameter is 10 mm or less (average normal is 12 mm)
4. If the anterior chamber is shallow and the iris seems to bow forward toward the cornea (check with flashlight illumination from the side)
5. If frequent, unsatisfactory changing of glasses suggests the possibility of eye disease
6. If there is unexplained aching around the eyes

Coexistence of age over 40 years and any other one of the factors just listed should strongly suggest the desirability of referral to an ophthalmologist. Tonometric measurement of intraocular pressure is required for accurate diagnosis. This is done routinely by most ophthalmologists in the examination of elderly patients. The intraocular pressure in open-angle glaucoma is usually *not* elevated enough to permit detection by finger tension. Finger tension is easily confused with compressibility of orbital tissues and even when done by an expert may be in error by more than 10 mm Hg.

Open-angle glaucoma is caused by gradually increasing resistance to the outflow of aqueous due to aging changes in the angle of the anterior chamber. The anatomic predisposition to glaucoma is genetically transmitted, and it is therefore desirable to include inquiry about familial blindness in the routine family history. A concrete example of the value of genetic counseling is provided by the pedigree illustrated in Fig. 15-1. Patients III 6, 8, 9, 11, and 13 became completely blind from glaucoma. Through genetic search, patients IV 13, 23, 27, and 35 were detected as having glaucoma and were placed under therapy early in the course of the disease. These patients were followed for years without evidence of visual loss. By contrast, patients IV 10 and 24 refused to submit to examination. Both suffered advanced visual loss and then began treatment—too late.

Certain anatomic features markedly predispose their possessors to glaucoma. However, the great majority of patients with open-angle glaucoma do *not* show grossly visible changes of any sort. Nevertheless, it is well known that eyes with a reduced corneal diameter or shallow anterior chamber have a great disposition to the development of glaucoma.

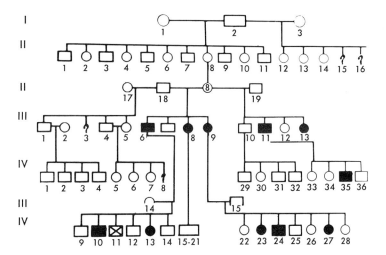

Fig. 15-1. Familial transmission of glaucoma is recorded in this pedigree. As described in the text, genetic knowledge permitted early detection of glaucoma and prevention of visual loss in several of these patients. (From Havener, W.H. Published with permission from The American Journal of Ophthalmology **40**:828-831, 1955. Copyright by The Ophthalmic Publishing Company.)

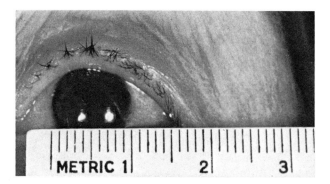

Fig. 15-2. This patient with glaucoma had a 10 mm corneal diameter bilaterally (normal, 12 mm). Persons with small eyes are markedly predisposed to develop glaucoma and should have tonometry performed annually to detect pressure elevation before serious damage occurs.

The normal adult corneal diameter is 12 mm. Inadequate development of the anterior segment of the eye, including the aqueous outflow mechanism, betrays itself by a small corneal diameter (Fig. 15-2), 10 mm or even less. This small cornea is present throughout the patient's life but ordinarily does not cause elevation of pressure until degenerative changes after the age of 40 years further embarrass aqueous outflow. No matter at what age these patients with small corneas are seen, it is wise to advise them that ophthalmologic consultation may avert serious eye damage.

Shallowness of the anterior chamber refers to a reduced distance between the cornea and the iris. This characteristic is not seen in early life and becomes most pronounced in old age. It is partially caused by an increase in size of the lens, which pushes the iris into a forward position, thereby embarrassing outflow. The forward bulging of the iris may easily be recognized as a domelike protrusion. Oblique illumination will cast a characteristic crescent shadow on the peripheral iris, as illustrated in Fig. 15-3.

Sometimes it is possible to make a relatively early diagnosis of glaucoma through suspicion of vague symptoms. Prominent among this group are the patients who have gotten two or three pairs of unsatisfactory glasses within a short period of time. Such a history often means simply that the patient suffers from eye disease rather than from refractive error. (Psychoneurosis is, unfortunately, another cause for such complaints. Many patients with glaucoma are tense, nervous individuals and may at first be misdiagnosed as having a functional disorder.) Another group of patients may have vague ocular aching or discomfort, sometimes referred to the occipital region. Glaucoma should be considered as a possible cause of such unexplained discomfort in the older patient.

Regrettably, the textbook emphasis on glaucoma suggests that it should be detected by findings such as the following:

1. Reduced visual acuity uncorrectable with glasses
2. Visual field loss

Normally deep anterior chamber

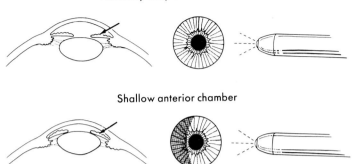

Shallow anterior chamber

Fig. 15-3. Shallowness of the anterior chamber occurs when lens growth displaces the iris forward toward the cornea (or if a penetrating wound permits aqueous loss). Oblique illumination casts a crescentic shadow on the far portion of the iris, as illustrated. This sign is easily observed and indicates a pronounced predisposition to develop angle-closure glaucoma. A shallow anterior chamber is also present in glaucoma caused by pupillary block.

3. Cupping and atrophy of the disc as recognized with the ophthalmoscope (see Plate 26) (Refer to the description of the physiologic cup in Chapters 5 and 8. Recognition of a C/D ratio greater than 0.5 is one of the most effective screening criteria for glaucoma.)

4. Markedly elevated pressure, detectable through finger tension estimation

Undeniably, the diagnosis can be made under these circumstances, but it is *too late!* Such a patient will already have sustained some irreversible eye damage. For maximum benefit to the patient, open-angle glaucoma should be discovered by suspicion of the disease in the group over 40 years of age—suspicion that is increased by a family history of eye disease, by anatomic changes such as a decreased corneal diameter and shallow anterior chamber, or by vague symptoms of discomfort that may lead to repeated unsatisfactory refraction checks. Confirmation of the early diagnosis is possible only though tonometry (Fig. 15-4).

Ideally, tonometric screening should be done by every physician. This will never happen, because of the demands of time and because of the great reluctance of many physicians to manipulate instruments about the eye. The most practical solution is referral of suspected patients to an ophthalmologist. Referral, of course, costs the patient money, and the referring physician is loath to incur this expense merely because of a suspicion. Bear in mind, however, that presbyopic symptoms manifest themselves in this age group. For maximum visual efficiency, most people require about three changes of glasses between the ages of 40 and 55 years. If these lenses are prescribed by an ophthalmologist, the patient will simultaneously receive careful examination of his eyes for disease, including screening for glaucoma.

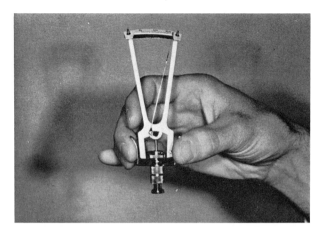

Fig. 15-4. A tonometer is necessary for accurate measurement of intraocular pressure. It is held as shown and gently rested on the anesthetized cornea. This examination is simple, nontraumatic, and sight-saving.

With great frequency, both ocular and systemic diseases manifest themselves through visual disturbances and eye fatigue. The patient has no way to differentiate these symptoms from those of refractive error. The ophthalmologist can diagnose the true nature of the patient's difficulty and initiate proper and immediate treatment, frequently avoiding the prescription of unnecessary spectacles.

Cup/disc ratio. You probably look at the optic discs as a part of all your routine physical examinations. Why? What are you looking for?

Disc edema is the usual answer to the above question. Disc edema is certainly a finding of enormous significance and should be looked for in all patients complaining of headache, neurologic symptoms, recent head injury, severe hypertension, or recently reduced visual acuity. Still, you will not see very many patients with disc edema.

Disc atrophy is another answer. This disc pallor may be caused by any disorder that can damage the optic nerve. The color of the disc should be carefully observed in every patient, especially if reduced visual acuity is present. Again, you will not see very many white discs.

Cup/disc ratio is the best answer. As you look at each disc in every patient, you should note and then record its C/D ratio. This record is important because an increase in the ratio in subsequent years means death of many nerve fibers has occurred. Only 5% of normal patients will have a C/D greater than 0.5. An increasing C/D ratio is characteristic of glaucomatous nerve damage. Eyes with a C/D greater than 0.5 should be evaluated by tonometry. If other suspicious findings are present, perimetry is also indicated. Normal eyes have bilaterally similar C/D ratios. A difference between the two eyes of 0.2 or more is highly suspicious of glaucoma. Refer to Plate 29 for illustrations of C/D ratios of 0.2 *(A)*, 0.3 *(B)*, 0.5 *(C)*. 0.6 *(D)*, 0.8 *(E)*, and 0.9 *(F)*. Another feature of glaucomatous cups is that the vertical diameter is longer than the horizontal one. The most certain feature of a glaucomatous cup is that its margin reaches the edge of the disc; that is, the disc does not have a rim of normal pink tissue throughout its entire circumference (see Figs. 8-8 and 8-10).

Please, when you use the ophthalmoscope, always consciously measure the C/D ratio. If it is greater than 0.5 or differs between the two eyes by 0.2 or more, consider the patient to be a glaucoma suspect.

Therapy. In most patients simply the instillation of miotic drops several times daily will control pressure adequately. Various combinations and concentrations of timolol, pilocarpine, eserine, carbachol, and echothiophate iodide are used, depending on the patient's response. Just as no given dose of insulin can be predicted in advance for a patient with diabetes, so also the medical requirements of a patient with glaucoma are subject to regulation by clinical trial. Glaucoma is *not* cured by medications but is controlled only so long as therapy is maintained. The patient with glaucoma ordinarily requires lifetime treatment. During vacations and hospitalizations, as well as during everyday life, miotic drops must not be neglected.

Timolol, epinephrine, and carbonic anhydrase inhibitors act by decreasing the rate of formation of aqueous humor. All the miotic drugs act by increasing the rate at which aqueous traverses the trabecular meshwork, thereby escaping from the eye.

Should systemic atropinization be necessary, as for preoperative medication or for treatment of peptic ulcer, the ocular effect of belladonna drugs may be effectively counteracted by increasing the frequency or concentration of therapeutic drops. There is no relation between systemic arterial hypertension and ocular hypertension.

Whether a case of glaucoma is being adequately controlled is determined by regular checks of visual acuity and intraocular pressure, by tonometry and tonography, by perimetry and ophthalmoscopy, and with the aid of gonioscopy and other specialized techniques. These same examinations are also necessary in the initial evaluation of a patient before the diagnosis of glaucoma is made. Obviously, proper management also requires knowledge of the pharmacologic properties of the various drugs and the ability to determine when or if surgery is indicated. Treatment of glaucoma is a great deal more complicated than simply prescribing 2% pilocarpine three times a day and should *not* be attempted without adequate experience.

Since the site of outflow resistance in open-angle glaucoma is in the trabecular meshwork, iridectomy (as performed for acute glaucoma) is not a useful operation. If medical control of open-angle glaucoma is inadequate, a filtering type of operation must be done. Filtering operations create a fistula between the anterior chamber and the subconjunctival spaces, thereby permitting aqueous humor outflow to bypass the trabecular block. Filtering operations include trabeculectomy, iridencleisis, and trephining. Trabeculectomy is performed by dissecting up a 5 mm flap of sclera overlying the limbus. Beneath this flap the trabecular meshwork is excised, creating an opening into the anterior chamber. The dissected flap is then loosely apposed to its normal position with sutures and covered with

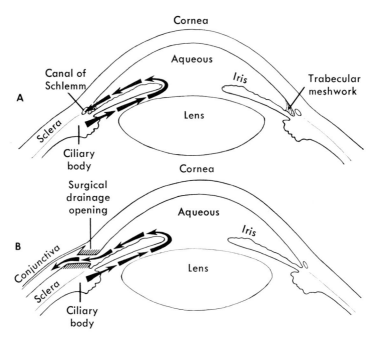

Fig. 15-5. A, Originating from the ciliary processes, the aqueous flows through the pupil into the anterior chamber and normally leaves the eye via the canal of Schlemm. **B,** In glaucoma, the normal aqueous outflow is blocked. The purpose of glaucoma surgery is to create a new channel through which aqueous can leave the eye.

the conjunctiva. In iridencleisis, a wick of iris is incarcerated in the scleral incision with the intent to prevent its closure. In a trephine operation, a 1.5 mm button of sclera is excised, thereby creating a tunnel for aqueous outflow (Fig. 15-5). Most persons with open-angle glaucoma do not require surgery.

Laser trabeculoplasty is a very effective new procedure for open-angle glaucoma inadeqately controlled by medical therapy. This consists of placing 50 to 80 laser burns around the circumference of the trabecular meshwork. The laser heat shrinks the collagen, thereby reducing the circumference and diameter of the trabecular circle. The resulting inward pull opens the trabecular meshwork and enhances aqueous outflow from the eye. In most cases, medical therapy is still necessary following laser trabeculoplasty. However, pressure will be controlled in as many as 90% of cases, thereby avoiding the more dangerous filtering operations.

Summary. Two percent of people over 40 years of age are estimated to have open-angle glaucoma. This is an insidious disease that causes serious ocular damage before the patient is aware of his disability. It should be diagnosed by suspicion in patients over 40 years of age, especially if there is a family history of eye disease, if structural defects such

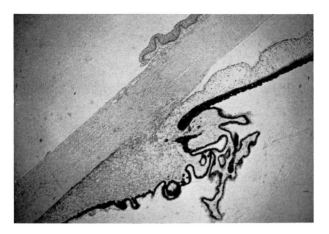

Fig. 15-6. Acute glaucoma is entirely different from chronic glaucoma in that the peripheral iris is the cause of blockage of aqueous flow. In this section of an eye with acute glaucoma, the base of the iris completely occludes the filtration angle and prevents aqueous from leaving the eye. In open-angle glaucoma the angle is open, the iris does not touch the cornea, and the outflow obstruction is within the trabecular spaces themselves.

as a small cornea or a shallow interior chamber are present (most persons do *not* show these structural changes), or if there are vague ocular symptoms.

Since C/D ratios greater than 0.5 occur in only 5% of normal individuals and are characteristic of glaucomatous optic atrophy, detection of such a defect is an important consideration during routine ophthalmoscopic examination of the optic disc.

Confirmation of the early diagnosis must be made by tonometry. It is best done as routine screening by the ophthalmologist during his examination of the presbyopic patient with suspected glaucoma.

ACUTE GLAUCOMA (CLOSED ANGLE)

Acute glaucoma is one of the most dramatic and rapidly destructive diseases of the eye. It characteristically produces severe pain, at first localized to the eye but later radiating to any part of the head. Nausea and vomiting are common and sometimes mislead the patient and physician into believing that the primary complaint is abdominal. Corneal edema causes vision to become blurred. The many tiny droplets in the edematous cornea disperse light into its spectral components and result in the rainbow-colored halos seen around lights. Untreated, a severe attack of acute glaucoma may cause permanent blindness within a few days.

Acute glaucoma can occur only in a structurally predisposed eye. In such an eye the processes of aging result in a progressive narrowing of the peripheral angle of the anterior chamber. Ultimately the iris approaches so closely to the trabecular structures that slight dilatation of the pupil caused by darkness, excitement, or a mydriatic results in apposition of the iris to the filtration spaces, with complete block of the aqueous outflow mechanism (Fig. 15-6). Aqueous secretion continues, and intraocular pressure rises rapidly. The extreme hardness of such an eye can easily be recognized by finger tension estimation. Death of the nerve fibers results when the intraocular pressure reaches such heights that the central retinal artery can no longer maintain circulation.

Acute glaucoma is a relatively rare disease, and fear of its existence should not deter the physician from using dilating drops as a valuable aid in diagnosis. It is, however, unwise to dilate the pupil of a patient who is known to have glaucoma, who has elevated finger pressure, or who has recognizably shallow anterior chambers.

Subacute angle-closure glaucoma refers to a series of relatively mild attacks of acute glaucoma occurring early in the course of the disease. They spontaneously subside, usually when the patient goes to sleep. (The pupils become miotic during sleep.) Recurrent attacks of severe ocular pain in an adult certainly deserve careful evaluation for the presence of glaucoma.

Therapy of acute angle-closure glaucoma is surgical and consists of excision of a portion of the peripheral iris (Fig. 15-7). Such an iridectomy provides an opening through which aqueous can escape and is an effective and permanent cure. Most ophthalmologists recommend surgery for any eye that has had an attack of acute glaucoma, even if emergency medical therapy controls the pressure. Such persons are likely to suffer another attack and often lose a great deal of vision through only a few hours of delay. Indeed, prophylactic surgery on the fellow eye is often advised, because this disease is bilateral.

The iridectomy may also be made with a laser beam. This has the advantages of much

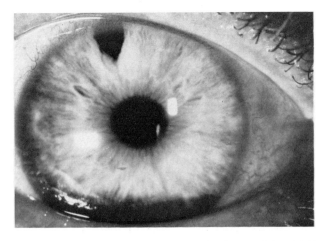

Fig. 15-7. The dark spot on the upper portion of the iris is a peripheral iridectomy. Surgical treatment of acute glaucoma consists of removal of part of the iris periphery, thereby eliminating the cause of blockage of the trabecular spaces.

greater safety and ease of performance. Since no surgical incision is necessary, the dangers of hemorrhage and infection are almost nonexistent. No anesthetic is required, not even local anesthetic drops. The light beam traverses the transparent cornea and burns a tiny hole through the opaque iris.

Osmotic therapy (glycerol, 1 to 2 g/kg of body weight, orally) combined with miotic therapy (1% pilocarpine, one drop every 5 minutes for three doses and then one drop four times daily) and aqueous secretory inhibitors (0.5% timolol, one drop; acetazolamide, 250 mg) will often reduce the pressure of acute glaucoma. (Do not use the pilocarpine more often; it will cause systemic parasympathomimetic poisoning.) If this treatment is successful, it is best to defer surgery for a day or so until the eye is less inflamed. Should intraocular pressure remain high, emergency surgery is urgently indicated. The general physician who encounters a person with acute glaucoma should administer such treatment and immediately refer the patient, not waiting to see whether the pressure drops. Morphine will relieve pain and aid in producing miosis. Delay is disastrous. If recognized as such, precipitation of an attack of acute glaucoma through use of mydriatics is beneficial to the patient, for it results in definitive treatment at an optimal early stage. Such an occurrence should therefore be considered to be a provocative test and not an accident.

CONGENITAL GLAUCOMA

Because of abnormal development of the filtration angle, increased intraocular pressure may be present at birth or develop within the first few months of life. Congenital glaucoma is extremely rare, but it is mentioned because blindness (inevitable if untreated) can be prevented by early recognition and surgery. The two signs that usually lead to diagnosis are cloudiness of the cornea (Fig. 15-8) and an increased corneal diameter (Fig. 15-9). Infants with congenital glaucoma have marked photophobia and may be mistakenly thought to have an ocular inflammation.

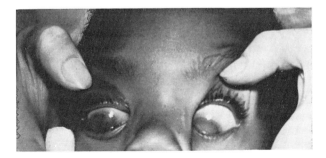

Fig. 15-8. This advanced stage of congenital glaucoma has produced dense blue-gray corneal opacities. Surgical care is urgently indicated.

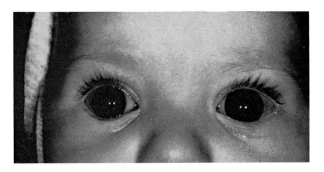

Fig. 15-9. Congenital glaucoma has caused stretching of this infant's corneas until they are obviously enlarged. This appearance of an infant's eyes should cause great concern and requires prompt, careful, thorough examination. Do not share the parents' admiration of the "pretty big blue eyes."

SECONDARY GLAUCOMA

Secondary glaucoma refers to a rise in intraocular pressure due to some other ocular disorder. This increased pressure occurs because of blockage of the normal channels of aqueous outflow.

The presence of secondary glaucoma is always of serious significance because it indicates that the underlying disease process is of considerable magnitude and because it may damage the optic nerve. Periodic measurement of intraocular pressure is therefore done in the management of eye diseases that are often found to produce secondary glaucoma.

Predisposing conditions

Some of the conditions resulting in secondary glaucoma are iridocyclitis, trauma, severe diabetic changes, total occlusion of the central retinal vein, intraocular tumors, dislocation of the lens, operative complications, and encephalotrigeminal angioma.

Iridocyclitis. Inflammation of the iris may result in adhesions between the pupil margin and the lens (posterior synechiae), thereby blocking the normal flow of aqueous through the pupil. Pupillary block results in a bulging forward of the iris (iris bombé), which is readily recognized by the use of oblique illumination. Oblique illumination of an iris bombé produces the crescent-shaped shadow characteristic of a shallow anterior chamber (see Fig. 15-3). The adhesions may themselves be visible and sometimes are extensive enough to form a dense membrane entirely covering the pupil and destroying sight.

Inflammatory adhesions may also develop between the iris periphery and the cornea (peripheral anterior synechiae). If extensive enough, these adhesions will prevent aqueous access to the angle of the anterior chamber, trabecular spaces, and canal of Schlemm, resulting in secondary glaucoma. The complication of secondary glaucoma in iridocyclitis indicates prompt consultation with an ophthalmologist. Intensive cycloplegic, corticosteroid, and timolol or acetazolamide therapy will usually control pressure; if not, filtering surgery may be necessary.

Trauma. Injury may cause outpourings of fibrin and blood, which are deposited on the angle structures and block aqueous outflow. Particular hazard exists if secondary glaucoma develops when the anterior chamber is filled with blood. Under these conditions hematogenous pigment may be forced into the cornea, resulting in corneal blood staining. Blood staining of the cornea may develop within a few days, appearing as a dense gray corneal infiltration that reduces vision to light perception and usually requires years to clear enough to permit useful vision. For this reason and because of the existence of many other complications, it is wise to seek ophthalmologic consultation in management of traumatic intraocular hemorrhage of any magnitude.

Severe diabetic changes. Severe diabetic changes within the eye are characterized by connective tissue proliferation and neovascularization. Occurring on the retina, this condition is termed retinitis proliferans; occurring on the iris, it is termed rubeosis iridis. This vascular and connective tissue may completely occlude the outflow angle, producing an intractable form of secondary glaucoma. Frequently, spontaneous bleeding occurs from the contraction of newly formed connective tissue. Such cases are termed neovascular glaucoma. Blindness and recurrent, severe pain commonly result. Surgery is sometimes helpful.

Rubeosis iridis is recognized by the presence of dilated vessels on the iris surface. Such vessels are sometimes grossly visible but more often require the magnification of a slit lamp. Hemorrhage from these thin vessels commonly settles into the inferior part of the anterior chamber (hyphema). Diabetes and total occlusion of the central retinal vein are the common causes of rubeosis iridis. Such eyes will show the limbal distribution of redness that indicates serious eye disease.

Total occlusion of the central retinal vein. Total occlusion of the central retinal vein (see Plate 7) causes neovascularization and connective tissue proliferation closely resembling diabetic retinopathy except that it is more uniformly distributed throughout the retina rather than being concentrated posteriorly as in diabetes. In about one third of persons with total venous occlusion, after a period of some months there develops blockage of the outflow angle through membrane formation similar to that of diabetic rubeosis iridis. These secondary glaucomas are intractable. Partial venous occlusions affecting one or more branches of the central retinal vein are a great deal more common than total venous occlusion. Partial occlusions almost never cause secondary glaucoma.

Intraocular tumors. Intraocular tumors can cause monocular glaucoma. Approximately 5% of eyes enucleated for monocular blindness, pain, and degeneration are found to contain malignant melanoma. This tumor may be unrecognized clinically because of cataract, corneal scar, or vitreous opacities that prevent ophthalmoscopic examination of the interior of the eye. Metastatic tumors, advanced retinoblastomas, hemangiomas, and other tumors may also cause secondary glaucoma.

Dislocation of the lens. Dislocation of the lens may cause mechanical occlusion of the

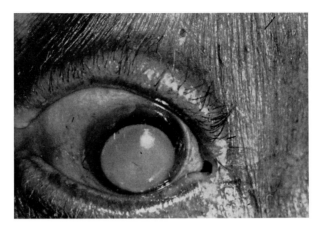

Fig. 15-10. Dislocation of this cataractous lens into the anterior chamber caused secondary glaucoma through blockage of the pupil.

pupil, thereby preventing aqueous flow. Lens dislocation may be caused by trauma and occurs spontaneously in several developmental and degenerative syndromes. (Marfan's syndrome is the most common.) Secondary glaucoma is particularly likely to occur if the lens enters the anterior chamber (Fig. 15-10). In this position the lens is readily seen by simple inspection, especially if it is cataractous. Dislocation of a perfectly clear lens may be overlooked unless examination is careful and aided by a bright flashlight. (Bright, diffuse room illumination is not nearly as revealing as oblique, moving flashlight illumination.) Tremulousness of the iris is diagnostic of loss of the normal support of the lens and is seen in posterior dislocation or absence of the lens. It is readily observed after cataract extraction. Small movements of the aphakic eye result in easily visible undulating movements of the iris.

Operative complications. Operative complications such as wound leakage, hemorrhage, or inflammation predispose the eye to secondary glaucoma. Similar problems are often encountered with penetrating eye injuries. Contusion angle glaucoma is due to trabecular damage.

Facial angioma. Unilateral glaucoma frequently accompanies the hemifacial angioma of Sturge-Weber syndrome. Since advanced glaucomatous optic atrophy may occur as soon as the second decade of life, tonometric measurement of these patients should be done at least every few years after the age of 10 years.

Summary. A variety of intraocular diseases may produce secondary glaucoma. When they do so, they obviously exist in a serious degree and require prompt, skilled attention for their own sake and for the prevention of glaucomatous damage to the eye. Detection of the complication of secondary glaucoma is the responsibility of the physician treating these eye diseases. Knowledge that secondary glaucoma commonly occurs indicates periodic measurement of intraocular pressure during the course of such eye diseases.

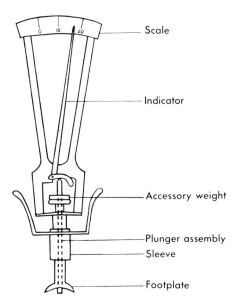

- Scale
- Indicator
- Accessory weight
- Plunger assembly
- Sleeve
- Footplate

Fig. 15-11. Schiøtz tonometer. This diagram of tonometer construction illustrates how the sleeve by which it is held simply maintains the tonometer erect, neither lifting nor pressing down. The full weight of the tonometer rests on the cornea. The plunger slides freely within the tonometer and indents the cornea a variable degree, depending on the intraocular pressure.

TONOMETRY

Measurement of intraocular pressure is an easy and safe procedure that requires only a few minutes of time. The technique consists simply of resting a tonometer vertically on an anesthetized cornea and observing the scale reading (Fig. 15-11).

Technique. As usual, description of the technique takes considerably longer than the procedure itself. This description considers in detail tonometry technique, interpretation, instructions to the patient, indications for tonometry, contraindications to tonometry, and maintenance of the tonometer. A few minutes of demonstration by an ophthalmologist will make tonometry seem simple.

1. The patient must keep his head facing straight upward, either by leaning his head back over the chair or by lying flat on a couch.
2. The eyes are anesthetized by instillation of one drop of 0.5% proparacaine. (Tetracaine burns slightly, whereas proparacaine feels like a drop of plain water.) Anesthesia is adequate in 1 minute. It is helpful to instill an additional drop in the eyes of apprehensive patients and wait another minute to be absolutely certain of good anesthesia.
3. During the waiting period, tonometer accuracy should be checked on the metal test

block, on which the scale reading should be exactly zero. The indicator arm must swing freely, without sticking. Proper weights must be in place (see step 7).

4. With *both* eyes open, the patient should look exactly vertically. Vertical gaze is aided by having him look at a spot on the ceiling directly above his head. He must hold his eyes steady and avoid squeezing his lids.

5. The physician gently separates the lids with his thumb and forefinger applied to the upper and lower orbital rims. If pressure is exerted into the orbit, a falsely high reading will register.

6. The sterile tonometer footplate is placed gently on the center of the cornea in a perpendicular position. Placement in this position must be accurate. Tilting or eccentric positions readily produce erroneous readings. If the patient sees the tonometer approaching, he will tend to blink. This problem may be avoided by bringing the tonometer in from the side, so close that the patient cannot focus clearly on it. The footplate should not be scuffed from side to side on the cornea, because scuffing may cause abrasions. Resting the fourth and fifth fingers on the patient's forehead will help steady the physician's hand. The tonometer sleeve, which is the part held, slides freely up and down for a certain distance on the shaft of the tonometer. The sleeve serves simply to balance the tonometer and should be held in midposition, neither lifting nor pressing down the tonometer. The tonometer is calibrated to measure intraocular pressure when its own weight is resting on the eye.

7. The scale reading is read off and checked against the table (Table 10). The table transposes the scale readings to millimeters of mercury. You will note that the tonometer may be used with three weights (5.5, 7.5, and 10 g), which give different readings on the table. The tonometer plunger assembly alone weighs 5.5 g. Accessory weights are provided to slip on the plunger shaft and are marked by the total weight of the plunger assembly when they are added (7.5 and 10 g). The most useful weight is 7.5 g, and it may be left on the tonometer constantly during all screening examinations. Measurement of pressure in very soft eyes is more accurate with the 5.5 g weights; in hard eyes, with the 10 g weight.

8. The pressure of the second eye is recorded in the same fashion.

9. Standard recording is as follows:

$$\text{TT} \Big\langle \begin{array}{c} \overset{\text{7.5 g}}{20} \\ 18 \end{array}$$

TT is the abbreviation for tonometer tension. By custom, the record of the right eye is always above and that of the left eye always below. If the examiner customarily uses different weights from time to time, the weight used should be recorded. If the 7.5 g weight is always used in screening examination, this figure may be omitted.

Interpretation. Pressures of 24 mm Hg or higher suggest the possibility of glaucoma.

Table 10. Calibration scale for Schiotz tonometers (1955)

Tonometer reading	5.5 g	7.5 g	10 g	15 g
0.0	41.5	59.1	81.7	127.5
0.5	37.8	54.2	75.1	117.9
1.0	34.5	49.8	69.3	109.3
1.5	31.6	45.8	64.0	101.4
2.0	29.0	42.1	59.1	94.3
2.5	26.6	38.8	54.7	88.0
3.0	24.4	35.8	50.6	81.8
3.5	22.4	33.0	46.9	76.2
4.0	20.6	30.4	43.4	71.0
4.5	18.9	28.0	40.2	66.2
5.0	17.3	25.8	37.2	61.8
5.5	15.9	23.8	34.4	57.6
6.0	14.6	21.9	31.8	53.6
6.5	13.4	20.1	29.4	49.9
7.0	12.2	18.5	27.2	46.5
7.5	11.2	17.0	25.1	43.2
8.0	10.2	15.6	23.1	40.2
8.5	9.4	14.3	21.3	38.1
9.0	8.5	13.1	19.6	34.6
9.5	7.8	12.0	18.0	32.0
10.0	7.1	10.9	16.5	29.6
10.5	6.5	10.0	15.1	27.4
11.0	5.9	9.0	13.8	25.3
11.5	5.3	8.3	12.6	23.3
12.0	4.9	7.5	11.5	21.4
12.5	4.4	6.8	10.5	19.7
13.0	4.0	6.2	9.5	18.1
13.5		5.6	8.6	16.5
14.0		5.0	7.8	15.1
14.5		4.5	7.1	13.7
15.0		4.0	6.4	12.6
15.5			5.8	11.4
16.0			5.2	10.4
16.5			4.7	9.4
17.0			4.2	8.5
17.5				7.7
18.0				6.9
18.5				6.2
19.0				5.6
19.5				4.9
20.0				4.5

Approved by the Committee on Standardization of Tonometers of the American Academy of Ophthalmology and Otolaryngology.

Patients with such elevated pressures require further evaluation by a number of tests and should be referred to an ophthalmologist. A single elevated reading does not by itself make the positive diagnosis of glaucoma. Conversely, a single normal reading does not rule out the possibility of glaucoma. A patient with symptoms or findings strongly suggestive of glaucoma deserves further study than just a single normal pressure reading. Pressures as low as 10 mm Hg are entirely normal. Ordinarily the two eyes have quite similar pressures, and a difference of 8 mm or more indicates disease. Approximately 2% of patients over the age of 40 years will be found to require further examination because of increased pressure.

Patient instructions. The patient should understand that tonometry is an important test to detect the presence of a serious eye disease that affects 2% of people over 40 years of age.

He must cooperate by looking straight up, holding his eyes steady, and avoiding squeezing his lids.

He must not rub his eyes for 15 minutes after tonometry, because he could scuff the anesthetized cornea without feeling it.

Indications for tonometry. All patients over the age of 40 years should be considered candidates for routine tonometric screening, since the incidence of open-angle glaucoma is 2% in this group. Patients over 40 should certainly have their intraocular pressure checked annually if there is a family history of blindness or of treated glaucoma, if they have unexplained headaches or other symptoms about the eyes, if repeated changes of glasses do not produce satisfactory vision, or if they have anatomic characteristics sometimes associated with glaucoma, such as a shallow anterior chamber or reduced corneal diameter. Most ophthalmologists routinely check the intraocular pressure in all their patients over 40.

During the care of eye diseases known to produce secondary glaucoma, pressure estimation is important. Such diseases include trauma with anterior chamber hemorrhage, severe iridocyclitis, and dislocation of the lens.

Contraindications to tonometry. Superficial infection, whether bacterial, viral, or fungal, is practically an absolute contraindication to tonometry. The reason is that the minute abrasions produced by the tonometer may serve as portals of entry through which infection may reach the cornea. Furthermore, the tonometer becomes contaminated and may carry infection to the next patient.

Corneal edema renders the epithelium much more susceptible to damage by the tonometer. Corneal degenerative conditions, which produce edematous blebs beneath the epithelium, may be made temporarily worse by any manipulation. Such eyes are readily recognizable as abnormal by the presence of redness, corneal haziness, tearing, and discomfort.

The eye with corneal exposure damage, such as may occur in Bell's palsy or unconscious patients, should not be further injured by tonometry.

If a patient is so uncooperative that constant eye movements are present, a reliable reading will not be obtained and the cornea is particularly likely to be abraded.

Maintenance of the tonometer. *Sterility* is the most important consideration. If the tonometer is used infrequently and kept in its case, the footplate should be thoroughly wiped with benzalkonium chloride, 1:1,000 solution, before and after each use. If used frequently, the footplate should be suspended in a solution of 1:5,000 benzalkonium chloride constantly between use. Tonometry should never be done on an obviously infected eye.

Protection is important, because the tonometer is a relatively fragile instrument. The tonometer case or a special stand (many types are commercially available) affords adequate protection. The tonometer must not be handled roughly.

Cleaning is necessary to prevent sticking of the plunger. The tonometer is easily disassembled and cleaned by running a pipe cleaner soaked with ether through the barrel. Afterward, a thin coat of very light antirust oil should be applied. Frequency of cleaning is determined by the amount of use and by the type of sterilizing solution used.

Calibration is necessary to ensure accuracy and is ordinarily done at the factory. Should your instrument fail to register zero on the test block, it may be necessary to send it away for adjustment.

Applanation tonometry. Most ophthalmologists do not routinely use a Schiøtz tonometer but prefer the Goldmann applanation tonometer. This device measures the amount of pressure required to flatten 3.06 mm of the corneal surface. This delicate measurement requires use of the magnification of a slit-lamp microscope.

Although applanation tonometry is more accurate, its cost is prohibitive to the non-ophthalmologist; hence, my recommendation of Schiøtz indentation tonometry—a reliable method for general medical use.

Summary. Despite the length of this description, it requires only a few minutes to perform tonometry, the simple test that is the key to prevention of blindness from glaucoma—the present cause of 12% of all blindness in this country and one of the most readily preventable causes!

chapter 16 Strabismus

Deviation of an eye (strabismus) is a readily observed and common sign of ocular, central nervous, or general systemic abnormality (Fig. 16-1). During evaluation of every new patient, the physician should check the straightness of the patient's eyes. Simple observation can be supplemented, if necessary, by study of the corneal light reflex and the cover-uncover test (see Chapter 5).

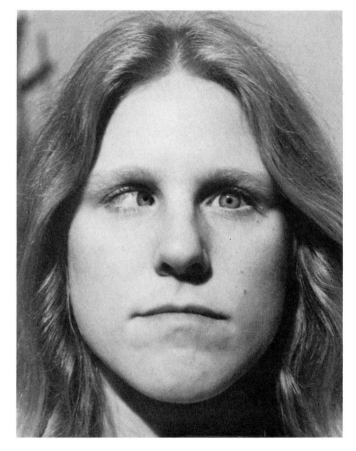

Fig. 16-1. Right esotropia.

Two major types of strabismus, *paralytic* and *nonparalytic,* are quite different in their characteristics and significance. Paralytic deviations of the eyes are usually due to *nerve damage* (cranial nerves III, IV, and VI), although the lesion may be of the extraocular muscle itself. Obviously, therefore, the presence of paralytic strabismus arouses suspicion of such diseases as brain tumor, encephalitis, intracranial aneurysm, vascular accident, thyrotropic exophthalmos (Fig. 16-2), myasthenia gravis, and orbital cellulitis. As the name implies, nonparalytic strabismus is not caused by a paralyzed muscle but by a defect of the position of the two eyes relative to one another. The tendency to develop nonparalytic strabismus is usually inherited, but this type of ocular deviation may *also* be caused by serious disease of the eye or brain (Fig. 16-3).

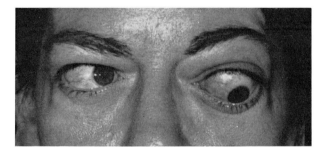

Fig. 16-2. This patient with thyrotropic exophthalmos (note that it is unilateral) is attempting to look up and to her left. Limited movement into the left superior rectus position is conspicuous. Strabismus is best detected by having the patient look as far as possible in each of the six cardinal positions.

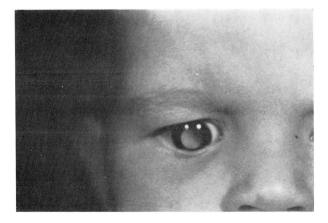

Fig. 16-3. One third of children with retinoblastoma are first seen for the complaint of strabismus. This patient also shows the yellowish pupil reflex caused by growth of a tumor within the eye. Thorough examination of the eyes themselves is necessary in all cases of strabismus.

PARALYTIC STRABISMUS

Recognition of extraocular paralysis and identification of the responsible muscle(s) require rotation of the eyes into the six cardinal positions. A cardinal position is one that the eye cannot reach without the action of a specific extraocular muscle—paralysis of which is identified by failure to attain this position. Fig. 5-16 shows the six cardinal positions. In a neurologic examination, the physician should always have the patient rotate his eyes as far as possible into each of these six positions in order to detect extraocular muscle paralysis.

Rather than blindly following a "cookbook" routine ("Look this way, look that way"), the examiner should take into consideration innervations during study of extraocular muscle movements. If one muscle innervated by the third nerve is found to be weak, the thoughtful physician will closely examine the other muscles having the same innervations (superior rectus, inferior rectus, medial rectus, inferior oblique, levator, and pupil constrictor). *Minimal changes recognized through such specific examination* may clearly indicate the diagnosis of an early third-nerve weakness at a stage when the careless examiner might disregard a slight ptosis, minimal enlargement of the pupil, and a tendency toward outward deviation of the eye. Since the nuclei of the third, fourth, fifth, and sixth nerves are closely positioned within the brainstem, superior oblique function (cranial nerve IV), lateral rectus function (cranial nerve VI), and corneal and facial sensation (cranial nerve V) are also all to be examined closely if any one of these nerve actions is impaired.

The following description of the physiology of eye movements is necessary to explain the methods of identification of partial paralyses of the extraocular muscles.

The eye rotates as if it were attached to a universal joint located near its center. This "universal joint" effect results from ocular suspension by multiple tendons, ligaments, fasciae, vessels, nerves, and fat. Pull of an extraocular muscle does not displace the eye by any great amount but mainly causes a rotation about this central "universal joint."

Up, down, nasal, and temporal rotations of the eye are easily observed and understood. In addition, the eye may rotate as a wheel turning in the plane of the iris. Rotation of the top of the iris toward the nose is termed intorsion. Rotation of the top away from the nose is extorsion.

The direction toward which a given extraocular muscle rotates the eye is determined by its origin and the position of its insertion on the eye. Fig. 16-4 illustrates the origin of the superior rectus from the orbital apex, its insertion on the top of the eye, and the outward angle of 23 degrees between the direction of the muscle and straight ahead. A similar drawing would illustrate the direction of pull of the inferior rectus, which parallels the superior rectus and inserts on the bottom of the eye. All four recti originate at the back of the orbit near the optic foramen. They are called superior, inferior, medial, or lateral, corresponding to their insertion on the eye (see frontispiece).

Fig. 16-5 shows the functional origin of the superior oblique from the trochlea near the upper nasal orbital rim (although its actual muscular origin is from the orbital apex), its

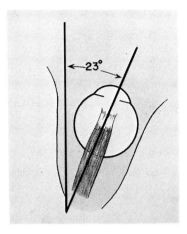

Fig. 16-4. The pull of the superior rectus (and inferior rectus) is exerted at an angle of approximately 23 degrees from the anteroposterior axis of the head.

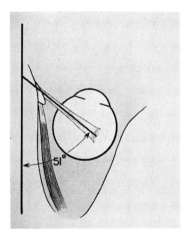

Fig. 16-5. The pull of the superior oblique (and inferior oblique) is exerted at an angle of approximately 51 degrees from the anteroposterior axis of the head.

insertion on the top of the eye, and the outward angle of 51 degrees between the direction of the tendon and straight ahead. A similar drawing would serve to illustrate the direction of pull of the inferior oblique (originating near the lower nasal orbital rim), which parallels the superior oblique and inserts on the bottom of the eye. Note that both oblique muscles insert behind the equator of the eye, whereas all four recti insert anterior to the equator.

Although contraction of a given extraocular muscle will always rotate its insertion point on the eye toward its origin, how this rotation affects the eye may vary considerably, depending on the position of the eye (direction of the cornea) at the time of muscular contraction. The student should not, therefore, memorize complicated tables of primary, secondary, and tertiary functions of these muscles but should think geometrically, considering what will happen when the eye rotates toward the muscle origin.

The change in function of a given muscle with changing eye position may be illustrated by use of the superior oblique muscle as an example. (In similar fashion, rotation of the eye by the other extraocular muscles causes different effects, depending on the starting eye position.)

If the eye looks toward the nose at an angle of 51 degrees (Fig. 16-6, *A*), rotation of the top of the eye toward the upper inner orbital rim (superior oblique function) will cause the eye to look down (Fig. 16-6, *B*) and nasally (which is the cardinal position for the superior oblique). However, if the eye looks temporally 39 degrees (90 degrees minus 51 degrees) (Fig. 16-7, *A*), rotation of the top of the eye toward the upper inner orbital rim (superior oblique function) will not change the direction of gaze but will wheel-rotate the

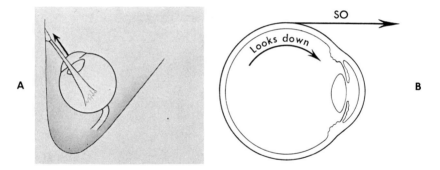

Fig. 16-6. When the eye is turned nasally, the superior oblique acts to turn the cornea downward.

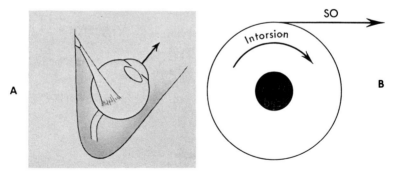

Fig. 16-7. When the eye is turned laterally, the superior oblique will intort the eye.

eye (intorsion) (Fig. 16-7, *B*). When the eye is in an intermediate position (for example, looking straight ahead), rotation of the top of the eye toward the upper inner orbital rim (superior oblique function) will cause a combination of intorsion and downward gaze.

An understanding of the preceding description of ocular rotation will explain the following three difficulties commonly encountered in interpretation of faulty movements in the cardinal positions:

1. If only the *medial rectus* is paralyzed, the eye will not turn fully to the up-nasal and down-nasal cardinal positions corresponding to inferior oblique and superior oblique function. Vertical movement is not impaired, but the eye does not move nasally. This failure should not be misinterpreted to indicate oblique weakness.
2. If the *lateral rectus* is paralyzed, comparable loss of lateral movement prevents the eye from attaining completely the up-temporal and down-temporal positions of the superior or inferior rectus. This deficiency should not be misinterpreted to indicate weakness of the vertical recti.
3. If there is a complete third-nerve paralysis, the eye is positioned laterally, somewhat as in Fig. 16-7, *A*. *Superior oblique movement* in this position causes intorsion (Fig. 16-7, *B*) rather than down-nasal movement. If the patient is asked to try to look down and nasally, wheel rotation of the iris may easily be observed and confirms function of the fourth nerve, although the eye will remain directed laterally.

Because the extraocular muscles are 100 times as strong as necessary to move the eye, a muscle that has lost more than 90% of its strength will still be able to move the eye into its cardinal position. Hence, failure of one eye to achieve cardinal positions will occur only in almost complete muscle paralysis, and early partial loss of innervation will not be detected by this test. Study of muscle function in the six cardinal positions should always be done with *both eyes simultaneously,* because observance of the movement of both eyes will result in a much more sensitive evaluation than observance of the movement of one eye alone.

The coordinated movement of both eyes together requires almost perfect muscle function and is recognizably disrupted by even slight weakness of an extraocular muscle. Clinical recognition of these slight weaknesses requires understanding of the yoke muscle concept. Yoke muscles are the two muscles (one in each eye) that move both eyes into a given cardinal position. For example, movement of both eyes up and to the right requires the action of the right superior rectus and the left inferior oblique, which are the yoke muscles for this cardinal position. The pairs of yoke muscles are easily identified by superimposing the cardinal positions (see Fig. 5-16) of right and left eyes, as shown in Fig. 16-8.

To cause coordinated turning of the two eyes in a given direction, the brain always sends an exactly equal innervation to each of the yoke muscles. If faulty nerve or muscle function affects one of the yoke muscles, the muscle will be unable to turn its eye as far as can its healthy mate. Usually this deficient movement can be recognized by observing with the aid of the *corneal light reflexes* that one eye does not turn as far as the other.

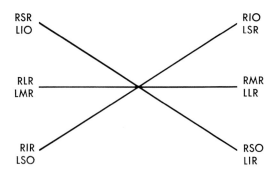

Fig. 16-8. The pairs of muscles (yoke muscles) that act simultaneously in turning both eyes into each of the cardinal positions.

Faulty binocular alignment of less than 5 degrees' magnitude is difficult to recognize by observation alone. The *cover test* (described in Chapter 5) will reveal movements as small as 2 degrees. Even more sensitive is the patient's own observation of *diplopia,* which accurately recognizes displacement even smaller than 0.5 degree.

Diplopia occurs when the eyes are not straight and the brain therefore sees two overlapping pictures. The symptom of diplopia means that the eyes are not both pointing at the same object and requires the physician to evaluate extraocular muscle function. Study of diplopia in the cardinal positions is a valuable method for identification of very early and slight muscle weakness.

In diplopia testing for a weak muscle, a fixation light is held in turn in each of the cardinal positions. If one yoke muscle is weak, the eyes will not be properly aligned in this direction, and the patient will see two lights. To identify which light is seen by which eye, hold a red glass before either eye, thereby coloring the light seen by that eye. The light farther away from the straight-ahead direction of the eyes is the one seen by the eye with the weak muscle.

The direction in which the diplopia image from the paretic eye is seen is always toward the position that the eye fails to attain. *The diplopia image is where the eye is not.* The reason is that light rays cross as they pass within the eye, so that the temporal retina sees in the nasal direction and the nasal retina sees temporally (Fig. 16-9). If the eye diverges, the image of the object being observed by the fixing eye will stimulate the temporal retina of the deviating eye (Fig. 16-10). The temporal retinal stimulation is interpreted by the brain as representing an object situated nasally (where the eye is not).

Because a given muscle relaxes when the eye is turned away from the corresponding cardinal position, a paralysis of its function will cause least binocular disturbance in this turned-away position. If a muscle is only partially paralyzed, the eyes may be straight in all positions except the corresponding cardinal position. The patient with a paralyzed muscle will often turn his head to avoid the diplopia caused by moving his eyes in the direction of the paralyzed muscle. When questioning a patient with diplopia, always ask whether

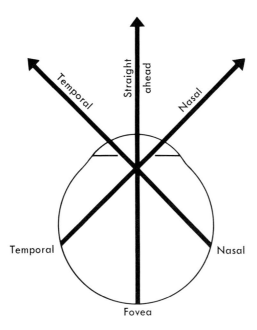

Fig. 16-9. The nasal retina normally sees the temporal field of vision; hence, stimulation of the nasal retina is interpreted by the brain to signify position of the stimulus in the temporal field. Similarly, temporal stimuli are projected into the nasal field. Normally, foveal stimulation is interpreted as originating directly in front of the eye.

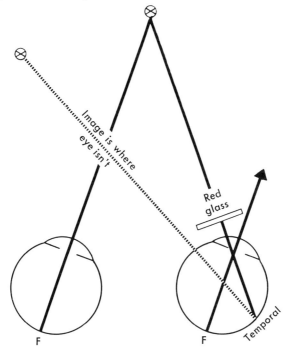

Fig. 16-10. The purpose of a red glass in examination of a patient with diplopia is to identify by which eye each of the two images is seen. (The red glass does not necessarily have to be placed over the deviating eye.) In exotropia, the image of the fixation point falls on the temporal retina of the deviating eye and is therefore identified by the brain as being displaced in the nasal direction. A diplopia image will always be perceived to be displaced in the direction toward which the eye fails to turn.

separation of the two images is more marked on gaze in any particular direction—this direction will correspond to the cardinal position of the weak muscle. Diplopia is the classic symptom of *paralytic* strabismus. (Nonparalytic strabismus practically never causes diplopia except very transiently at the time of onset.)

Physiologic diplopia can be observed by all normal persons and must not be confused with the diplopia caused by muscle paralysis. Hold your two forefingers directly in front of you, one 6 inches from your face and the other 2 feet away. If you look at either finger now, the other finger will appear double (and out of focus). Although diplopia of this sort can be perceived for any object at a different distance from the fixation point, it is generally ignored unless accidentally recognized by an apprehensive patient. Diplopia that is very transient (a few seconds only), that is accompanied by blurring of the object, and that disappears when the patient looks attentively at the object can be considered to be physiologic and of no serious significance. *Physiologic diplopia is always horizontal;* that is, the images are side by side. Vertical diplopia almost always signifies muscle paresis.

Management of paralytic strabismus consists of careful search for the underlying disorder and appropriate specific treatment. Recent onset of diplopia caused by paralytic strabismus always demands a thorough evaluation of the patient. After the underlying cause is treated, annoying diplopia sometimes persists. Occlusion of one eye (either eye or the one with poorest vision) may be necessary to relieve confusion. Sometimes muscle surgery is helpful but usually should not be done in less than 6 months because of the possibility of spontaneous recovery.

NONPARALYTIC STRABISMUS

Nonparalytic strabismus is a defect of the position of the two eyes relative to one another. It is as if the front wheels of an automobile were out of alignment. No matter which way the steering wheel is turned, the abnormal relationship of the front wheels to each other will not be corrected.

In nonparalytic strabismus the amount of crossing does not change as the eyes are rotated through the six cardinal positions. The amount of deviation of the crossed eye may be estimated in degrees (Fig. 16-11) by observing *displacement of the corneal light reflex.* When an eye looks straight at a light, its reflection is seen to be in the center of the cornea (Fig. 16-12), provided the examiner is positioned directly behind the light. As illustrated in Fig. 16-13, the corneal light reflex of an eye deviating 45 degrees is positioned at the edge of the cornea. In a 15-degree deviation, the light reflex is positioned at the edge of the pupil (provided pupil size is about 3 or 4 mm). A 30-degree deviation causes the light reflex to be positioned midway in front of the iris surface. Corneal displacement of 1 mm is caused by each 7 degrees of strabismus (Fig. 16-13). Corectopia (pupil displacement) may cause the central corneal reflex to be misaligned. A small amount of corectopia, equal in the two eyes, is a not uncommon normal variant (Fig. 16-14).

In ophthalmologic practice more precise measurements of the amount of ocular deviation in nonparalytic strabismus are made with the aid of prisms. A prism is a triangular

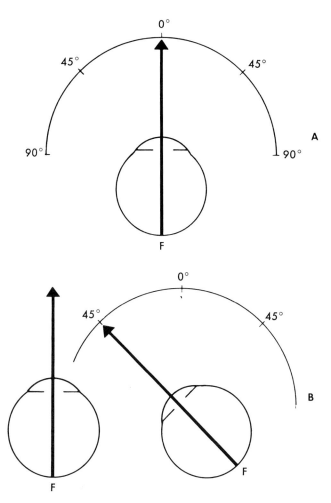

Fig. 16-11. The amount of deviation of an eye with strabismus may be measured in degrees. **A,** The zero point is situated where the nondeviating eye is fixing. **B,** Forty-five–degree right esotropia during distance fixation by the left eye.

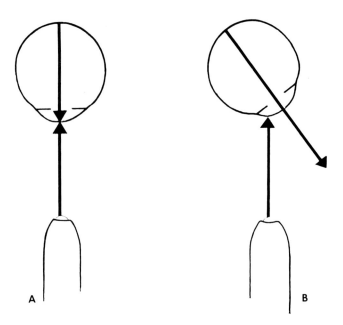

Fig. 16-12. A, When an eye looks directly at a light, its reflection will be in the center of the cornea. **B,** When an eye does not look directly at a light, its reflection will be displaced away from the corneal center.

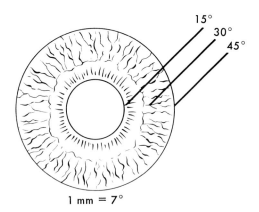

Fig. 16-13. Deviation of an eye by 15, 30, or 45 degrees will cause displacement of the corneal light reflex to the edge of the pupil, the midportion of the iris, or the limbus, respectively. For each millimeter of displacement of the corneal light reflex, approximately 7 degrees of ocular deviation exist.

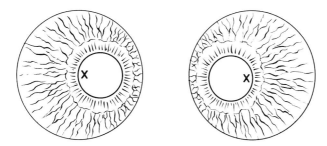

Fig. 16-14. Nasal displacement of the pupil (exaggerated for purposes of illustration) causes the corneal light reflexes to be symmetrically displaced. This is normal in some patients. A different amount of asymmetrical displacement of the reflex in the two pupils is abnormal.

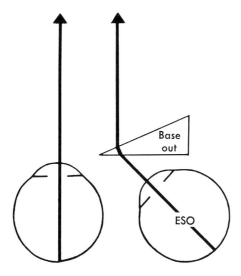

Fig. 16-15. The angle of nonparalytic strabismus is measured by the prism strength required to neutralize the deviation. In measurement of esotropia the prism base is directed temporally; for exotropia it is directed nasally.

lens that changes the direction of light passing through it (Fig. 16-15). Although prisms could be calibrated in terms of degrees of angular displacement, a smaller unit of measurement (the prism diopter) is generally used. A prism diopter corresponds to 0.5 degrees of arc. The general physician will ordinarily not require measurements of the accuracy obtainable with prisms and will record estimates of the angle of deviation made with the aid of the position of the corneal light reflex. (The amount of deviation in *paralytic* strabismus, if recorded in degrees, must be accompanied by a notation of the position of the eyes at the time of measurement, because the amount of deviation is greatest in the cardinal position of the affected muscle and least in the opposite direction.)

The cause of nonparalytic strabismus is an abnormal convergence-divergence relationship in the brain. Normally, the convergence reflex will maintain both eyes pointing straight at the fixation point, whether it is at infinity or only several inches away. (Note that the term "straight" eyes does not necessarily mean parallel gaze. When a patient is looking at a point several inches away, his eyes should be markedly convergent, although they are considered to be straight because both foveas are directed at the same object.) The eyes of almost all normal patients will be able to converge considerably closer than 10 cm from the nose. The near point of convergence is measured by bringing a fixation object slowly closer to the patient's nose until his eyes can no longer converge. At this distance one eye will suddenly diverge, and the patient may experience diplopia.

Measurement of convergence is not a particularly vital part of a general medical examination. Brainstem lesions may cause simultaneous loss of convergence and vertical binocular movement. Faulty convergency may be found in some patients complaining of reading difficulty and is common in neurasthenic individuals.

The convergence abnormality in many children with nonparalytic convergent strabismus (esotropia) is related to an inherited farsighted refractive error. Because of this hyperopic refractive error, the child must accommodate more than normal. Since accommodation and convergence are interdependent, the child also has a tendency toward excessive convergence. The onset of this type of esotropia is usually before the age of 4 years, because farsightedness (hyperopia) gradually increases in these children during the early years of life. One may imagine a struggle between binocular vision and the tendency to deviate. (As long as the binocular reflexes are stronger, the eyes remain straight, but when these reflexes are overcome, strabismus suddenly appears.) Accidents or childhood illness (for example, whooping cough) may handicap the normal reflexes and *precipitate* nonparalytic strabismus; however, the strabismus is not truly caused by the illness.

When treated early, this accommodative type of esotropia may be eliminated simply by the wearing of proper glasses. Accurate refraction of a cross-eyed child requires cycloplegic drops and therefore cannot be done by an optometrist. The glasses are to be worn constantly, usually for several years, until the eyes remain straight unaided (because of strengthened normal fusion reflexes and the spontaneous decrease in hyperopia after childhood).

Nightly instillation of parasympathomimetic drops (for example, 0.06% echothiophate [Phospholine] iodide) may correct the convergence abnormality and straighten the eyes, either alone or in combination with the wearing of glasses.

Only about one third of the cases of childhood esotropia can be corrected by glasses and/or drops. The remaining two thirds are said to be "nonaccommodative" and are due to other types of convergence anomalies. If esotropia is present from birth, it will always be nonaccommodative.

The fact that serious disease of the eye or of the brain may cause nonparalytic strabismus is often overlooked. Strabismus is the presenting complaint in one third of all persons with retinoblastoma (see Fig. 16-3). Destructive inflammation, injury, or cataract of one eye often results in its deviation. The neurologic deficit of brain tumor, subdural hematoma, or congenital anomalies may cause nonparalytic strabismus. Thorough medical examination of the dilated eyes is mandatory in the study of a cross-eyed child. The time for medical evaluation of strabismus is as soon as the strabismus is recognized! Delay may result in serious consequences (Figs. 16-16 and 16-17).

Unless strabismus is corrected during childhood, normal binocular vision usually cannot be achieved. The synthesis of two ocular pictures into one cerebral picture is termed "fusion." Fusion requires perfect alignment of the two eyes, so that both foveas are aimed exactly at the same point. The fine adjustments of ocular position necessary to maintain this perfect alignment are made automatically in response to visual reflexes. In other words, the act of seeing with both eyes reflexly guides the eyes into perfect alignment.

If the vision of one eye is blocked (as by disease or during the cover test), fusion is impossible. Deprived of the corrective fusional reflexes, the covered (or blind) eye drifts out of alignment. Deviation of a covered eye is normal and occurs in almost everyone (Fig. 16-18). "Phoria" is the term describing ocular deviation that occurs only when fusion is interrupted (as by the cover test). If the eyes are spontaneously not straight (no cover used to interrupt fusion), this condition is termed "tropia" (synonym for strabismus). Tropia occurs if the tendency to deviation is greater than can be overcome by fusion.

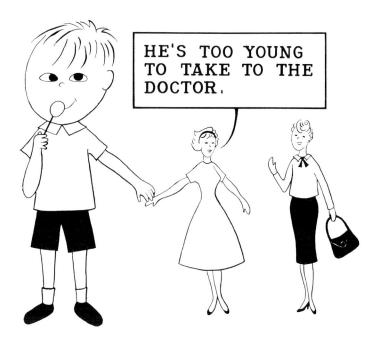

Fig. 16-16. Since strabismus may be caused by serious eye or brain disease, prompt medical evaluation of this condition is essential as soon as the strabismus is recognized.

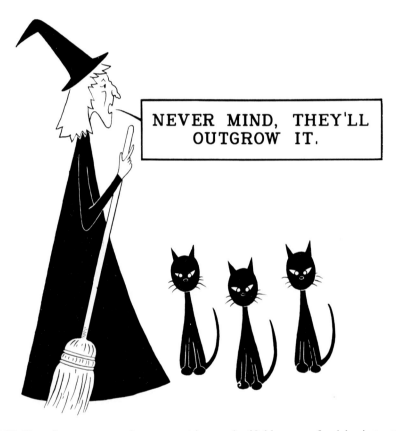

Fig. 16-17. Hope for spontaneous improvement is an unjustifiable reason for delay in treatment of childhood strabismus.

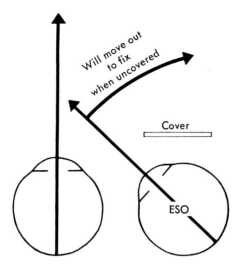

Fig. 16-18. Covering an esophoric eye causes it to deviate inward. The eye may be observed to move out to normal position when it is uncovered.

Convergent deviation is called esotropia, divergent deviation is called exotropia, and vertical deviation is called hypertropia. Nonparalytic strabismus may be monocular or alternating. In monocular strabismus, the deviating eye is always the same one. The designation "left" or "right" refers to the horizontally deviating eye; for example, left esotropia means that the left eye turns inward. In alternating strabismus, either eye may be used in turn for fixation. Whichever eye is not used deviates. Alternating strabismus is not classified as "right" or "left." In the description of vertical deviation, "right" or "left" designates the higher one of the two eyes and does not indicate which eye is used for fixation; for example, left hypertropia means that the left eye is directed higher than is the right eye and does not imply preferential use of either eye.

The brain may use the two pictures received from the eyes in three different ways: *fusion, diplopia,* or *suppression.* Fusion occurs if the eyes are functioning normally. Diplopia occurs in paralytic strabismus. Suppression occurs in nonparalytic strabismus.

Although diplopia may be experienced initially in nonparalytic strabismus, it is transitory and disappears completely after a few days. Absence of diplopia is due to suppression of the deviating eye. Suppression of the image from one eye is a common and normal cerebral phenomenon that may be activated whenever the eyes send two different pictures to the brain. For example, with both eyes open we can look into a monocular microscope and see the magnified field, undisturbed by the suppressed picture of the tabletop seen by the other eye. Unfortunately, suppression becomes habitual in nonparalytic strabismus and interferes seriously with binocular vision. At its worst, suppression irreversibly damages the vision of the deviating eye, resulting in the condition known as *suppression amblyopia* ("lazy eye") (Fig. 16-19).

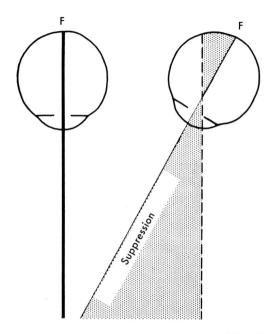

Fig. 16-19. An eye with suppression amblyopia is not entirely blind but has a visual defect extending from the fovea to the part of the retina that is usually directed straight ahead. The retina on either side of this suppressed *(dotted area)* area sees normally.

Suppression amblyopia is common! About 0.5% of patients have lost good vision in one eye because of suppression amblyopia. Usually by the age of 6 years the brain has developed suppression of such severity that it will not respond to a reasonable amount of treatment. Most tragic is the fact that this visual loss could have been prevented by simple treatment. If detected in early childhood (measurement of visual acuity with the letter E is possible by 4 years of age), suppression amblyopia may be reversed simply by occluding the good eye (see Fig. 16-27), thereby forcing the child to use the suppressed eye. (Although the principle of occlusion is simple, in practice expert supervision is necessary.)

The visual acuity of a deviating eye with suppression amblyopia may be estimated with reasonable accuracy even though the child is too young to indicate the direction the E is facing. This estimate is made from the *fixation behavior of the deviating eye*. In general, the less the deviating eye is used, the less is its acuity. The test consists of having the child look at a light while the good eye is covered and then while it is uncovered. If the deviating eye is unable to look directly at the light even when the good eye is covered, its vision is very poor (20/200 or less) (Fig. 16-20). If the deviating eye can fix the light monocularly but cannot hold fixation when the good eye is uncovered, vision is probably between 20/100 and 20/50 (Fig. 16-21). If the deviating eye fixes monocularly and holds fixation fairly well when the good eye is uncovered, acuity is probably between 20/50 and

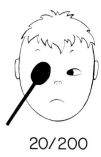

20/200

Fig. 16-20. A child with severe amblyopia may not be able to fixate an object even when the good eye is covered. Vision of such an eye is 20/200 or less.

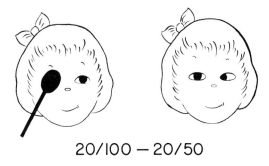

20/100 — 20/50

Fig. 16-21. If the child with an amblyopic eye can fix when the good eye is covered but cannot hold fixation when the cover is removed, vision of the poor eye is usually from 20/100 to 20/50.

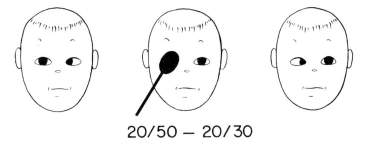

20/50 — 20/30

Fig. 16-22. If covering the fixing eye causes fixation with the other eye, and if this second eye maintains fixation for some time even when the cover is removed, the second eye will usually have vision between 20/50 and 20/30.

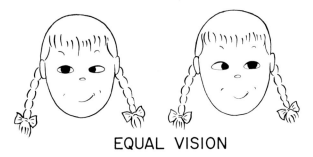

EQUAL VISION

Fig. 16-23. Spontaneous alternation of fixation between the two eyes occurs if vision is equal (no suppression amblyopia).

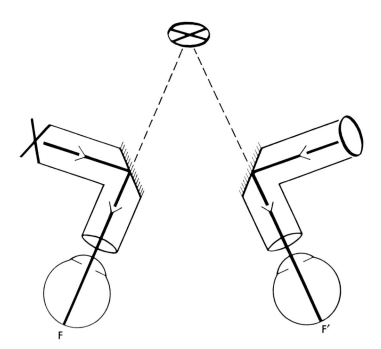

Fig. 16-24. The stereoscopic instruments used in orthoptics consist of movable tubes with which mirrors are used to deflect the line of sight so that different images are presented to each eye at varying angles. As illustrated, an X and O would be perceived as a combined image of a cross within a circle. This instrument can be adapted to the amount of ocular deviation present in the patient.

20/30 (Fig. 16-22). If the child spontaneously alternates fixation between the two eyes, then the vision is equal (20/20 in both eyes if no other defects are present) (Fig. 16-23).

By observation of these fixation characteristics, the physician can recognize the severity of amblyopia and evaluate the progressive improvement of vision obtained through occlusion.

Nonparalytic strabismus does *not* cause symptoms such as headache, eyestrain, or reading difficulty. However, the emotional aspects of childhood strabismus are important. Almost without exception, a cross-eyed child will be sensitive about his obvious deformity. Withdrawn, belligerent, or other antisocial behavior is common. Strabismus should be cosmetically corrected before school age to avoid schoolmates' cruel jibes.

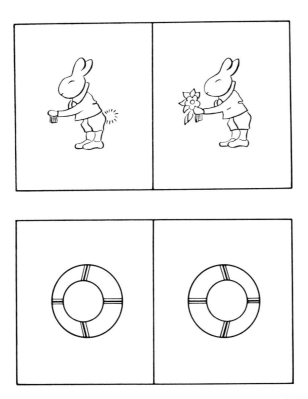

Fig. 16-25. During orthoptic evaluation and training of a patient, stereoscopic slides may be used. Each of the upper two pictures is incomplete, and failure to use both eyes can therefore be recognized if a part is perceived as missing. Many people can combine these pictures without the aid of a stereoscope simply by holding the picture about 2 feet away and looking at a finger that is held about halfway between the picture and the eyes. The right eye then observes the left picture, and the left eye observes the right picture. If this procedure is done properly, a bunny complete with flowers and tail will be seen between the two pictures. The stereoscopic impression of depth (as if looking into a bucket) results from fusion of the lower two pictures.

Therapy. Treatment of nonparalytic strabismus is complex and requires ophthalmologic supervision. A brief outline follows:

1. Thorough evaluation to rule out major cerebral and ocular disease
2. Cycloplegic refraction to detect and correct refractive errors
3. Orthoptic evaluation (Figs. 16-24 to 16-26) to measure the angle of strabismus under different conditions (necessary to determine the method of surgical correction or to evaluate progress under nonsurgical management) and to encourage fusion ability
4. Occlusion (Fig. 16-27) to restore good vision if suppression amblyopia has developed
5. Surgery (Fig. 16-28) if the previous steps are not sufficient

The objective of surgery is to alter the position of the eye by moving the muscle insertions appropriately backward or forward (Fig. 16-29). Surgery neither strengthens nor weakens the extraocular muscles but simply rotates the eye to a different position in respect to the muscle involved.

The function of a muscle is determined by the location of its attachment to the eye, the direction in which the muscle pulls, and the position of the eye at the time of muscle action. It is almost always possible to achieve a cosmetic straightening of the eyes; however, several operations may be necessary. Commonly, one muscle in each eye will be resected or recessed, because this procedure results in more symmetrical binocular movements. Since the parents consider only one eye to be crossed, they are often surprised that surgery is to be done on both eyes. It is important to recognize that *surgery will not benefit amblyopia.*

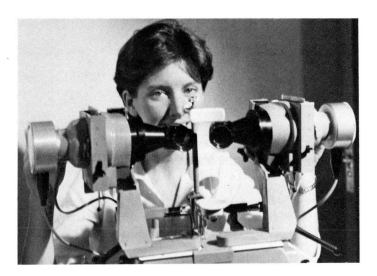

Fig. 16-26. Orthoptic instrument for evaluation and training of binocular functions.

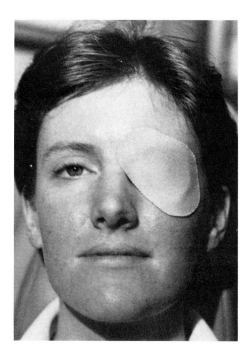

Fig. 16-27. Constant occlusion of the *good* eye in a child with suppression amblyopia will often restore vision to the bad eye. Ideally, suppression should be avoided through prompt referral of a child when squinting is noticed. The sooner occlusion is begun, the more rapid the restoration of lost vision. Occlusion is useless after the age of 6 years, a fact that underscores the importance of preschool vision testing in detection of suppression while it can still be treated. Proper management of occlusion is complicated and should be supervised by an expert. Occlusion of an adult eye, as shown here, is a waste of time.

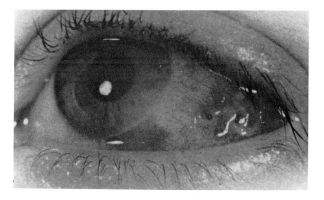

Fig. 16-28. Six days earlier, the lateral rectus was moved backward (recessed) in treatment of exotropia. The suture and postoperative tissue reaction are visible. Within 1 month, no scar will be visible except on very close inspection. Subconjunctival hemorrhages follow most types of ocular surgery, are of no significance, and clear within several weeks.

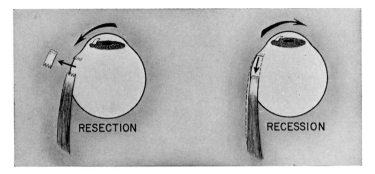

Fig. 16-29. In surgery for strabismus, the tendon of the extraocular muscle may be *resected*. This has the effect of rotating the eye toward the resected tendon, the cut end of which is reattached at the original point of insertion on the sclera. *Recession* moves the point of insertion backward on the sclera, thereby permitting the eye to rotate away from the recessed tendon. Appropriate combinations of these procedures on the various extraocular muscles will cosmetically correct most cases of strabismus.

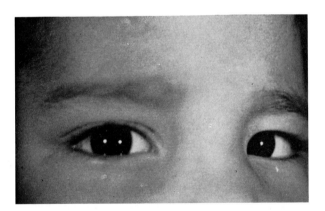

Fig. 16-30. Epicanthus is a fold of skin running from the upper lid to the nose. It tends to conceal the eye, especially on adduction, giving the false appearance of esotropia. Note that the corneal light reflex is symmetrically positioned on the left edge of each pupil, indicating that the eyes are perfectly straight. Under these circumstances other tests, such as the alternate cover examination, should be employed to confirm the diagnosis of straight eyes.

PSEUDOSTRABISMUS

Epicanthus (Fig. 16-30), a minor congenital anomaly in which the lids have an oriental slant and conceal the inner portion of the eyes, may closely simulate esotropia, particularly when the child is looking to the side. If a child with epicanthus is reported by the parents to have crossed eyes at irregular intervals unrelated to fatigue, ask them to observe him while his head is turned to one side so as to exaggerate the concealment of one eye by the lid-nose skin fold. If now, while you know the eyes to be straight, they say

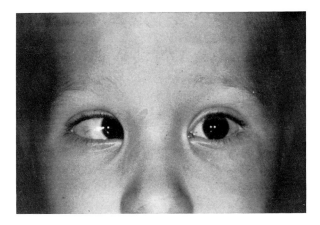

Fig. 16-31. Epicanthus and strabismus may coexist. Recognition of an eccentric corneal light reflex will establish the presence of strabismus.

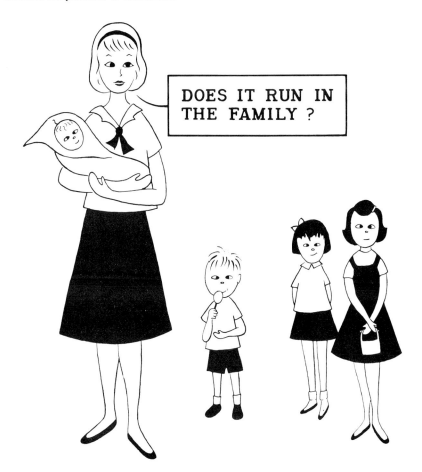

Fig. 16-32. Patients informed of the hereditary nature of strabismus may be able to bring subsequent children for earlier medical care, thereby avoiding the development of severe suppression amblyopia.

"That's it!" you may safely conclude that they have simply observed the epicanthus. Epicanthus and esotropia may coexist (Fig. 16-31).

Although the physician recognizes the presence of epicanthus and finds the eyes to be straight at the time of office examination, the possibility of intermittent esotropia has not yet been excluded. Intermittent esotropia is an early stage of accommodative esotropia in which fusion is still strong enough to maintain straightness except when the child is tired or during activity requiring intensive accommodation at a near distance. Do not disregard the mother's positive statement that the child's eyes cross when he is tired. Bringing a small picture very close to the patient's nose may induce a recognizable esotropia. Sometimes the cover test, done as the child looks intently at a near object, will disclose esodeviation. If one eye is suspected of deviating, the other eye is covered. If the suspected eye is actually deviating, a compensatory movement of the deviating eye will occur in order to fixate the light. Suspicion of strabismus is greatly increased by a family history of this disorder (Fig. 16-32).

Hypertelorism (lateral displacement of the orbits) may be mistaken for exotropia. The cover test will permit differentiation of these two conditions.

SUMMARY

Understand clearly the difference between normal "straightness" of the eyes (with binocular fusion), paralytic strabismus (results in diplopia), and nonparalytic strabismus (causes alternating suppression or suppression amblyopia).

Strabismus is a serious finding, resulting in loss of vision or even death. Therefore, do not ignore deviation of the eyes but evaluate the problem promptly and adequately to permit accurate etiologic diagnosis and appropriate management. Childhood strabismus should be referred to an ophthalmologist as soon as it is identified. Strabismus is never normal, not even in the youngest infant.

chapter 17 Cataract

The development of contact lenses and intraocular lenses has dramatically changed the practice of cataract surgery. As a result, the number of cataract operations has tripled within a decade. The correction of aphakia by these new methods is so much better than the use of cataract spectacles that the legitimate and proper indications for surgery are greatly expanded. More than 400,000 cataract extractions are performed annually in the United States. A conservative estimate of the cost per operation is $3000. This multiplies to $1.2 billion. The socioeconomic importance of cataract is so enormous that physician and patient alike require an understanding of the condition and its correction.

Cataract is the most common cause of blindness; however, this statement must be qualified by knowledge that normal visual acuity may be restored through surgical removal of uncomplicated cataracts. The clinician will be aware that laymen often designate as "cataract" any disease causing visual loss in old age. Because of this inference of blindness, the diagnosis of cataract terrifies many persons. Awareness of such fear will permit a considerate physician to accompany the diagnosis of cataract with the reassurance that the patient can anticipate effective correction of the problem when necessary.

SYMPTOMS

As the lens becomes opaque, it scatters light instead of transmitting a sharply focused image. "Glare" is the term describing the visual disability resulting from light scatter. A winter-frosted windshield provides the best understanding of glare. One can easily see through a lightly frosted windshield to drive if it is barely dawn and very little light strikes the windshield. However, an oncoming headlight from another vehicle will transform the frost into a sheet of light that obscures all detail. In exactly the same way, light striking a cataract causes glare to reduce visual acuity. Inability to drive at night because of glare is almost pathognomonic of cataract.

Patients with cataract rapidly learn to avoid extraneous light. Strategies for this include reading with the light behind their head, using a shaded light source that shines on the reading matter but not on the eye, lowering the automobile visor when driving during the day, wearing a cap or wide-brimmed hat during the day, and using dark glasses (but *not* for night driving).

The importance of glare as a symptom is that it distinguishes cataract from the multiple other causes of reduced visual acuity.

A second symptom very characteristic of cataract is a gradual change in refractive error in the direction of increasing myopia, occurring in adult life. (Childhood myopia normally increases during growth—this is *not* indicative of cataract.) This adult onset of myopia is due to the increased refractive index of a nuclear cataract. Such a change is not all bad, for the myopia permits the presbyopic patient to see near detail and to read without glasses. Some fortunate patients develop a nuclear cataract in one eye and can read with it, and they can also see in the distance with the other eye.

A third symptom characteristic of cataract is monocular double vision. This is fairly uncommon, but it is diagnostic of cataract.

TYPES OF CATARACT

Important varieties of cataract include senile, congenital, developmental, traumatic, endocrine, and uveal types.

Senile cataract. Senile cataracts (Fig. 17-1) are genetically determined lens opacities that occur frequently at all ages past 40 years. Rarely, an individual in his twenties or thirties will develop senile cataract. Typically, the onset is noted as a gradual visual loss that requires from a few months to many years to become incapacitating. It is not possible to predict accurately the rate of development of a given cataract, although in some instances an expert may be able to give a rough estimate.

In general, nuclear cataracts progress slowly, often requiring years before surgery becomes necessary. Posterior subcapsular cataracts cause an unusually severe and handi-capping glare and usually grow rapidly (in months). The best way to predict the rate of cataract growth is to suggest that when the second eye becomes affected, its rate of

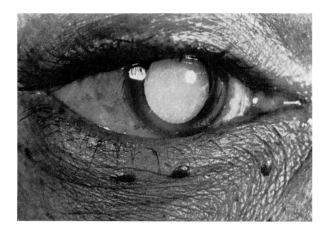

Fig. 17-1. A dense cataract is readily recognizable as a gray mass behind the pupil. It is not desirable to permit a cataract to become this mature without ophthalmologic supervision, because it may produce acute inflammatory or glaucomatous changes of great severity. Note the sessile papillomas on the lower lid. In blacks, such benign lesions closely simulate melanomas.

progression will probably be about the same as that of the first eye. (More often than not, one cataract will begin considerably earlier than the other.) Almost all senile cataracts are bilateral, although they are usually unequal in density.

Occasionally, sudden visual loss is said to occur from cataract. This loss is invariably due to gradual, unnoticed development of unilateral cataract that is accidentally brought to the patient's attention. If the visual loss truly happens rapidly, it is almost certainly due to some other problem (such as embolus into retinal arterioles, hemorrhage affecting the macula or vitreous, or retinal detachment). Quite commonly, an elderly person who is aware of having a cataract will conclude that the new symptom is simply progression of the cataract and will fail to seek medical attention.

Examination. Next to the slit lamp, the ophthalmoscope is the best instrument for the clinical study of lens opacities. Obviously, examination is greatly aided by good mydriasis. Study of the type of cataract is best done by observing the defects in the red reflex as seen from about 1 foot away through a +5 lens. With this method, the examiner can easily distinguish the gradually increasing central density of a nuclear cataract and the cuneate (wedge-shaped) spoke of cortical cataracts (the two most common senile types) from the rounded peripheral clubs seen in nonprogressive developmental cataracts. Posterior subcapsular cataract, the third—and least frequent—type of senile cataract, appears ophthalmoscopically as a vacuolated, very well circumscribed opacity located near the visual axis (center of pupil).

The ophthalmoscope is also the best instrument with which to determine how much visual loss a given cataract should cause. If the examiner can see in clearly, the patient should be able to see out. Marked visual loss suffered by a patient whose retina is clearly visible *cannot* be due to cataract (except for the rare condition of "double-focus" lens).

Although a dense cataract is easily observable by oblique illumination, a flashlight is not a reliable instrument for determining the density of less advanced lens opacities. Older lenses frequently become relucent (disperse and reflect light as if they were opaque), appear quite gray when observed with a flashlight, and yet transmit light perfectly, as proved by good visual acuity and clear ophthalmoscopic visualization of the fundus.

Therapy. The only effective treatment of senile cataract is surgical removal, which should be done when the patient's vision no longer meets his needs. Although postoperative vision should be excellent in the great majority of patients with uncomplicated cataract, the patient may be completely dependent on a pair of heavy spectacles (Fig. 17-2). The patient and surgeon must judge when the handicap of the cataract is worse than the risks of surgery and the problems of aphakia. In general, a healthy patient with an eye normal except for the cataract should have better than a 95% expectation of successful restoration of vision. Other problems, such as myopic degeneration, corneal dystrophy, and diabetic neovascularization, for example, may greatly reduce this percentage and require individualized consideration. Hemorrhage, infection, accidental falls, retinal detachments, and other evil problems do happen sometimes, and the surgical prognosis is absolutely not 100% guaranteed.

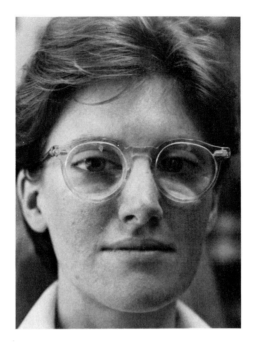

Fig. 17-2. Cataract lenses. Note the magnifying effect of strong convex lenses.

Aphakia (*a,* without; *phakos,* lens) requires optical correction with cataract glasses, a contact lens, or an intraocular lens. Cataract glasses magnify 25%, which causes marked difficulty in distance judgment and precludes binocular vision unless both eyes are aphakic. Most patients are very unhappy with the distorted vision obtained with cataract glasses.

Contact lenses give excellent quality of vision but require considerable maintenance. Many older persons lack the manual dexterity required to insert and remove contact lenses. Extended-wear lenses are oxygen permeable and can be worn without removal for several months by most persons. On the average, an extended-wear lens breaks or is lost every 6 months. At a price of $300 per lens, this can be expensive. Perhaps 10% of patients cannot tolerate contact lenses at all.

Intraocular lens implants have become the most popular means to correct aphakia. These are plastic lenses designed to be supported within the anterior or posterior chamber of the eye. The implant is usually inserted immediately following removal of the cataract. Secondary implantation may be performed as a subsequent operation, but this timing risks the hazards of a second surgical operation. Without any doubt, the insertion of an implant adds to the expense and risk of a cataract operation. These problems are counterbalanced by better vision and the absence of maintenance nuisance (Fig. 17-3).

The optimal time for cataract surgery depends on the occupational needs of each

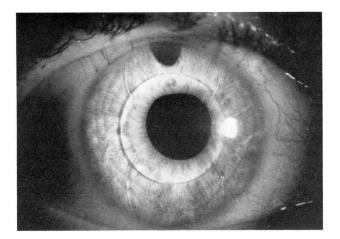

Fig. 17-3. Intraocular lens implant. Such a lens is virtually invisible except on the very closest inspection.

patient and is therefore a matter of good judgment. Although I have just stated that surgical removal should not take place until vision has become insufficient for the patient's needs, this is not to say he should not be referred until that stage. Because of the many serious diseases affecting the eyes of older persons, the elderly patient who notes gradual reduction of vision should be seen by the ophthalmologist unless the diagnosis is completely evident to the examining physician. Remember that glaucoma and cataract may coexist!

Medical therapy of cataract is practically synonymous with placebo treatment or quackery. With the exception of the very rare hypoparathyroid, galactosemia, or acute diabetic cataracts, no medication has proved effective in preventing or retarding cataract formation. The ''success'' of ''anticataract'' regimens is due to the very slow development of many types of cataract and to the stationary nature of others.

Congenital cataract. The growth of the lens is similar to the growth of a tree; new rings of tissue are constantly added peripherally. The developing fibers are sensitive to an unfavorable environment, and under adverse circumstances a layer of opaque fibers may be deposited. The external appearance is a gray mass of varying density, situated in the inner portions of the lens (Fig. 17-4). Congenital cataracts are usually bilateral. Most such cataracts are hereditary, and the exact enzymatic cause of their development is unknown. Deficiencies of calcium or hypoparathyroidism may also cause such an opaque layer within the lens. Depending on the extent and density of the cataract, a quite variable amount of visual loss will occur. Surgery (Fig. 17-5) should be done only in patients with cataract of handicapping severity, because there is a high incidence of serious complications, such as retinal detachment. Not infrequently other ocular anomalies may coexist with congenital cataract. There are many varieties of minor developmental lens

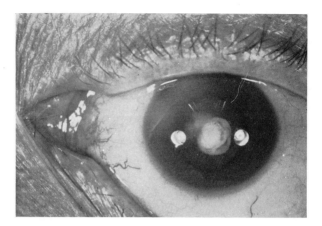

Fig. 17-4. A congenital cataract is situated in the central portion of the lens because new, clear fibers are added to the lens from outside during its growth. When the pupil is widely dilated, the congenital cataract seems to be floating freely behind it because the peripheral lens is clear.

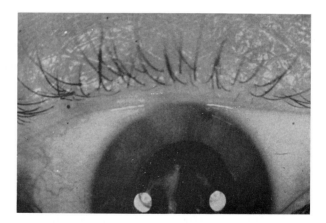

Fig. 17-5. These gray membranes in the pupil are remnants of a congenital cataract that has been "needled." An extremely thin, needle-shaped knife with a cutting tip is employed to cut an opening into the cataract, which may then be washed out by irrigation and aspiration. Repeated needlings may be required, which is the reason why modern surgery aspirates the cataract with special irrigation-aspiration devices.

opacities that cause no visual difficulties whatsoever, although they are technically termed "cataracts."

Developmental cataract. Developmental cataracts are those in which the growing lens fibers have failed to remain transparent. The most serious is the *zonular cataract,* in which the central portion of the lens is opaque. It develops at about the time of birth and is the type of opacity found in almost all congenital cataracts requiring surgery.

Minor developmental lens opacities are present in most eyes. These opacities are either too small to be of optical significance or are situated in the equatorial periphery of the lens. The most prominent representative of this group is the *coronary cataract,* which causes large rounded peripheral opacities that are easily seen when the pupil is dilated. Since coronary cataracts are commonly seen, the physician should be aware that they do not progress to the center of the lens and therefore will not disturb vision. Such patients should not be told they have "cataract," because they will become unnecessarily alarmed.

Traumatic cataract. Subsequent to either a penetrating injury or contusion, the lens may lose its transparency. The time required for cataract development depends on the severity of injury to the lens and may vary from hours to many years. Rapidly developing cataracts may swell to such size that they impede aqueous outflow and cause secondary glaucoma. The prognosis for an eye with traumatic cataract is guarded, because other major complications (for example, macular damage, retinal detachment, glaucoma, vitreous opacity, or corneal scarring) may be present.

The lens is very sensitive to radiation injury. As little as 600 roentgens may cause a slowly developing cataract, first recognized a year or so after exposure.

Ordinary senile cataract is sometimes asymmetrical and may be mistakenly considered the result of trauma.

Endocrine cataract. Endocrine cataracts are those associated with acute diabetes mellitus and hypoparathyroidism, and are closely related to the cataracts seen in mongolism, severe neurodermatitis, and some types of poisoning. In these cases characteristic punctate opacities laid down in the lens cortex may readily be observed with the slit-lamp microscope. Their appearance is only one of many ways in which careful ophthalmologic examination of the eye may provide clues to the diagnosis of obscure medical diseases.

Uveal cataract. Severe or prolonged intraocular inflammation commonly results in cataract. The trauma of surgery may reactivate the uveitis. Inflammatory damage to the vitreous, macula, or optic nerve may also compromise the visual result.

SUMMARY

A cataract causes reduction of vision comparable to the blur of the ophthalmoscopic view. Its presence is usually identifiable by a history of glare or of increasing myopia in adult life. Ophthalmoscopic recognition of the opacity confirms the diagnosis. Because other disorders commonly exist in an eye old and sick enough to have a cataract, referral to an ophthalmologist is proper, even though it is too early for surgery.

Surgery, the only effective therapy for cataract, should not be performed until the patient's vision is sufficiently reduced to warrant the discomfort, inconvenience, time, expense, risk, and postoperative aphakic problems that will inevitably accompany the operation.

RECOMMENDED READING

Havener, W.H., and Gloeckner, S.L.: Atlas of cataract surgery, St. Louis, 1972, The C.V. Mosby Co.

chapter 18 Retinal Detachment

You, as a physician, should be interested in retinal detachment because it is a preventable cause of blindness. Early detection and prompt surgery can maintain excellent sight in eyes that would otherwise become irretrievably blind.

DETECTION

Your detection of a retinal detachment will be made possible by the patient's complaints. The most common preliminary symptom is the sudden appearance of a great many floating spots in the vision of one eye. Such floating spots are caused by the entry of red blood cells or retinal pigment cells into the vitreous humor. These cells gain entry into the vitreous when a retinal tear occurs.

Because most retinal tears do not cause an immediate detachment, no further symptoms may appear for some time. These retinal tears are almost always so far peripheral as to be entirely out of the field of vision—that is, the patient does *not* have a defect of vision corresponding to the tear. This phenomenon is possible because the far peripheral retina is normally nonseeing.

The multiple floating spots may disappear rapidly from the patient's sight because the red cells and the pigment cells sediment inferiorly in the vitreous. Such clearing of the visual disturbance is reassuring to the patient and physician, who usually assume (wrongly) that it represents spontaneous cure of the problem. The rate of vitreous clearing depends on the structure of the individual vitreous body. A relatively fluid vitreous will permit rapid sedimentation and clearing, whereas a more solid vitreous structure may maintain the cellular suspension much longer. Hence, the floaters from a retinal tear may last only for days, or they may persist for many months.

From days to years after the floaters have appeared, the patient will note a visual field defect, beginning in the periphery and gradually extending. This field defect corresponds to the advancing retinal detachment, which slowly extends from the tear as the intraocular fluid leaks through the tear and extends underneath the retina. Separation of the retina from its nutritive source, the choroid, arrests the metabolism of the visual cells; therefore, the part of the retina that is detached cannot see. Because of the left-right and up-down crossing of the light rays as they enter the eye, the location of the visual field defect will be exactly opposite the portion of the retina that is detached.

326

Surprisingly often, the field defect does not greatly alarm the patient, perhaps for the following reasons: No pain is present. Central visual acuity is normal as long as the central retina (macula) remains unaffected. A gradually progressive peripheral field defect may be completely unnoticed by the patient. The gravitational effects of bed rest may cause marked improvement in the detachment overnight, leading the patient to believe that a few more nights of rest will spontaneously correct the problem. Also, some patients seem unaware of the significance of blindness affecting only the first eye.

The typical symptoms of retinal detachment are, therefore, the sudden onset of many floating spots followed, after a variable interval, by a progressive field loss. Not all patients report such a typical history. Some simply say they cannot see, and others may even claim unawareness of the loss of sight until it is detected by measurement of visual acuity.

Confirmation of the diagnosis of retinal detachment requires ophthalmoscopy (see Plate 30). The pupil must be widely dilated for adequate examination. The detachment will be found in the part of the retina exactly opposite the field defect. Elevation of the retina, as measured by dioptric focusing of the lens wheel of the ophthalmoscope, is the diagnostic finding. Furthermore, the presence of subretinal fluid will conceal the background details of choroidal vessel and pigment markings that are normally easily visible.

In honesty, it must be admitted that almost all early retinal detachments are beyond the ophthalmoscopic talents of almost all physicians. These subtle changes are inconspicuous and are interpreted with difficulty. Retinal holes are even more elusive. A specialist in retinal detachment may spend a half hour or more in the examination of a single eye to be absolutely sure that he has identified all the holes in a difficult case. For practical purposes, therefore, attempted ophthalmoscopic confirmation of the diagnosis is appropriate, but a typical history requires referral to an ophthalmologist *whether or not* you can see any abnormality with the ophthalmoscope.

Your suspicion of the possibility of retinal detachment should be greatly increased if the patient has had cataract extraction. One third of all detachment patients are aphakic. Myopia substantially predisposes the patient to retinal detachment, as does preceding severe ocular injury (either contusion or penetrating wound).

ETIOLOGY

Retinal detachment is not due to retinal disease; rather, it is the consequence of vitreous traction. Focal vitreous traction is the cause of retinal tears. Use of the eyes, fatigue, heavy lifting or exertion, and comparable activities do not cause retinal detachment. The spontaneous vitreoretinal degenerative changes of age, perhaps aided by genetic predisposition or by environmental insults (inflammation, trauma), are the usual cause of retinal tears and detachment.

Severe diabetic retinopathy may result in proliferation and subsequent shrinkage of preretinal and vitreous connective tissue (see Plate 22). The prognosis of the detachments caused by diabetic traction damage is especially poor.

Rhegmatogenous (hole-induced) detachments are the type discussed so far. Nonrhegmatogenous (no hole present) detachments result from the leakage of fluid from choroidal or retinal vessels. Causes of nonrhegmatogenous detachment include metastatic and primary neoplasms, sympathetic ophthalmia and comparable severe inflammations, eclampsia, and similar causes of transudative or exudative fluid accumulation. Nonrhegmatogenous detachments are not amenable to the usual surgical techniques designed to correct retinal detachment by sealing the responsible retinal hole(s).

MANAGEMENT

From the practical standpoint, retinal detachment is a disorder that should be referred to and treated by a subspecialist. Most ophthalmologists prefer not to perform this type of surgery because of its complexity, although they do diagnose and follow patients. Patients with a typical floater-shadow historical sequence should be referred urgently to an ophthalmologist. After confirmation of the diagnosis, emergency hospitalization and surgery will usually be advised.

Gravity is an important principle used to protect a macula threatened by detachment. The retina is relatively heavier than the vitreous fluid and tends to fall downward. Positioning the eye so that the retinal hole is relatively downward will help prevent further detachment and may even cause some settling back of the retina into a more normal position. Decreasing eye movement by binocular patching is another method of preventing progression of the detachment.

Most retinal surgeons prefer general anesthesia. The patient will undergo the traditional preparation for such general anesthesia. Whether preoperative bed rest is required depends on the retinal status. If the macula is not yet detached, care is more urgent and protective restrictions will be more severe. The duration of hospitalization will vary according to the beliefs of the individual surgeon, but it will ordinarily be 2 or 3 days, in contrast to the long periods of the past. Similarly, the amount of allowable activity has been greatly extended, so that the average patient can be completely responsible for his own self-care as soon as he goes home. Restoration to normal physical activity may occur 2 to 4 weeks after surgery.

PROGNOSIS

The average relatively uncomplicated retinal detachment has a 70% to 90% chance of permanent reattachment by a single operation. Perhaps 5% to 10% of detachments considered operable will continue to develop new holes and problems. Some patients have far more serious problems and must decide whether they wish to undergo the risks of surgery for a slight possibility of regaining only limited vision.

In general, the quality of vision regained after a 3-month ocular convalescence will be determined by the status of the central retina (the macula). If uninvolved by the detachment, the macula may permit entirely normal vision after successful surgery. If involved, the macula is usually distorted or damaged sufficiently to preclude fully normal vision.

For this reason, early detection and care of a retinal detachment is important. For best results, surgery should be performed before the patient loses central vision—while the shadow is still to the side, rather than involving straight-ahead vision. Even better is prophylactic sealing of a retinal tear before the detachment occurs.

The peripheral retina is better nourished by the retinal vessels (the macula depends more on the choroidal circulation) and is able to withstand deterioration from detachment for a much longer time than can the macula. In fact, successful reattachment of a peripheral detachment will usually restore essentially normal peripheral vision.

GENERAL POSTOPERATIVE ADVICE

The patient who has recovered from a retinal detachment should have a sufficiently strong bond sealing his retinal hole so that this particular area is stronger than the normal eye. Unfortunately, other areas of the retina in the same or fellow eye may be affected by the same genetic vitreoretinal degenerative changes that are responsible for the great majority of retinal detachments. In fact, about 10% of fellow eyes will develop a future detachment, and perhaps 10% of apparently successfully operated eyes will suffer new holes and redetachment. Obviously, these figures are extremely general and subject to wide variation in individual cases. Nevertheless, the possibility of future detachment is so great that both the patient and his general physician must be aware of the importance of the two classic symptoms. Either the sudden onset of many new floating spots or the progression of a field defect from the periphery warrants emergency evaluation by an ophthalmologist. In addition, routine inspection of *both* retinas is proper at intervals determined by the condition of the vitreous and retina (perhaps every 6 to 12 months).

Restriction of physical activity or of use of the eyes after convalescence is not warranted. Subsequent retinal detachments, if any, will result from internal vitreoretinal stresses and are unlikely to be caused by normal activity.

SUMMARY

Every year 1 in 10,000 persons will develop a blind eye from retinal detachment—unless the condition is detected and treated sufficiently early. This uncommon and insidious condition usually succeeds in blinding the eye unless it is foiled by an alert physician.

RECOMMENDED READING

Havener, W.H., and Gloeckner, S.L.: Atlas of diagnostic techniques and treatment of retinal detachment, St. Louis, 1967, The C.V. Mosby Co.

chapter 19   Uveitis

The uveal tract is composed of the choroid, ciliary body, and iris. It is highly vascular and contributes significantly to the nutrition of the eye, being solely responsible for aqueous secretion and maintenance of the rods and cones. Inflammation of the uveal tract (uveitis) is a common and serious disease, leading often to blindness (see Plate 27). Unfortunately, it is poorly understood. Beyond doubt, granulomatous organisms, protozoa, nematodes, fungi, certain viruses, trauma, and allergic sensitization are all capable of producing uveitis. However, the overwhelming majority of cases of uveitis cannot be certainly diagnosed as to cause. The ophthalmoscopic appearances of uveitis are usually not sufficiently distinctive to permit etiologic diagnosis through observation. In general, the management of uveitis consists of a careful medical evaluation of the patient, specific therapy if a definite cause is uncovered, or nonspecific cycloplegic and corticosteroid treatment, which will usually reduce the extent of permanent scarring.

ETIOLOGY

The following is a brief description of the various possible causes of uveitis. It is appropriate to repeat that only a very small proportion of cases can be proved to be due to such a specific cause. Nevertheless, search for such causes is our responsibility when we are confronted with a severe case of uveitis.

Toxoplasmosis. Toxoplasmosis is believed to cause 10% to 15% of uveitis in the United States. It may be acquired transplacentally, as well as postnatally. It has a predilection to involve the macula (Fig. 19-1), often bilaterally, and may cause characteristic intracranial calcification and central nervous system disorders. Adults may also suffer from toxoplasmic chorioretinitis. Toxoplasmin skin tests and the methylene blue serum test are used in diagnosis, but they may be difficult to interpret, since a considerable proportion (up to one third of rural inhabitants) of the population have positive tests because of previous subclinical infection. Sulfonamide therapy and pyrimethamine (Daraprim) therapy are helpful, although pyrimethamine is quite toxic.

Histoplasmosis. Histoplasmosis is a widespread, usually asymptomatic disease that has been incriminated as the most frequent cause of uveitis in the midwestern United States. A typical patient with histoplasmosis has one or more small focal lesions, commonly near or affecting the macula. Localized choroidal hemorrhages may surround the active lesion. Recurrences may appear immediately adjacent to an old scar. The diagnostic value of a positive skin test is not great because of the high proportion of positive

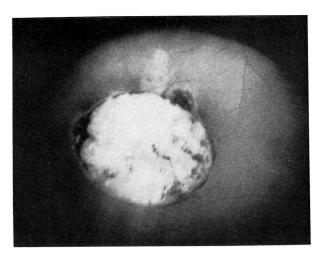

Fig. 19-1. This punched-out lesion in the macula is an old chorioretinitis originating in infancy. Within this scar the retina is destroyed. The patient has therefore irreparably lost her central vision.

tests among the general population. Although amphotericin B therapy is somewhat effective in treatment of systemic histoplasmosis, it is sufficiently toxic that the treatment may be worse than the disease. Systemic corticosteroid therapy is recommended for presumed histoplasmic maculopathy.

Syphilis. Syphilis, congenital or acquired, may cause a disseminated chorioretinitis or an iridocyclitis. Although it may be an isolated disorder, the cutaneous lesions of secondary syphilis may coexist and will be helpful in diagnosis. A serologic test for syphilis should be performed as part of the uveitis workup. Syphilitic uveitis sometimes responds dramatically to penicillin.

Tuberculosis. Tuberculosis causes destructive granulomatous intraocular lesions. Strangely, patients in tuberculosis hospitals rarely had uveitis. Formerly, every patient with uveitis who had a positive skin test or inactive pulmonary nodule was assumed to have a tuberculous uveitis. Obviously this assumption is invalid. Positive diagnosis is practically impossible without enucleation of the eye. If no other cause can be found, patients with positive skin tests or x-ray findings may be given isoniazid, streptomycin, or para-aminosalicylic acid as a therapeutic trial. Since the high doses of corticosteroids used routinely in nonspecific therapy for uveitis are contraindicated in patients with tuberculosis, evaluation for this disease assumes added significance.

Sarcoid. Sarcoid may cause a nodular iritis that is somewhat characteristic. Biopsy of involved lymph glands, x-ray examination of the chest and hands, and determination of the albumin/globulin ratio help in the diagnosis. Relatively small amounts of systemic corticosteroid often are markedly beneficial.

Nematodes. Nematodes, particularly the dog ascarid, have been demonstrated in eyes enucleated for severe uveitis. Children are more often found to be affected than adults (perhaps because their eyes are enucleated for suspicion of retinoblastoma, whereas this tumor does not occur in adults). The parasites are not found in the child's feces.

Fungi. Fungi cause a slow but inexorable destruction of the eye. The portal of entry is usually via trauma caused by a plant substance (such as a thorn) or a farm implement. Such injuries should *not* be treated with cortisone, inasmuch as such treatment markedly reduces the natural defense mechanisms against fungus growth.

Herpes zoster. Herpes zoster ocular involvement practically always includes a severe iritis. Diagnosis is easily made from the characteristic skin lesions. The side of the tip of the nose is often affected simultaneously with the eye, since the nasociliary nerve innervates both structures. The severe surface scarring may be reduced considerably by antibiotics (to prevent secondary bacterial corneal and skin infection), cycloplegics, and corticosteroids. Although corticosteroid therapy is contraindicated in acute herpes simplex corneal infection, herpes zoster seems to respond favorably to corticosteroid treatment.

Traumatic uveitis. Traumatic uveitis is extremely common and follows almost all ocular contusions of any magnitude, intraocular operations, severe corneal lacerations or burns, and so on. It responds rapidly to cycloplegic treatment, so that the shorter-acting cycloplegics such as homatropine may be used (four times daily until recovery) rather than atropine. Neglected corneal injury is a particularly common cause of traumatic iritis, which is recognized by the small pupil, limbal flush, excessive photophobia, or pain not relieved by topical anesthetics. Obviously, if possible, the primary cause (for example, corneal foreign body) must be eliminated before routine treatment methods are followed.

Rheumatic uveitis. Rheumatic uveitis is frequently seen in association with severe arthritic disorders. Its management does not differ from that of other cases of uveitis of unknown cause. The infection theory of rheumatism and uveitis formerly led to the extraction of innumerable teeth, tonsils, and reproductive organs. Although careful examination of these and other parts of the body should be included in the uveitis examination, no surgery is warranted unless the diseased organ is so badly infected that its removal would be advised even if the patient did not have uveitis.

Sympathetic uveitis. Sympathetic uveitis is an extremely rare condition supposedly due to allergy of an individual to his own uveal pigment. It follows a penetrating injury of the uveal tract, especially if the ciliary body is involved (perhaps 0.5% of such injuries), and is bilateral. Enucleation of a hopelessly damaged eye within several weeks of the injury will prevent sympathetic disease of the good eye. If injury is not too severe, and if the eye can be salvaged with some hope of useful vision, enucleation is absolutely contraindicated. Once sympathetic uveitis has started, enucleation of the injured eye does not alter the course of the disease. Prolonged corticosteroid therapy is helpful in treatment of sympathetic uveitis; however, corticosteroid therapy should *not* be started immediately after penetrating injury in the mistaken hope of preventing sympathetic uveitis, because resistance to infection is significantly decreased by such treatment.

Other diseases. Numerous other diseases have been found in association with uveitis.

Certainly, if any significant illness is found, it should be treated appropriately. Assumption of a causal relationship with the uveitis may not be warranted. The ophthalmologist will often refer a patient with uveitis to his general physician for a thorough examination, including such special tests as have been mentioned.

THERAPY

The nonspecific therapy for iritis is primarily good *dilatation* of the pupil (Fig. 19-2). On the first visit the pupil is dilated (Fig. 19-3) and synechiae are broken (Fig. 19-4) by

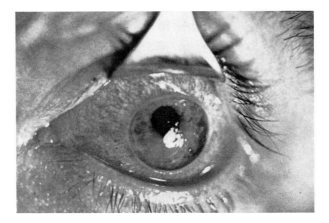

Fig. 19-2. This is a severe iritis with secondary glaucoma. The pupil is irregular and does not dilate well even with atropine. Obviously, it is most important to differentiate this condition from acute angle-closure glaucoma, the therapy for which is constriction of the pupil.

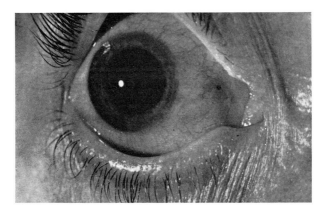

Fig. 19-3. On diagnosis of iritis, the pupil should be maximally dilated with atropine and phenylephrine hydrochloride, as illustrated. Dilatation should be maintained until all signs of inflammation have subsided, which usually requires several weeks.

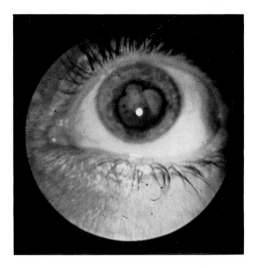

Fig. 19-4. In iridocyclitis, adhesions may develop between the pupil margin and the lens. These adhesions cause the pupil contour to be irregular, particularly when dilated. Intensive use of cycloplegics and mydriatics may break these adhesions and restore the pupil to normal. Inflammatory deposits may also be seen on the anterior lens and posterior cornea.

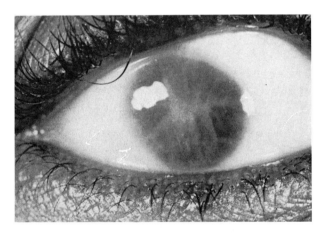

Fig. 19-5. This shrunken, blind eye is the end result of severe uveitis. Note the dense gray membranes that occlude the pupil and seal the iris to the lens. Proper cycloplegic and corticosteroid therapy will often avert such a tragedy. Other medications, such as antibiotics, are not helpful, and their use may delay proper therapy and permit serious scarring to develop.

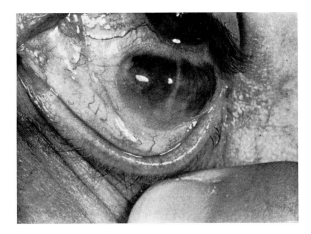

Fig. 19-6. Inflammatory thinning of the lower sclera has permitted herniation of the uveal tract (staphyloma), which appears as a bluish black bulge. A variety of such unpleasant complications accompany severe rheumatic uveitis, which is a disease one is well advised to refer to a specialist.

repeated office instillation of atropine, phenylephrine hydrochloride, or cyclopentolate hydrochloride. Thereafter, 1% atropine and 10% phenylephrine hydrochloride, three times daily, generally suffice. Topical corticosteroids administered every 2 hours while the patient is awake are very helpful. Unusually severe iritis may be helped by systemic corticosteroids. Except in the unusual cases with a specific cause, antibiotic therapy of iritis is absolutely worthless (Fig. 19-5). Cycloplegic therapy must be continued until the attack subsides. The physician who undertakes to treat a patient with severe iritis must be aware of the major complications of iritis (such as secondary glaucoma) that may contribute to an unfortunate outcome (Fig. 19-6).

Nonspecific therapy of chorioretinitis ordinarily requires fairly large doses of systemic corticosteroids. The size of the dose employed depends on the severity of the lesion, whether it is located near a vital structure (such as the macula), and whether a therapeutic response is obtained.

The duration and intensity of treatment are therefore guided by the ophthalmologic findings. Naturally, the patient with active tuberculosis, peptic ulcers, mental instability, or other corticosteroid contraindications will be treated with special precautions and only if absolutely necessary.

Cycloplegic and corticosteroid therapy for uveitis, although nonspecific, will greatly reduce the amount of permanent scarring and may make the difference between a seeing eye and a blind one.

chapter 20 Disorders of the Eyelids

With the exception of positional defects, diseases of the lids (and conjunctiva) are similar to general dermatologic disorders. Infections, allergies, dermatoses of unknown origin, degenerations, and neoplasms, as well as positional defects, affect the lids.

BACTERIAL INFECTIONS

Marginal blepharitis. Marginal blepharitis refers to inflammation of the lid edges, especially of the glands at the base of the lashes. It is common, persistent, irritating, and unsightly. Staphylococci are the most common offending organisms and are often superimposed on a *Pityrosporon ovale* infection of the lid margins. Characteristically, there is a fine crusting (Fig. 20-1) deposited at the base of the lashes, the lid edges are often reddened and slightly thickened, lashes may fall out, and the conjunctiva is often hyper-

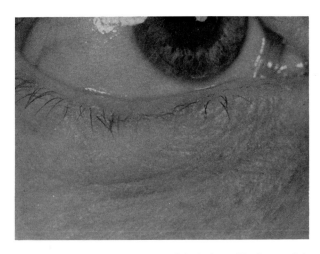

Fig. 20-1. Very slight granular crusting at the base of the lashes will often explain annoying chronic irritation of the eyes as being due to superficial infection.

emic. The severity of the process depends on the virulence of the organism and individual resistance. (Leukemic and diabetic patients sometimes develop severely destructive lesions.)

Therapy requires thorough cleaning and should include hot, moist soaks followed by removal of all crusts and discharge (Fig. 20-2) with a cloth or cotton applicator. Ointment vehicles are used for the antibiotic and should be applied to the entire lid margin. The choice of antibiotic depends on the general principles discussed in Chapter 23 and usually

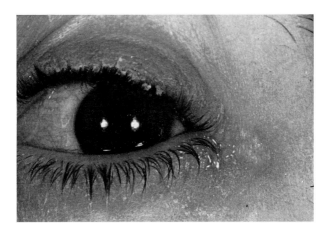

Fig. 20-2. Acute marginal blepharitis has caused this prominent crusting of the lid margins and lashes and the macerated area of the outer angle. Conjunctival redness and discharge are also present. Before antibiotic application, all these crusts should be scrubbed off mechanically. Hot soaks greatly facilitate removal of crusts.

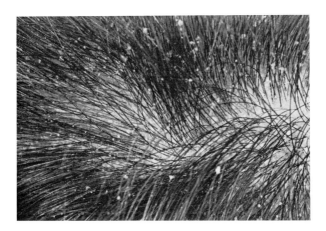

Fig. 20-3. Dandruff is often the source of reinfection in chronic marginal blepharitis and must be eliminated.

should be a broad-spectrum mixture of the drugs used externally only (for example, neomycin, bacitracin, and polymyxin). If dandruff (Fig. 20-3) is present, it will be a source of reinfection unless eliminated. Marginal blepharitis is a stubborn disease and requires morning and night treatment daily for at least 1 week. Recurrences are common and require treatment.

Sty. A sty (hordeolum) is a localized abscess of the glands about the hair follicles and therefore is located in the anterior part of the lid (Fig. 20-4). Most sties are found in patients with marginal blepharitis, treatment of which will be prophylactic against development of further sties. Prompt resolution of most sties will occur if hot compresses are used for 5 to 10 minutes every several hours, followed by application of antibiotic ointment. Because the thin skin macerates readily and permits spontaneous drainage, incisions are practically never necessary to evacuate a sty. In fact, cutting and squeezing is likely to spread the infection and produce a lid cellulitis (Fig. 20-5).

Chalazion. A chalazion (Fig. 20-6) results from blockage of the meibomian glands lying deep in the tarsal plate. Chalazia are often found in patients with marginal blepharitis and probably originate when the gland orifices are blocked by infection. Hot, moist compresses for 10 minutes four times daily will cure about half of the patients with acute chalazia of less than 1 week's duration. Topical antibiotics are not useful in the treatment of chalazia except in a prophylactic sense to cure obvious external infection and prevent new chalazia from developing. When the inflammation and pain have subsided, a persistent mass (Fig. 20-7), if present, will remain for many months and may need to be removed by incision and curettage.

Dacryocystitis. Dacryocystitis (Fig. 20-8) (inflammation of the lacrimal sac) causes

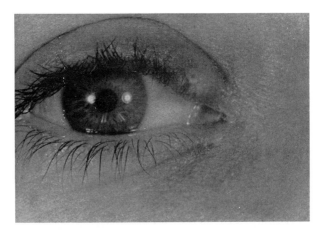

Fig. 20-4. This rather large hordeolum (sty) is simply an abscess of the glands at the base of the lashes. Note that infectious material has been deposited on the lower lid below the lesion. In this fashion, bacteria can be spread to adjacent glands and cause additional hordeola.

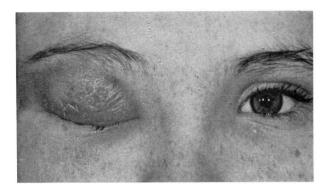

Fig. 20-5. Cellulitis of this lid resulted from unwise manipulation of a minor infection of the lid margin. The lid skin is very loose and permits free spreading of infection if the bacteria escape from infected glands. Squeezing or incising a hordeolum may provide the perfect opportunity for bacterial dissemination.

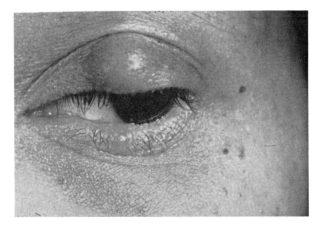

Fig. 20-6. Compare the appearance of the chalazion in the upper lid with the hordeolum in the lower lid. Note that the chalazion arises deep within the lid, whereas the hordeolum is situated on the anterior margin. Their locations directly opposite each other clearly indicate a common infectious origin.

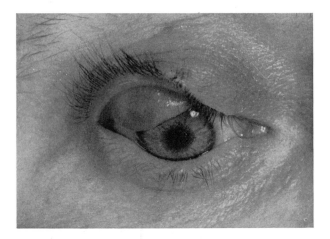

Fig. 20-7. The tarsal conjunctiva underlying a chalazion is red and inflamed. This confirmatory sign is useful in diagnosis. Eversion of the upper lid is the best way to inspect the upper tarsal conjunctiva.

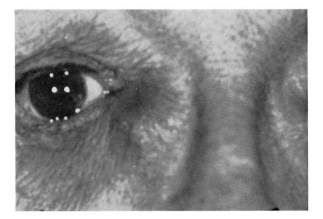

Fig. 20-8. Acute dacryocystitis is readily recognizable by the tender swelling below the inner canthus. Epiphora and mucopurulent discharge are present. Note the whiteness of the conjunctiva—this finding is important in differentiating dacryocystitis from conjunctivitis.

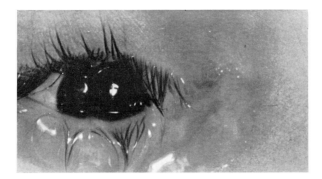

Fig. 20-9. This very large amount of mucopurulent discharge was expressed from an infected lacrimal sac by firm pressure directed into the lower inner corner of the orbit. Do not press on the side of the nose. The lacrimal sac is situated in the lacrimal fossa, which is posterior to the orbital rim. Confirmation of the diagnosis of suspected dacryocystitis is made through expression of purulent material from the sac.

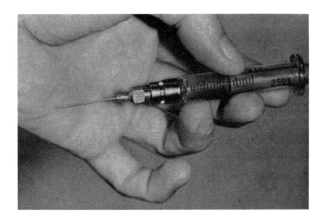

Fig. 20-10. A thin lacrimal cannula may be inserted into the punctum and threaded through the canaliculus into the lacrimal sac. Irrigation of the sac removes infected debris and permits instillation of an antibiotic solution. Often the question arises as to whether a block of lacrimal drainage exists. An attempt to irrigate through the sac into the nose will answer this question.

considerable tearing and discharge (Fig. 20-9) that may be mistaken for inflammation of the eyelids.

The swelling of dacryocystitis is located at the far nasal aspect of the lower lid, a position where no meibomian glands exist; hence, confusion should not arise in differentiating this type of swelling from a chalazion. Sinus tumors or mucoceles may cause a similar appearance.

The immediate treatment of dacryocystitis is application of antibiotics by topical instillation into the conjunctival sac or by direct irrigation into the lacrimal sac (Fig. 20-10). In most cases the infection is secondary to obstruction of lacrimal drainage through the nasolacrimal duct. Definitive treatment requires opening of free drainage into the nose, either by probing through the nasolacrimal duct (usually successful in children suffering from congenital stenosis of the lower end of the nasolacrimal duct) or by surgical creation of a new opening between the lacrimal sac and the nose (dacryocystorhinostomy, usually necessary in adults with acquired blockage of the nasolacrimal duct).

VIRAL INFECTIONS

Herpes simplex. Herpes simplex is an acute viral disease resulting in typical superficial clear cutaneous vesicles that heal without scarring. If these vesicles occur on the lid, care should be taken not to inoculate their contents onto the cornea, because a dendritic ulcer may develop.

A dendritic corneal ulcer is the zigzag surface lesion pathognomonic of herpes simplex. Herpes simplex corneal ulcers are common, and their presence should be suspected in any spontaneously developing, persistent red eye with corneal irregularity. Fluorescein staining is often helpful in recognition of such lesions. Dendritic corneal ulcers are stubborn, recurrent, scarring infections that cause a great deal of difficulty and are therefore best managed by referral to an ophthalmologist.

The differential diagnosis, as well as the proper treatment of corneal lesions, is difficult and complicated. Because even slight scarring of the central cornea will result in permanent visual handicap, referral of corneal disease is a wise policy.

A particularly serious mistake is the use of topical corticosteroids in the treatment of a red eye due to acute herpes simplex corneal infection (dendritic ulcer). Corticosteroid

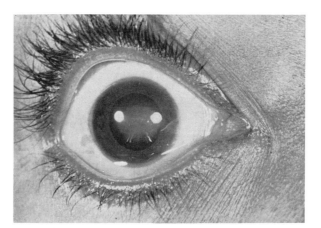

Fig. 20-11. Disciform keratopathy is a gray, opaque, corneal thickening usually caused by a severe herpetic infection. Corticosteroid therapy is contraindicated in herpes simplex keratitis because it tends to increase the severity of the lesion, with resultant extensive scarring.

treatment enhances corneal spread of the virus, resulting in extensive and disabling corneal scarring (Fig. 20-11).

Herpes zoster. Herpes zoster is best recognized by its typical unilateral trigeminal distribution (Fig. 20-12). The skin lesions are deeper than those of herpes simplex, are painful, and tend to become secondarily infected and to leave permanent scars. The eye is usually affected if the side of the tip of the nose is involved (nasociliary nerve distribution) (Fig. 20-13). Mydriatic, antibiotic, and corticosteroid ointment should be used vigorously

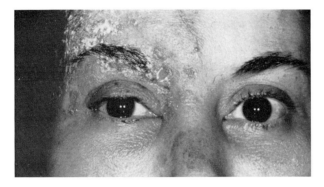

Fig. 20-12. Ophthalmic herpes zoster tends to form thick-crusted, infected lesions, with resultant deep scarring. Careful cleaning and application of antibiotic ointment will minimize this infectious scarring.

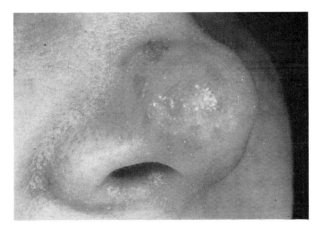

Fig. 20-13. Zoster of this portion of the nose usually means that the eye will also be involved. The nasociliary nerve supplies the side of the tip of the nose and the eye.

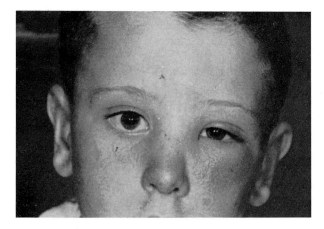

Fig. 20-14. Poison ivy dermatitis was spread to the left eyelid through rubbing with a contaminated finger. Disproportionately severe edema occurs when contact dermatitis affects the thin lid skin.

in such patients. The skin lesions should be kept clean of crusts and infection through hot soaks, mechanical cleaning, and antibiotic ointment.

Vaccinia. Vaccinia may become generalized if the patient has skin breaks (for example, scratches, eczema, or poison ivy) or may be autoinoculated through scratching. This condition may be prevented by protecting the vaccination site and by avoiding vaccination in the presence of generalized skin disorders. Should vaccinia occur on the lids, every effort should be made to avoid scuffing the cornea during cleaning and treatment, because permanent scarring results from corneal inoculation.

Acute exanthemas. The acute exanthemas of childhood often involve the lids and cause conjunctival redness. In fact, measles characteristically causes a superficial punctate keratitis.

ALLERGIES

Lid allergies are almost always of the contact type. They commonly result from such agents as cosmetics, soaps, eye medications, and industrial chemicals. Usually the typical reddened, rough, weeping, itching area is confined to the lids alone and does not extend to the rest of the face. Obviously, exceptions occur if the irritation is sufficient, as in the case of poison ivy (Fig. 20-14). Elimination of the allergen will cause symptoms to subside rapidly. Cortisone ointment will hasten relief from itching. Respiratory tract allergies, such as hay fever, may respond to desensitization and antihistamines, in contrast to contact allergies, which require identification and removal of the allergen.

DERMATOSES OF UNKNOWN CAUSE

Acne rosacea. Acne rosacea causes typical patches of dilated facial vessels and is likely to produce a keratoconjunctivitis. The result is a marginal vascularization and

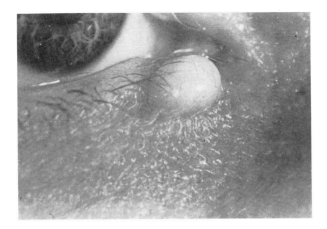

Fig. 20-15. This smooth, rounded, yellowish, discrete, subcutaneous mass is a sebaceous cyst. Excision of such a large cyst is usually desirable for cosmetic reasons. Sebaceous cysts are not malignant and do not interfere with lid function. This cyst lies immediately anterior to the lower canaliculus, which must not be damaged during removal.

scarring of the cornea, which progresses centrally with time and may eventually result in serious visual loss. The keratoconjunctivitis, as well as the skin condition, may be arrested by use of topical corticosteroids and systemic tetracyclines. Long-term therapy is necessary and must be particularly encouraged whenever the cornea is vascularized.

Atopic dermatitis. Atopic dermatitis results in annoying thickening of the lid skin. Surprisingly, it rarely interferes with lid closure. Occasionally these patients will develop rapidly maturing cataracts. In the early stages vigorous corticosteroid therapy may arrest progress of the skin disease and the cataracts.

Erythema multiforme. Erythema multiforme (Stevens-Johnson syndrome) often damages the conjunctiva severely, resulting in deficient lubrication and permanent corneal scarring. During the acute stage of such mucocutaneous diseases, any eye involvement should be treated vigorously with topical antibiotics (prophylactic against secondary infection) and corticosteroids.

DEGENERATIONS

Sebaceous cysts. Sebaceous cysts of the eyelids are common and appear as yellowish or gray, smooth, rounded subcutaneous nodules (Fig. 20-15). They are especially frequent near the lid margin. Simple incision is usually inadequate therapy, because recurrence is usual. These cysts may easily be dissected with the patient under local anesthesia. They tend to be adherent by means of vascular fibrous bands and require some sharp dissection. Except for the thinnest central portion, the overlying skin can be freed, preserved, and sutured (if necessary) to close the defect, leaving practically no scar.

Blepharochalasis. Blepharochalasis is a redundancy of the skin of the upper lid, which droops down, sometimes interfering with vision. This condition is *not* ptosis,

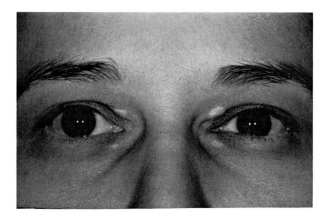

Fig. 20-16. Xanthelasma palpebrarum plaques are confined to the eyelids and are circumscribed, slightly elevated, yellowish, and slowly progressive. Multiple foci appear and are often roughly symmetrical. Xanthelasma palpebrarum causes no local damage except of a cosmetic nature.

because only the skin is involved, and not the tarsus. Blepharochalasis usually has a hereditary basis, although it may follow severe lid edema. Excision of redundant skin is curative. (In general, the inexperienced surgeon would do well to seek expert advice before excising lid skin in any given patient. Ectropion is a nasty complication of such surgery.)

Xanthelasma. Xanthelasma is characterized by slightly elevated, yellowish plaques situated often symmetrically in the lids (Fig. 20-16). A gradual increase in the size and number of lesions may occur. Cautery or excision is effective, but if the lesions are large, skin grafts may be necessary.

NEOPLASMS

Papilloma. A papilloma may be sessile or pedunculated and often arises near the lid margin (Fig. 20-17). Excision, including the base, will eliminate those of unsightly size. Until experience has taught the physician to differentiate benign from malignant lesions, a pathologic report is helpful in ruling out carcinoma (Fig. 20-18). Surgical procedures involving the lid margin are likely to leave unsightly notches if the precepts against excising more than half the lid thickness are violated.

Hemangioma. Treatment of a hemangioma of the lids may be unsatisfactory. Unless they are enlarging rapidly, such tumors in infants are best left alone, because they almost invariably spontaneously shrink. Carbon dioxide snow, injection of sclerosing solutions, and radiation are sometimes recommended but often cause more scarring and complications than allowing the lesion to regress by itself. Almost unbelievably large hemangiomas may virtually disappear within a few years.

Basal cell carcinoma. Basal cell carcinoma (Fig. 20-19) of the lids is easily treated surgically in the early stages, and any suspicious lesions should therefore be removed

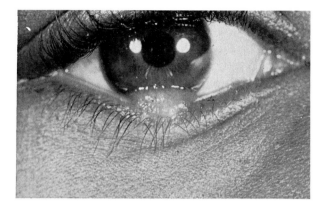

Fig. 20-17. The lower lid margin shows a recurrent benign sessile papilloma. Removal of papillomas must always include the base, or recurrence may be anticipated. If the full thickness of the lid margin is involved, simple excision of the papilloma may leave an unsightly notch, necessitating plastic reconstruction.

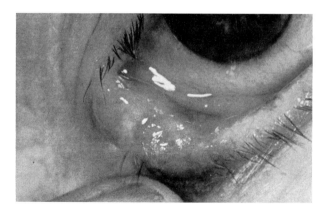

Fig. 20-18. Infiltrative lid tumors are usually malignant. This tumor is a malignant melanoma. If such a tumor is seen early, wide excision of the involved lid, with plastic reconstruction, is preferable to exenteration of the orbit. Such surgical specimens should always be sent for pathologic diagnosis.

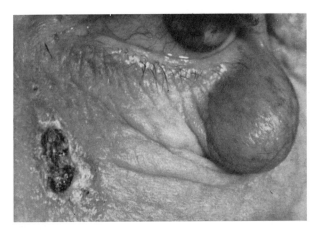

Fig. 20-19. The large lesion on the right is simply a huge sebaceous cyst. The left lesion has been present for over a year, is gradually growing, has indurated edges and a crusted surface, and tends to bleed when the crust is removed. Wide and complete excision should be done for such a typical basal cell carcinoma and should include a portion of the underlying orbicularis muscle. If the skin edges will not approximate without tension, a full-thickness skin graft will prevent ectropion.

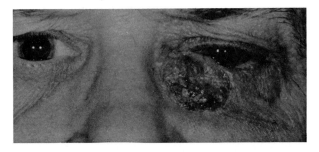

Fig. 20-20. Irritated areas on the side of the nose are often ascribed to spectacle pressure and may be neglected for unbelievably long periods of time. Although early removal of this carcinoma would have been quite simple, at this advanced stage radical excision of the lower lid and inner canthus is necessary for surgical cure. Radiation therapy is preferable to surgery in management of such a large carcinoma in this position.

while small. Persistent, crusting ulcerations should be strongly suspected of being neoplastic, especially if they occasionally bleed. Patients will often disregard a carcinoma on the side of the nose (Fig. 20-20), thinking that it is merely irritation from the spectacle nosepiece. This type of carcinoma often has a smooth gray surface supplied with multiple tiny capillaries, is slightly elevated and firm, and overhangs a central excavation if ulcerated.

Phakomatoses. Phakomatoses include von Recklinghausen's neurofibromatosis, tuberous sclerosis, and the encephalotrigeminal angiomatosis of Sturge-Weber syndrome. They involve the lids and facial skin with large, redundant neurofibromas, sebaceous

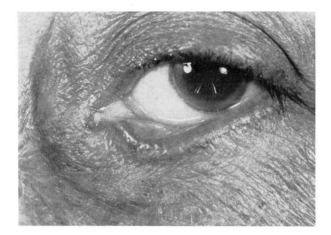

Fig. 20-21. This cicatricial ectropion resulted from a burn. The lower lid has been pulled away from the eye, and the punctum is not in proper apposition to the tear lake. The bright reflections along the lower part of the eye come from a pool of tears that have gathered in the lower cul-de-sac.

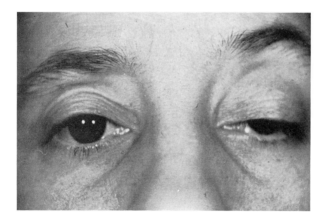

Fig. 20-22. Congenital maldevelopment of the levator muscle was responsible for this ptosis. Note the absence of the skin fold of the left upper lid. The normal skin fold is due to attachments of the levator muscle to the lid skin about a centimeter above the lid margin. The left eyebrow is raised in an attempt to lift the lid above the pupil.

adenomas, or capillary hemangiomas, respectively. Such lesion have more significance as indicators of general disease than local importance. The eyes and central nervous system are particularly likely to be involved by the phakomas.

POSITIONAL DEFECTS

Ectropion. Ectropion refers to an outward rolling of the lids (Fig. 20-21). It may be due to traction, as in cases of scarring, or to unwise excision of too much skin without grafting during removal of lid lesions, or it may be the result of severe burns. Relaxation of the lid structures with aging may permit the lids to sag outward. Paralysis of the seventh nerve will also cause ectropion. Regardless of the cause, poor apposition of the lower lid to the globe interferes with proper lacrimal drainage, causing epiphora and a tendency toward infection. Drying of the exposed conjunctiva and cornea occurs. Plastic surgical repair is indicted in ectropion of significant magnitude.

Entropion. Entropion, or inward rolling of the lid, is due to spasmodic contraction of the bundles of orbicularis muscle nearest the lid margin and is particularly likely to occur in the relaxed lids of elderly patients. Because of corneal abrasion by the in-turned lashes, entropion is uncomfortable and annoying to the patient. Pending surgical correction, the lid may be held in proper position by pulling it downward and fastening it to the cheek with a small piece of tape.

Ptosis. Ptosis is a drooping of the upper lid and is most often due to congenital defects of the levator muscle (Fig. 20-22). Third-nerve paralysis causes ptosis, as does interference with the sympathetic innervation (Horner's syndrome).

The ptosis of myasthenia gravis becomes worse with fatigue. Chronic progressive external ophthalmoplegia is a hereditary degenerative process that causes slowly developing weakness of the extraocular and levator muscles. Resection of the levator muscle will cosmetically and functionally improve many cases of congenital and acquired ptosis.

chapter 21 Errors of Refraction

Every person has some type of refractive error, muscle imbalance, or other slight ocular imperfection. Refractive errors are clinically significant only when they are severe enough to require correction. The purpose of refractive correction is to relieve symptoms. No secondary therapeutic benefits to the eye accrue from the wearing of glasses (with the exception of refractive correction of accommodative strabismus). The correction of the majority of small refractive errors would be purely a nuisance and an expense to the patient.

SYMPTOMS

Only two symptoms produced by refractive errors deserve correction, and these two symptoms may be used as reliable criteria for identification and referral of patients who are likely to benefit from such correction. These symptoms are *reduced visual acuity* and *chronic discomfort related to use of the eyes*. No other symptoms or problems are likely to be corrected by glasses.

Objective measurement of visual acuity by means of reading charts is the only reliable method. Asking the patient whether he has trouble seeing is completely unreliable, because gradual loss of vision is rarely recognized until acuity has declined to surprisingly low levels. Children, in particular, do not know whether their vision is subnormal, for they have no previous visual experience for comparison.

Measurement of visual acuity is an incredibly good screening test. It is easily, quickly, and accurately performed with simple and inexpensive equipment by personnel who require a very small amount of training. It will detect a great variety of ocular, central nervous system, or systemic diseases (in contrast to such a test as tonometry, which will identify only glaucoma). In a study of more than 1000 patients, I found that reduction of visual acuity to 20/40 or less in at least one eye was present in 80% of patients who had demonstrable visual field defects. Furthermore, a high proportion of patients will have correctable defects that can be detected in this simple manner.

Approximately 10% of college professors and business executives will fail a test requiring them to read (with their existing glasses) 20/30 with each eye and newspaper print held at a distance of 1 foot. Myopia sufficient to require correction occurs in over 10% of the population. When this frequency is compared with the incidence of positive urine tests for phenylketonuria, one wonders at the sense of perspective of physicians who do not include visual acuity as part of their routine examination. *Every physical examination should include visual acuity measurement.* Visual acuity of 20/40 or less in either eye requires evaluation.

The second symptom due to refractive error, chronic discomfort related to use of the eyes, may take many forms. Headache is common and may be ocular, orbital, frontal, occipital, or almost anywhere. Ocular fatigue, burning, and irritation (often referred to as "eyestrain") are also frequently produced by uncorrected refractive errors. Since refractive errors do not appear suddenly, they do not cause symptoms that are of definitely recent onset (for example, "The pain in my eye started last week"). An exception would be discomfort related to use of the eyes appearing simultaneously with greatly intensified ocular work, such as preceding an examination.

Reduced acuity and ocular discomfort are *not* to be considered solely symptoms of refractive error. Serious ocular, general, or functional disorders often cause such complaints. Frequently ophthalmologists see patients with these symptoms that have persisted despite the prescription of glasses after a nonmedical examination. If this delay in seeking medical care has been detrimental to the patient, the ophthalmologist may doubt the quality of the previous care.

ETIOLOGY

Refractive errors are due to faulty coordination of the curvatures of the cornea and lens, the refractive index of the lens, and the length of the eye. These factors of importance to the total refractive strength of the eye are subject to considerable physiologic variation, which is determined by inheritance. Disease, injury, and degenerative changes may also cause refractive errors.

Causes of refractive error include diabetes, sulfonamide toxicity, cataract, and the effect of tranquilizers. Uncontrolled diabetes causes rapid changes in refraction, myopia being associated with hyperglycemia, and hyperopia with hypoglycemia. Marked changes in refractive error occurring within days or weeks are not physiologic and arouse suspicion of diabetes or drug toxicity. New glasses should not be prescribed until diabetic control has been stable for at least several weeks.

A rare patient reacts to sulfonamide by developing a variable myopia. Acetazolamide (Diamox) may cause transient myopia. An osmotic imbalance of the lens is the presumed cause.

Nuclear cataracts increase the density of the central lens and commonly cause a slow increase in myopia. Usually this error can be corrected with glasses for several years before surgery becomes necessary. Cortical cataracts may cause hyperopia but are usually too irregular to permit correction with glasses.

Many of the tranquilizers and antihypertensive drugs reduce accommodative amplitude, thereby causing blurred near vision. If this blurring is sufficiently annoying, the drug must be given in a lower dosage or discontinued.

ACCOMMODATION

Accommodation, the increase in refractive power required to focus the eye on near objects, is achieved by increasing the strength of the lens. A young lens is enclosed within an elastic capsule that tends to force the soft lens structure into a more spherical shape, thereby increasing its curvature and refractive strength. Opposing the capsular elasticity is the constant pull of the zonular fibers, which are inserted around the lens equator and hold it in proper position before the pupil. Zonular traction tends to flatten the lens, thereby reducing its refractive strength. The amount of zonular traction may be varied by the

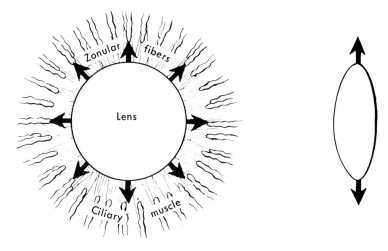

Fig. 21-1. When accommodation is relaxed, zonular pull flattens the lens.

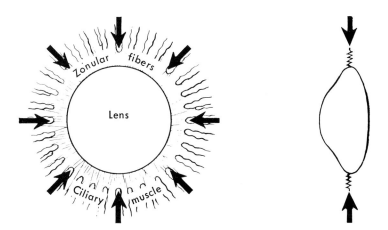

Fig. 21-2. Contraction of the ciliary muscle relaxes zonular tension and permits the lens to assume its more spherical, accommodated shape.

ciliary muscle, which encircles the zonular fibers. Contraction of the ciliary muscle relaxes zonular tension, thereby permitting the lens capsule to increase the lens curvature and strength (Figs. 21-1 and 21-2).

When the ciliary muscle is completely relaxed, the refractive power of an eye is at its lowest possible strength and cannot be further decreased. When the ciliary muscle is maximally contracted, the refractive power of an eye is at its greatest strength. Between these two extremes, the refractive strength of the eye is automatically adjusted for best vision. The amount of accommodation possessed by a person gradually decreases, and after 40 years of age becomes annoyingly inadequate for comfortable vision at different distances. By the age of 60 years, the lens has become so inelastic that no changes in its strength are possible.

EMMETROPIA

The refractive error of an eye is measured when accommodation is completely re-laxed, that is, when the ciliary muscle is not working. Without accommodation, an emmetropic eye is focused perfectly for distance; parallel rays of light striking the eye are focused to a point on the retina (Fig. 21-3). Such a person sees clearly in the distance with no effort, and with the aid of accommodation may focus on closer objects. Emmetropia causes no symptoms, although, of course, even the most perfect eye will tire with prolonged use and general bodily fatigue.

TYPES OF REFRACTIVE ERRORS

Myopia. A myopic (nearsighted) eye has an excessive amount of refractive power and hence brings light from distant objects to a focus in front of the retina. Since the eye cannot reduce this excessive power in any way, the person with myopia is unable to see

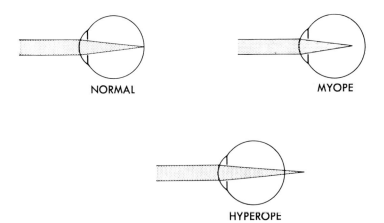

NORMAL   MYOPE

HYPEROPE

Fig. 21-3. Distant light focuses perfectly on the retina of an unaccommodated normal (emmetropic) eye but focuses in front of the retina in myopia and behind the retina in hyperopia.

clearly in the distance. Near vision requires greater refractive strength than distant vision; hence, the person with myopia will be in focus for some near point (depending on the amount of myopia) without the aid of accommodation. He may also accommodate, thereby focusing yet closer.

The only symptom caused by myopia is inability to see clearly in the distance without glasses. Myopia does not contribute to ocular discomfort, headaches, or fatigue with use of the eyes.

As children grow, their eyes tend to become less farsighted, or more nearsighted. Myopia usually first becomes evident in the first years of school and progresses at such a rate that new glasses are required every year or two. After adolescence, when the child stops growing, the myopia usually becomes relatively stationary. Use or nonuse of the eye does not affect the rate of development of myopia. About 1% of persons with myopia have serious ocular deterioration that may progress to retinal detachment or macular degeneration. This degenerative myopia is not identified by the strength of glasses required for correction but by its ophthalmoscopic appearance (see Plate 28). The eyeball has an elongated, egg-shaped contour that requires strong minus lenses to observe the posterior pole and less strong lenses to focus the periphery. A "washed-out," dirty gray-orange, irregularly pigmented chorioretinal appearance is seen in moderately advanced stages (Fig. 21-4). Selectively intense degeneration occurs about the disc, in the macula, and in the far peripheral retina. The "myopic crescent" is a zone of choroidal and retinal atropy that exposes the sclera to view. It is usually situated just temporal to the disc but may

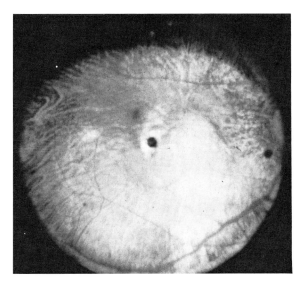

Fig. 21-4. Extensive chorioretinal pigmentary degeneration reveals markedly sclerotic choroidal vessels and leaves scattered, irregular, dirty pigmentation. Degenerative myopia is an ophthalmoscopic diagnosis and not a refractive designation.

extend entirely around it. Rather severe chorioretinal deterioration may gradually develop at the macula, which frequently appears as a very heavily pigmented black or reddish area. Peripheral cystic and atrophic changes, as well as vitreous liquefaction, contribute to the much higher incidence of retinal detachment in eyes subject to myopic degeneration.

No treatment for degenerative myopia is effective. It has a definite hereditary factor and progresses despite any known management. The misconception of providing weaker glasses than are required results only in poor distance vision. "Exercises" will not cure myopia, although they are widely heralded by quacks. Diet and vitamins are of no effect. Because his eyes are more fragile than normal, the uncommon patient with degenerative myopia is well advised to avoid blows on the head, such as occur in diving, boxing, or football. The patient with simple myopia and a healthy retina should *not* be subjected to any such restrictions, because such eyes are no more liable to injury than anyone else's.

Hyperopia. A hyperopic (farsighted) eye has insufficient refractive power to focus light on the retina, whether the light originates from distant or near objects. Without the aid of accommodation, a person with hyperopia is unable to see clearly at any distance. Fortunately, additional refractive power may be obtained through accommodation. Most young persons with hyperopia are able to see clearly in the distance or close up, but to do so, they must exert more accommodative effort than does a person with emmetropia. If the hyperopic refractive error is large enough, the constantly required excessive accommodative effect will cause discomfort and unduly rapid fatigue directly related to use of the eyes, especially for near work. Very large hyperopic errors may exceed available accommodation and cause reduced visual acuity. As accommodation is gradually lost in the late thirties and early forties, hyperopia becomes progressively less compensated and finally forces the patient to wear presbyopic correction earlier than would be required for a person with emmetropia.

Anisometropia. Anisometropia refers to a difference in the focus of the two eyes. Refractive errors tend to be symmetrical, so that a comparable degree of myopia or hyperopia will exist in each eye. An infrequent patient has considerable difference in the focus of his two eyes. Because accommodation cannot be exerted unequally by the two eyes, this difference in focus cannot be compensated, and the patient is forced to use one eye or the other but never both in clear focus simultaneously. The anisometropic patient commonly experiences discomfort and fatigue with use of his eyes. Suppression of the vision of one eye may develop.

Astigmatism. Optical surfaces in cameras, telescopes, and other precision instruments have spherical curves that are exactly equal in all meridians. Unfortunately, the human cornea often lacks this perfection and is more curved in one direction than another. This unequal curvature is called astigmatism (*a*, without; *stigma*, point) because it distorts the focus of light rays so that they are not clear at any point. Astigmatism cannot be eliminated by accommodation or by any other effort on the part of the patient. Either hyperopia or myopia may coexist with astigmatism. The symptoms of astigmatism are blurred vision and discomfort with use of the eyes.

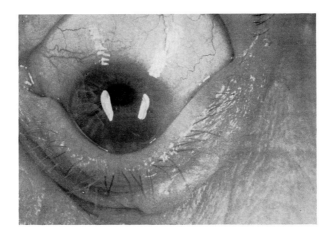

Fig. 21-5. The peculiar curvature of advanced keratoconus is best appreciated when the patient looks down. The lower lid then assumes the same conical curvature. Note also the peculiar appearance of the apex of the cornea, somewhat resembling a dark, translucent oil droplet.

The common, inherited form of astigmatism can be effectively corrected by optical lenses ground to neutralize the unequal curvature. Injuries to the cornea may cause, through scarring, irregular curvatures and distortions uncorrectable by lenses. This defect is termed irregular astigmatism. Another cause of irregular astigmatism is keratoconus.

Keratoconus. Keratoconus (Fig. 21-5) is an uncommon degeneration of the central cornea occurring during adolescence. Marked thinning occurs, and the cornea assumes a conical contour that causes serious optical distortion. In late stages the cornea may lose its transparency. No cause is known. The process is usually bilateral.

Ordinarily, spectacles do not adequately correct the high astigmatism of keratoconus. By substituting a smooth front surface for the irregular cone, contact lenses effectively restore vision as long as the cornea remains transparent. If corneal scarring develops, corneal transplantation is necessary.

Presbyopia. Presbyopia means ''the sight of age'' and refers to the problems caused by loss of accommodation. Presbyopia does not alter the preexisting refractive errors of myopia, hyperopia, or astigmatism but progressively reduces the ability to accommodate for near work. Since the person with presbyopia cannot change focus from distant to near, this change must be accomplished by glasses—hence the bifocal, with a lens of different top and bottom strength for far and near vision, respectively.

REFRACTION

Refraction is the clinical measurement of the optical faults of the nonaccommodated eye. A very close objective estimate of the refractive error of an eye may be made with the aid of *retinoscopy* (Fig. 21-6). Retinoscopy is the observation of the movement of focused

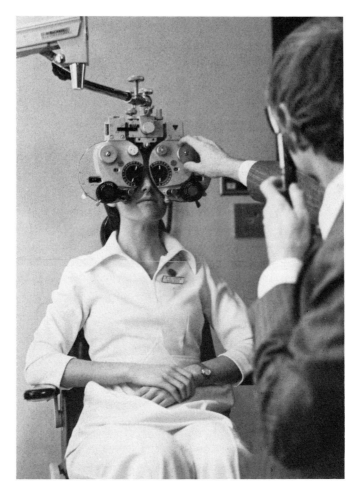

Fig. 21-6. Use of a retinoscope and a phoropter (a mounting of lenses that will permit any desired refractive correction to be rotated into position).

light emerging from the patient's eye. These patterns of movement are easily observed and are characteristic of myopia, hyperopia, and astigmatism. With the aid of retinoscopy, the proper lenses (Fig. 21-7) to correct the refractive error can rapidly and accurately be determined. Hence, the refractive error of even the youngest infant can be measured precisely.

Subjective refraction measures the refractive error by permitting the patient to choose the best of a series of lenses. In practice, retinoscopy is used to determine the approximately correct lens strength, and the subjective check is used for final refinement of accuracy.

The technique of refraction is really quite simple. Probably the main source of error

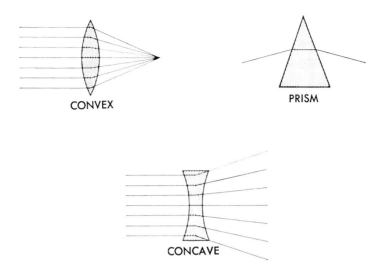

Fig. 21-7. Light is converged by a convex lens (used for correction of hyperopia or presbyopia), diverged by a concave lens (used for correction of myopia), and changed in direction by a prism (used for correction of minor deviations of ocular alignment).

arises from the unknown amount of accommodation exerted by the patient during examination. Special optical techniques have been devised to reduce the possibility of error due to accommodation. In general, these techniques work well in most adults, although they are time consuming. Hyperopic patients, being constantly accustomed to excessive accommodation, are frequently not suitable candidates for these optical techniques, particularly if they are younger than 25 years of age. Accurate refraction of hyperopic children is impossible by these methods. Particularly in the case of accommodative esotropia, accurate determination of the entire amount of hyperopia is vitally important.

Cycloplegic drugs (atropine, homatropine, cyclopentolate, and tropicamide) greatly enhance the accuracy of refraction of hyperopic patients and are essential for proper refraction of children. Cycloplegics block accommodation and dilate the pupil. Aided in this way, an expert retinoscopist can easily determine the average uncomplicated refractive error in less than 30 seconds.

Performance of only a refraction is an incomplete and potentially dangerous examination. Symptoms of disease mimic those of refractive error. Any patient with eye symptoms sufficient to bring him for examination requires careful fundus examination through an adequately dilated pupil.

CORRECTION

Glasses. Often patients with a relatively slight refractive error are happier without glasses, because their disadvantages (weight, reflections, dirty lenses, and expense) outweigh the benefits. The association of a significant refractive error with appropriate symptoms (in the absence of other cause for symptoms) indicates prescription of glasses.

Contact lenses. The development of strong, optically perfect plastics and of methods for precise machining and polishing to form extremely thin lenses has resulted in the modern contact lens boom. Corneal contact lenses are tiny discs about half the diameter of a cornea. They are precisely contoured to fit the anterior cornea, and the optical correction is ground into their front surface. They float freely on the precorneal tear film. After a period of adaptation, a high proportion of patients can wear accurately fitted contact lenses with minimal or no discomfort.

The optical quality of visual correction by contact lenses is good. A person with severe myopia or hyperopia (especially a patient who has undergone cataract extraction) is particularly benefited by the better field of vision and the absence of peripheral distortion attained through contact lenses. Keratoconus cannot be corrected except by contact lenses. The annoyance of frames and dirty glasses is eliminated. Contact lenses may be worn during athletic activity. However, the desire to look more attractive is the reason for the purchase of most contact lenses.

Disadvantages of contact lenses are many. Considerable training in their insertion and removal is necessary. Definite and prolonged minor discomfort must be endured during the development of corneal tolerance. Occasional acutely painful corneal abrasions or erosions are almost inevitable. Very rarely, permanent corneal scarring may result from some misfortune connected with contact lenses (such as *Pseudomonas* contamination of the lens storage case). They are expensive—the cost of a pair of contact lenses approaches that of surgery for strabismus. A lens is easily dropped—and not easily found. Bifocal contact lenses are not satisfactory. Finally, not everyone can wear contact lenses successfully. Because of the potential hazards of contact lenses, they should be fitted only under medical supervision.

SUMMARY

Refractive errors needing correction are recognized by the symptoms of reduced vision and chronic discomfort related to eye use. Because identical symptoms can be produced by eye diseases, a complete eye examination must accompany refraction.

chapter 22   Evaluation and
Management of
Reduced
Vision

IMPORTANCE OF REDUCED VISION

Reduced vision is important to you as a physician and to your patient as a person for the following reasons:

1. It is a seriously handicapping impairment of a particularly valuable sense.
2. It may be a manifestation of major central nervous system or general disease.
3. It may be an early stage of an ocular condition that will progress to blindness unless adequately and promptly treated.
4. If due to disease of the eye or body, it may often be improved by timely medication or surgery.
5. If due to refractive error, it may easily be corrected by proper spectacles.
6. It is extremely common. For example, 10% of university professors or business executives have significantly reduced vision.
7. It may be detected both quickly and easily, with complete safety, and at less expense than any laboratory test.

Consideration of the above seven facts would suggest that the medical profession routinely evaluates vision, the most priceless of all our senses. Alas, this is not so. The average hospital patient will certainly have tests performed for a half dozen varicties of serum rhubarb, but no visual acuity will be recorded on his chart. Does the patient fare better when he visits the office of a pediatrician, an internist, a neurologist or neurosurgeon, or a general practitioner? Rarely.

The following may explain this almost universal failure on the part of the medical profession:

1. Habit. Measurement of visual acuity has never become customary. The breaking of ingrained habit patterns is as unlikely as apostasy from church or desertion of a cherished political party.
2. Lack of time. Because there just is not time to do everything, the "less important" details are skipped. But what is less important to you—detection of an early and

asymptomatic inguinal hernia or detection of the glaucoma that is destined, if untreated, to blind you a decade from now?

3. Unfamiliarity. Eye disorders seem remote and forbidding to most physicians, who fail to appreciate the importance of visual acuity measurement and the ease with which reduced acuity may be evaluated.

The purpose of this chapter is to present in a simplified and orderly manner the approach to evaluation and management of reduced vision. Ideally, it will overcome the obstacle of unfamiliarity. The obstacles of habit and supposed lack of time can only be overcome by the resolve of the individual reader to include eyesight in his own physical examination routine. How about *you?* Will you do it?

CAUSES OF REDUCED VISION

Although the etiology of a medical problem is traditionally classified as congenital, degenerative, metabolic, traumatic, inflammatory, or neoplastic, it is clinically more helpful to think of reduced vision in terms of the anatomy of the visual system. Each portion of the visual system has easily recognizable characteristics that may be identified by the typical history and physical findings. From a practical standpoint, the visual system may be divided into the following parts:

1. The transparent focusing and light-transmitting media, which may be further sub-divided into the cornea, lens, and vitreous
2. The fundus structures, which include the optic disc, retina, and choroid
3. The transmitting system—the visual pathways, which consist of the optic nerve, chiasm, tract, and radiation
4. The cortical centers of recognition

Which of the four main parts of the visual system is responsible for a patient's reduced vision? This question is one of the first to be answered by the physician as he reviews the differential diagnosis. A reliable answer to this question should be supported by *both* a typical history and characteristic physical findings. Incompatibility of the history and physical findings indicates possible error in obtaining the history or in evaluation of the physical findings, or suggests that more than a single disorder may be present. The anatomic classification of visual problems is logical and straightforward and is definitely within the capability of every practicing physician.

Specific etiologic classification of visual disorders is considerably more complex than anatomic classification and requires more extensive knowledge of the significance of the history and the physical findings, but it is fortunately not necessary in determining proper management of many types of visual problems. For example, recognition of the central nervous system origin of a given case of reduced acuity and proper neurosurgical referral will effectively meet the patient's needs. The referring physician need not know the exact type and location of the intracranial neoplasm; he has adequately discharged his responsibility by making the anatomic diagnosis and initiating the proper referral.

METHODS OF EVALUATION

The clinical information required to diagnose the cause(s) of reduced vision is obtained by the *history* and by the techniques of *physical examination.* Physical examination of the eye is, naturally, somewhat different from that of other parts of the body and requires the following specialized techniques:

1. Subjective methods
    a. Measurement of visual acuity
    b. Perimetry
2. Objective methods
    a. Flashlight inspection
    b. Ophthalmoscopy
    c. Refraction
    d. Tonometry
    e. Others (for example, biomicroscopy)

Obviously, all abnormal findings will be carefully recorded. In addition, it is desirable to document negative findings pertinent to the patient's complaints. For instance, since glaucoma causes 12% of blindness, measurement of intraocular pressure cannot be disregarded when a patient complains of reduced vision.

History

1. What is the nature of the patient's reduced vision? Give details.
2. Describe its onset and course.
3. Are there any related symptoms?
4. Does serious eye trouble affect members of the family? What is the nature of this trouble?

Careful and detailed answers to the above four questions will include virtually all information of historical value in a case of reduced vision. Often a history will be so typical as to be almost diagnostic of a specific cause for visual loss. A few classic examples follow.

Classic symptoms

Myopia. The patient has good near vision but is unable to see in the distance. Reduced vision is slowly progressive, usually beginning during the early years of school. No other symptoms are associated. Other members of the family commonly have myopia.

Retinal detachment. The classic history describes a sudden appearance of a great many small floating spots (vitreous hemorrhage from the retinal tear), which briefly increase in number and then over a period of days may decrease in number. Often a framework of vitreous strands, described as a "cobweb" or "hair net," floats persistently and annoyingly in front of the patient. Sudden movement of the eye or head induces vitreous shifts that stimulate the retina to perceive "lightning flashes" in the periphery. When the retina begins to detach, the corresponding visual field is progressively lost, beginning in the periphery and advancing centrally. This field loss may be described as a dark curtain gradually encroaching on and destroying vision. During sleep the retinal detachment may partially subside—this improvement is dangerously misleading, because it often falsely suggests to the patient and the unwary physician that only a little more rest and patience will spontaneously cure the problem.

Migraine. Not only is the history of migraine characteristic, but it is also the sole evidence of the existence of the disorder. No abnormal physical findings are present. Migraine causes rapidly appearing homonymous (affecting *both* eyes) field loss that is often bordered by a bright zigzag line. The loss is brief (some minutes), with a gradual and recognizable decrease in the involved area, and is commonly followed by headache and nausea. Migraine is often familial.

Presbyopia. Over a period of years the patient gradually loses the ability to focus on near objects; yet he retains clear distant vision. This normal aging phenomenon has its onset during the forties. Since the older individual is more subject to a variety of insidious health problems affecting vision (for example, diabetes), the physician cannot safely ascribe sight problems of the middle-aged individual to presbyopia until adequate examination has excluded other problems.

Occlusion of a retinal arteriole. Within a minute the involved portion of the visual field goes blank. There is no pain or any other associated symptom.

Anatomic localization

An accurate description of reduced vision will often permit anatomic localization of the problem by means of dividing the visual system into separate parts, as in the preceding discussion of the causes of reduced vision.

Transparent focusing and light-transmitting media. Opacities of the cornea, lens, or vitreous are perceived as an obstruction to clear vision. Corneal and lens opacities are *fixed* in relationship to the eye, whereas vitreous opacities drift or float about within the eye and may be made to *shift* considerably by rapid eye movements. The closer an opacity is to the retina, the more sharply will its shadow be imaged on the retina. Hence, posterior vitreous opacities are perceived as distinct lines or spots, whereas cataracts never cause sharply defined retinal shadows.

Glare, or the scattering of light from translucent opacities, somewhat resembles the glare seen through a winter-frosted automobile windshield when sunlight strikes the frost. Usually the patient clearly recognizes that facing a bright light (for example, automobile headlights at night) causes glare and reduced vision. Less discerning patients may simply report that they see better at some times than at others. The history of glare localizes the problem in the anterior eye, in either the cornea or the lens.

Fundus structures. Damage to the retina or choroid causes a corresponding visual loss that maintains a fixed relationship to the eye (it does not float about, as do vitreous opacities). The area of visual loss is a positive scotoma, a term that signifies that the patient is aware of the defect. (Cerebral cortical disease may cause a negative scotoma, an area of visual loss of which the patient is totally unaware.) An intelligent patient can often describe accurately the difference between obstruction to vision (for example, cataract) and inability to see in a localized portion of the visual field (for example, focal chorioretinitis).

Transmitting system. Knowledge of the characteristic perimetric findings of visual pathway lesions (see Chapter 12) will explain the interpretation of historical complaints in this area. As an example, the patient who says that he "can't see on the right" should be questioned in more detail. Is it that he is unable to see with the right eye but does retain normal vision in the left eye? If so, the defect is localized in the right eye or optic nerve. Or is it that he is unable to see in the right field of vision with either eye but does retain vision in the left field of both eyes? The anatomic fault then lies in the left hemisphere of the brain, behind the optic chiasm.

Cortical centers of recognition. Although cortical defects may extensively damage vision, this loss is often completely unrecognized by the patient (negative scotoma). He therefore has no visual complaints.

For want of a better place, I will describe hysterical loss of vision in the cortical category. The important feature of hysteria from the historical standpoint is the peculiar attitude of the patient. With the aid of a compatible history, the perceptive physician will often sense the diagnosis of hysteria from this attitude. The patient never seems to be in the least bit alarmed by his visual "loss," a symptom that should cause realistic concern. Conversely, the parents or other relatives are usually greatly distressed and agitated. (It should be understood that familial attitudes are presumed to be a common basic cause of hysteria.) Usually there is considerable discrepancy between the rather severe amount of claimed visual loss and the apparent lack of handicap in moving about in the office or other unfamiliar place.

The student may have the impression that the hysterical patient will immediately relate some type of conflict or problem that confirms the diagnosis. This is not true. Usually everyone concerned denies any such problems, at least during the initial discussion. The other common misconception about hysteria is that its diagnosis is negative, made by exclusion of all other possibilities. Actually, hysterical visual loss is a positive diagnosis, reached because of the complete incompatibility of the subjective findings with the objective findings. For example, the unphysiologic "tunnel" visual fields, which can, surprisingly, be easily modified by suggestion, are virtually pathognomonic.

Malingering is similar to hysteria, except that the alleged cause of the symptoms is always stressed by the patient, who stands to gain financially if he can prove his contentions.

Summary

An adequate history is of enormous importance to patient evaluation. In practice, no patient ever receives a "complete" examination that includes all known diagnostic procedures—probably no one could survive the ordeal! A good history identifies the area or function of the body that requires special attention from the physician. Furthermore, the history should be sufficiently complete to exclude with reasonable probability other major or related disorders, provided, of course, that a physical examination of practicable thoroughness discloses no obvious defects in the historically negative areas.

In this era of intensive drug therapy, one other question should be asked of every patient whom you may treat: "Are you allergic to any medications, and if so, which ones?" Writing prescriptions before asking this question will, sooner or later, certainly result in trouble.

Physical examination

Measurement of visual acuity. The procedure for measuring visual acuity is so simple that any conscientious office assistant can rapidly learn it. No more time is required than is needed to weigh the patient and measure his height, and the necessary equipment (cardboard acuity chart) is less expensive than the weight scales. Unfortunately, we tend to equate the complexity, difficulty, and expense of an examination with the value. So evaluated, determination of visual acuity is so simple as to be totally worthless, and I suppose this is one ridiculous reason why most physicians never measure visual acuity as part of a "complete" physical examination.

Actually, visual acuity is almost the ideal screening test. This simple test will detect reduced acuity of every cause—whether it is refractive error, cataract, diabetes, brain tumor, or whatever. Although measurement of central visual acuity would not be expected to disclose purely peripheral field defects, in a considerable series of patients seen in our clinic for various disorders affecting the visual fields, 80% could have been detected as having abnormal fields simply because they were unable to read the 20/40 line with one or both eyes.

Furthermore, measurement of visual acuity is an accurate quantitative determination. It establishes clearly the amount of loss and the amount of remaining function. Subsequent visual acuity measurements will show whether sight is improving in response to treatment, or whether the disorder is progressively worsening. Knowledge of visual acuity permits partial prediction of the school capability of a child and whether an adult can meet industrial or driver's license requirements.

Measurement of the visual acuity of each eye separately should be part of every complete physical examination. Naturally, if the patient already has corrective spectacles, measurement of acuity should be done while he is wearing them as recommended (for example, reading glasses should not be used for measurement of distant acuity, because they will commonly blur distant vision).

Perimetry. Measurement of the extent of the visual fields is of no value in the clinical study of patients with defects of the transparent focusing and light-transmitting media.

Visual field studies may, however, be of great help in diagnosing and subsequently following patients with defects of the fundus or the brain pathways. The evaluation of many such patients with reduced vision is dangerously incomplete without the recording of the visual fields. For example, bitemporal hemianopia, easily demonstrable by perimetry, is not uncommonly the *only* abnormal physical finding that will betray the presence of an early neoplasm that is compressing the optic chiasm. Perimetry is particularly indicated if the optic disc is recognizably abnormal.

Techniques and the interpretation of confrontation field examination and of simplified perimetry are discussed in Chapter 12.

Flashlight inspection. Gross abnormalities of the cornea or pupil can easily be seen on inspection with a flashlight. Any recognizable loss of luster or perfect transparency of the central cornea may be responsible for decreased vision. Similarly, gross blocking of the pupil by iris adhesions is detectable by inspection. If the pupil is adequately dilated, the axial portion of the lens can be seen, and perhaps also any opacity of the far anterior vitreous. More posterior details within the eye are not ordinarily recognizable with a flashlight.

The optically important front surface of the cornea can be more accurately examined with the help of oblique, moving flashlight illumination in a darkened room. According to the laws of mirror reflection (angle of incidence equals angle of reflection), the glistening corneal reflection of the flashlight may be moved about on the corneal surface. An imperfection in the optical surface of the cornea causes distortion and faults in the reflections that are much more conspicuous than the defect itself when the defect is not outlined by the reflection technique (see Fig. 13-2).

Except in the case of extensive corneal or lenticular opacities, the expected visual acuity cannot be accurately assessed on the basis of flashlight inspection. A considerably more precise estimation of expected visual acuity can be made from examination of the ophthalmoscopic red reflex.

Ophthalmoscopy. Since it permits direct recognition of many causes of reduced vision, ophthalmoscopy is absolutely essential in the evaluation of all cases of reduced acuity. Examination of the ophthalmoscopic red reflex and anterior focusing with plus lenses permit examination of the normally transparent media. Through an adequately dilated pupil, all parts of the retina can be observed, except for the extreme periphery. (With special techniques such as scleral depression, one can see even beyond the retinal periphery and inspect the pars plana of the ciliary body.) Although the visual pathways cannot be seen with the ophthalmoscope, their state of health may often be inferred from the appearance of the optic disc. For example, papilledema suggests increased intracranial pressure. Optic atrophy not due to recognizable ocular cause indicates a lesion anterior to the lateral geniculate body, which is the termination of the axons from the ganglion cells of the retina.

Routine ophthalmoscopic examination should follow an orderly sequence—for example, red reflex, disc, vessels, macula, periphery. Such a routine sequence guards against overlooking a fundus finding because of incomplete examination. Examples of causes of reduced vision, corresponding to the above sequence, are cataract, optic atrophy, retinal arteriolar embolus, senile macular degeneration, and detachment of the peripheral retina.

Information concerning the use of the ophthalmoscope and the interpretation of observed details may be found in Chapters 5 to 12.

Refraction. Refraction, the accurate measurement of the optical faults of the eye, is of both diagnostic and therapeutic importance in the management of patients with reduced vision. Diagnostically, refraction determines the type and amount of optical error, permits decision as to whether the error is enough to account for the patient's problems, and demonstrates whether correction of the refractive error will improve vision to normal, as is expected if no other problem is present.

Although the technique of refraction requires optical equipment and skills with which the average physician is not familiar, he should be aware of the history and physical findings typical of cases of refractive error. To establish proper perspective, the student should know that by far the most common cause of reduced vision is refractive error. However, *no* case of reduced vision may safely be assumed to be due to refractive error until careful and complete examination of the eye has excluded the presence of disease. Furthermore, the failure of accurate refractive correction to improve vision excludes refractive error as the cause of reduced vision.

When should a patient with reduced vision be referred for refractive correction? Naturally, the presence of acute or major eye or general disease requires proper attention before correction is even considered. Premature refractive correction, provided during active disease, is usually a waste of the patient's time and money. For example, during periods of poor diabetic control, refractive error may fluctuate markedly. When a disease has become stationary, correction is indicated even if the patient retains only a little sight. I recall one patient with advanced optic atrophy and 20/200 vision whose vision improved to 20/30 with myopic correction.

The following generalizations are worth knowing and will help in proper evaluation of a patient's history. Refractive error does not cause the following.

1. Any symptoms of sudden onset (unless the patient suddenly greatly increases the use of his eyes)
2. Symptoms completely unrelated to use of the eyes
3. Floating spots or visual field defects
4. Redness, discharge, and crusting of the eye and eyelids
5. Abnormalities evident on physical examination of the eye (except changes of ophthalmoscopic focus on the fundus)

Tonometry. Because glaucoma is one of the more common diseases causing reduced vision, measurement of intraocular pressure is certainly part of the complete evaluation of reduced vision. If the optic nerve is pale, and particularly if it is excavated, the physician may not be satisfied by a single normal pressure reading but will recheck pressures at future examinations, or he may undertake special glaucoma procedures such as provocative tests or tonography. Greater suspicion of glaucoma will exist if other members of the family have suffered from this disease (the portion of the history dealing with the genetic background of the individual should certainly include questioning as to familial glaucoma), or if the patient is over 40 years of age.

Detailed information concerning glaucoma and the technique of tonometry is found in Chapter 15.

Other methods of examination. That the patient complains primarily of reduced vision should not blind the physician to the need for examining other parts of the body. For instance, it may be evident from the history and ocular physical findings that the function of the other cranial nerves should be checked, or that blood pressure should be measured.

Many specialized eye instruments are often helpful. As an example, the biomicroscope (slit-lamp microscope) and its various accessories permit the high-power microscopic examination of most parts of the interior of the eye.

MANAGEMENT

Obviously, the recommendations given to a patient with reduced vision will depend on the diagnosis. For illustration, the management of six different conditions that may present almost identical histories are briefly discussed in the following hypothetical situation.

The patient is middle-aged and complains of gradual reduction of visual acuity. Near vision has slowly deteriorated over a period of some years, despite the prescription of several pairs of glasses, each of which gave temporary improvement. Distant vision, also, has gradually decreased. The vision of one eye is recognizably worse than the other. The patient also has occasional headaches, complains of minor vague eye discomfort, is a little overweight, and has some arthritis.

The history is not specific, and it is compatible with many diseases, including cataract, glaucoma, senile macular degeneration, meningioma, diabetes, and presbyopia. Please note that the patient cannot determine from the nature of his complaints whether he suffers from an eye or a general disease, or whether he simply needs a better pair of glasses to correct presbyopia.

Cataract. If our hypothetical patient suffers from cataract, he may have surgery when his vision is sufficiently poor to handicap him. Within 3 months postoperatively, proper glasses will restore vision in 95% of cases.

Glaucoma. If the glaucoma patient waits until he cannot see adequately for his needs (as the cataract patient was advised), he has forever lost his vision. Glaucoma treatment usually consists of daily instillation of miotic drops, supervised by periodic tonometric and perimetric evaluation. Inadequate pressure control will permit further loss of vision.

Senile macular degeneration. Neither surgery nor medical treatment will prevent loss of central vision from senile macular degeneration. Fortunately, peripheral vision is never affected, and the patient will not become completely blind. He will need to adapt his activity to the handicap of being unable to read or drive.

Meningioma. The pressure of a benign brain tumor on the visual pathways causes gradual loss of vision that may initially be reversible but later becomes permanent. Successful neurosurgical removal of the tumor will prevent further damage to the vital intracranial structures.

Diabetes. Nutritional damage to the retina is only a local manifestation of the metabolic disorders associated with diabetes mellitus. Laser therapy may benefit diabetic retinopathy.

Presbyopia. Presbyopia is the most common cause of reduced vision in middle age and is easily corrected with bifocals. It is surprising to what extent the handicap of gradually progressive visual loss is accepted by the patient, to the detriment of his occupation and pleasure.

●   ●   ●

Obviously, the proper management of a patient is to entrust his care to a physician who thoroughly understands the particular problem involved. The first physician consulted may or may not possess this specialized treatment knowledge, but it is reasonable to expect all physicians to be capable of making the anatomic differentiations described in this chapter, which will permit accurate and timely referral, if necessary.

SUMMARY

Reduced vision is a common and important disability that will be discovered by the physician through history taking or by measurement of visual acuity (which should be a routine part of every complete physical examination). Every physician should be able to determine the anatomic location of the cause of reduced vision. This determination is useful in deciding management—for example, whether the patient simply needs refractive correction, or whether neurosurgical, ophthalmologic, or specialized medical evaluation is necessary

Ophthalmoscopy is by far the most useful and important single examination procedure for determining the cause of reduced vision. Ophthalmoscopy identifies not only ocular disease but also systemic and central nervous system disorders. Proficiency in ophthalmoscopy will adequately repay the general practitioner, the specialist in internal medicine, the pediatrician, and the neurologist for their time spent in learning skillful use of the ophthalmoscope and intelligent interpretation of fundus findings.

chapter 23　Ocular Therapy

The great majority of the common minor eye complaints can easily be managed by the general physician. Characteristic case histories, followed by a discussion of their proper management, are given in this chapter.

COMMON MINOR EYE COMPLAINTS
Case 1: Bacterial conjunctivitis

An 8-year-old child has had obvious diffuse bilateral conjunctival redness for 2 days. Considerable crusting discharge is deposited on the lashes and canthi. The corneas and media are clear. Visual acuity is 20/15 in both eyes. The pupils are round and equal, and there is no appreciable photophobia.

Discussion. These findings are characteristic of acute bacterial conjunctivitis (pink-eye). Proper management includes mechanical cleaning, topical antibiotics, and avoidance of spreading the infection to other children. Most superficial infections tend to deposit bacteria-laden crusts around the lid margins. These deposits should be thoroughly removed as often as necessary by using moist cotton swabs. Firm, adherent crusts may be softened by use of hot, moist compresses (Fig. 23-1). This material is infectious and should be disposed of in a sanitary fashion. Use of washcloths in common by several individuals will readily spread bacterial conjunctivitis. A topical antibiotic should be instilled three or four times a day. Topical use of penicillin should be avoided because of the high incidence of sensitivity (Fig. 23-2).

Case 2: Foreign body

With local anesthesia, a superficially imbedded cinder has just been removed from the patient's left cornea. The conjunctiva is slightly reddened, the pupils are equal, and vision has been recorded as 20/30 in both eyes. Still under anesthesia, the eye is comfortable without photophobia; however, there is some tearing.

Discussion. Whenever the corneal epithelium has been damaged, it is desirable to use topical antibiotics until healing occurs. Liquid vehicles are preferable, and the drops should be instilled three or four times a day (Fig. 23-3). Healing of a healthy cornea usually requires only a day or so and is recognized through failure of the cornea to stain with fluorescein and by the patient's comfort. Topical anesthetics should *not* be prescribed

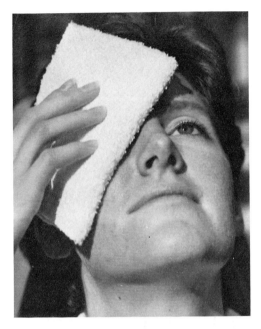

Fig. 23-1. Application of warm compresses. Wring out a clean washcloth from hot tap water and apply to the eye for 5 minutes or more. This is comforting and aids in cleaning debris from the eyelids.

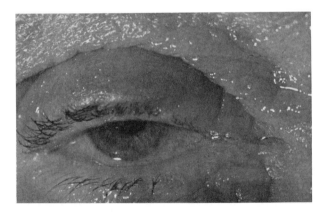

Fig. 23-2. Penicillin allergy caused this swollen, reddened, itching, macerated lid. Approximately 5% of adult patients are allergic to penicillin; therefore, topical use of this antibiotic should be avoided.

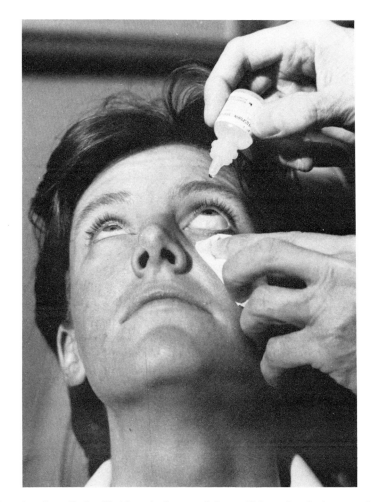

Fig. 23-3. A drop is easily instilled into the lower cul-de-sac if the patient looks up as the lower lid is gently everted. Use a tissue to catch any excess fluid, which would otherwise run annoyingly down the face. Instill the drop on any part of the conjunctiva rather than on the more sensitive cornea.

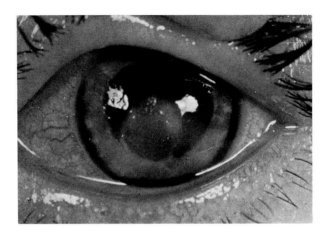

Fig. 23-4. This corneal ulcer resulted when a physiologist self-treated a small corneal abrasion with tetracaine to relieve pain. Repeated anesthetic instillation devitalized the corneal epithelium and resulted in a large ulcer that required several weeks to heal. Anesthetics should *not* be prescribed for home use.

for home use, because they inhibit epithelial regeneration (Fig. 23-4). Use of an eye pad is optional. It is my practice to bandage such an eye for an hour after removal of the foreign body and then begin antibiotic instillation. The eye pad is not replaced unless it makes the patient more comfortable.

Atropine should *not* be used, because it will cause prolonged inability to read. The presence of mild traumatic iritis indicates use of 2% homatropine three times a day; iritis is recognized by the presence of limbal redness, a smaller pupil on the injured side, and excessive pain and photophobia.

Corticosteroids should *not* be used for minor corneal injuries that are expected to heal within 1 or 2 days. They serve no useful purpose, reduce ocular resistance to infection, and are unnecessarily expensive.

Case 3: Chemical burn

Ten percent sodium hydroxide splashed into a student's left eye 2 hours previously. He washed it within 2 minutes, and it has just been irrigated with normal saline solution for 20 minutes. A few small areas on the lid show superficial chemical excoriation, and the lower half of the cornea stains with fluorescein and is faintly gray—enough to obscure partially the view of iris details. The entire lower cul-de-sac is discolored with red and gray mottling and is edematous.

Discussion. Immediate, prolonged irrigation with plain water will prevent more blindness from chemical burns than will all other medical care combined. The management of a patient with a chemical burn of this severity requires antibiotics and cycloplegics. Antibiotics should be selected as described in the subsequent discussion of antibiotics. One of the most neglected medications in cases of this sort is homatropine. Whenever extensive corneal injury or inflammation occurs, there will invariably be some iritis. This inflammation is easily recognized by smallness of the pupil, limbal redness, and photophobia. Symptoms of iritis are alleviated with 2% homatropine three times a day. The use of an ointment vehicle is important in preventing adhesions between apposing raw surfaces. In severe chemical burns, it is necessary mechanically to separate the lids from the globe several times daily in order to break these adhesions, which form surprisingly rapidly. The pain from an ocular burn is severe and usually prevents the patient from working. This pain is best relieved by codeine and sedatives. Topical anesthesia is not desirable, because it inhibits epithelial healing.

Patients with severe chemical burns should be referred immediately to an ophthalmologist, because there will usually be permanent damage.

Case 4: Penetrating injury

A 6-year-old boy fell off his stilts and broke his glasses this morning. He is frightened and will not cooperate for visual acuity measurements. A small bruise about 1 inch in diameter is on his right forehead. The lids show no evidence of trauma. The cornea of the right eye is crystal clear and is of normal contour, but the *iris appears to bow forward to touch the cornea.* The pupils are round and equal, and a slight amount of diffuse conjunctival redness is present in the right eye.

Discussion. Although antibiotics should be used freely in the management of superficial eye abrasions, it is extremely important not to treat only prophylactically and overlook an inconspicuous penetrating injury. The criteria for recognition of such injuries are stated in Chapter 13. Note that the anterior chamber has been lost in this patient.

This patient provides a classic example of an injury that can be cured by suturing the penetrating wound (which may be completely invisible in the cornea). Regrettably often, a patient with this type of injury is dismissed with topical antibiotic therapy, only to return in a week with serious and irreversible complications. Prompt referral to an ophthalmologist is urgent for all such patients.

Case 5: Marginal blepharitis

A 9-year-old child is brought for treatment with the chief complaint of "granulated eyelids" of 6 months' duration. She is a reddish-haired, freckled child. On the margins of both lids are many readily visible, small grayish scales loosely adherent to the skin about the base of the lashes. When dislodged, the scales do not leave a bleeding or ulcerated base. The conjunctiva is normally white. No previous therapy has been tried.

Discussion. One of the common superficial infections is marginal blepharitis. The fundamental requirements for successful treatment include thorough mechanical cleaning and effective antibiotic application. The use of warm, moist compresses for 5 minutes will soften these crusts so that they are readily removable. A cotton swab on a small stick is effective for mechanical separation of the scales. After thorough cleaning, antibiotic ointment should be applied to the lid margins. Such treatment should be repeated several times daily and continued for at least several days. Antibiotics should not be used for prolonged periods (more than 1 week) prophylactically. All this accomplishes is to ensure development of a flora of resistant organisms.

Marginal blepharitis is a stubborn infection that tends to recur and may require repeated periods of therapy. The most common source of reinfection is the bacterial flora on the body surfaces. A frequent type of marginal blepharitis is a combination of *Pityrosporon ovale* and staphylococci. Elimination of dandruff is an important step in minimizing recurrent infection. Sebaceous dermatitis also contributes to continuing infection and should be treated if present.

Case 6: Exposure keratopathy

Following general anesthesia for appendectomy, a 35-year-old man complains of severe and constant pain in the left eye, with some photophobia and blurring of vision. There is diffuse conjunctival redness, somewhat more marked about the limbus. Oblique, moving illumination shows irregular reflections from the lower cornea. This area stains with fluorescein. The pupils are approximately equal in size.

Discussion. Exposure damage of the cornea is extremely common and is usually preventable. Attention should be paid to the use of lubricant ointment and drops in unconscious patients and in individuals whose eyelid closure is not adequate. Once exposure damage has occurred, it is necessary to prevent further exposure through lid closure and ointment application. Use of an antibiotic ointment will prevent secondary infection. Neglect of chronic exposure damage may result in severe corneal scarring with permanent visual loss.

Case 7: Allergic conjunctivitis

A 9-year-old child has had chronic irritation and slight redness of both eyes during the past 2 months (June and July) and rubs them frequently. There is *no* crusting of lids, limbal flush, or corneal or intraocular opacity. Vision is 20/20 in both eyes. A few tiny glistening, round nodules are present on the tarsal conjunctiva.

Discussion. Minor allergic conjunctivitis is one of the most common eye complaints. If it is associated with systemic manifestations such as hay fever, antihistaminic tablets will give considerable relief of eye symptoms. If the conjunctivitis is an isolated complaint, as in vernal catarrh, topical sympathomimetic drugs, such as 0.12% phenylephrine, are much more effective. Frequency of instillation depends on the severity of symptoms. Use of drops two or three times a day will usually suffice. The patient's parents should be advised that treatment is not curative but simply alleviates symptoms. The child will eventually outgrow vernal conjunctivitis. There are commercially available many sympathomimetic preparations that seem to differ very little in their effectiveness.

Use of topical corticosteroids is unsafe, because glaucoma and cataract may develop. Corticosteroids should not be used at all for minor diseases such as allergy.

Case 8: Acute iritis

A 29-year-old patient spontaneously developed a red, painful eye beginning gradually about 1 week ago. Photophobia is pronounced. Her vision has been blurred. The pupil on the involved side is significantly smaller. The conjunctiva is diffusely quite red, with slightly more severe involvement about the limbus.

Discussion. Recognition of these symptoms and signs as indicating a serious cause of the red eye is obvious by the criteria given in Chapter 14. Reduced vision, excessive discomfort, pupil changes, and limbal flush clearly indicate that this is not a benign conjunctivitis. In treatment of recurrent iritis, it is desirable to evaluate the patient medically in an attempt to determine a specific cause that might be amenable to treatment (Chapter 19). The nonspecific treatment of iritis fundamentally requires good dilatation of the pupil by means of 1% atropine and 10% phenylephrine, which are ordinarily instilled three times a day. (Although atropine cycloplegia may last as long as several weeks in a normal eye, it certainly will not do so in an inflamed eye.) When the patient is initially seen in the office, an intensive effort should be made to dilate the pupil before she leaves. Dilatation is achieved by means of mydriatic and cycloplegic instillation repeated every 10 minutes. After initial dilatation of the pupil, the patient is sent home on routine treatment. Topical corticosteroid instillation every 2 hours will help considerably in quieting the inflammation. Systemic corticosteroids are helpful in severe iritis. A nonspecialist will be well advised to refer to an ophthalmologist the patients with more serious cases of iritis, which may be recognized through continuing discomfort, progressive and severe visual reduction, and destructive intraocular inflammatory changes. One example of these serious complications is secondary glaucoma, which requires urgent treatment to prevent permanent damage to the optic nerve.

Case 9: Dry eye syndrome

A 49-year-old patient with nervousness, minimal arthritis, mild hypertension, and moderate obesity complains of chronic irritation of both eyes, present for 6 to 8 months. She not infrequently awakens at night with a burning sensation of the eyes. Examination shows slight relaxation of the orbital septa inferiorly, moderate exophoria, the very slightest conjunctival redness, a few strands of stringy gray mucus in the lower cul-de-sacs, clear corneas and media, equal pupils, and 20/40 vision in each eye uncorrected.

Discussion. The great popularity of "eyewash" can be traced to a number of chronic ocular irritations. One of the best defined of these irritations is keratoconjunctivis sicca, which occurs as a syndrome of dry eyes and mouth, associated with arthritis in menopausal women. A great deal of relief is obtained from the use of 0.5% to 1% topical methylcellulose (or comparable tear substitute) as often as required in the individual patient. Endocrine preparations or drugs affecting the autonomic nervous system are not effective. Lubricant treatment is often one way in which a patient with multiple untreatable difficulties can be made more comfortable.

COMMON OPHTHALMIC MEDICATIONS

Brief descriptions of the commonly used ophthalmic medications follow.

Anesthetics

Most ocular diagnostic and surgical procedures may be performed with the patient under local anesthesia. Superficial manipulations (for example, tonometry, inspection of an abraded cornea, and removal of imbedded corneal foreign bodies) require only topical instillation of a surface-active anesthetic. More extensive procedures (such as incision and curettage of a chalazion or repair of lid laceration) require injection anesthesia. The surgeon should be aware that an inflamed eye is more difficult to anesthetize with local agents, because they are rapidly carried away by the increased circulation of blood.

Topical anesthetics. The various drugs used for topical ocular anesthesia have many characteristics in common. All act readily on mucosal surfaces but are relatively ineffective when applied to the less permeable skin surfaces. The surface-active anesthetics are relatively toxic and should not be injected. Severe systemic reactions may result from application of excessive amounts of topical anesthetics to mucosal surfaces. For instance, 100 mg of tetracaine is regarded as a potentially lethal dose—and it is only 5 ml of 2% solution! Such problems are not encountered when a few drops of anesthetic are used for ocular procedures, but they can occur when large mucosal surfaces are anesthetized—for

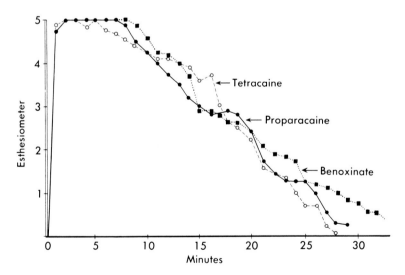

Fig. 23-5. Comparison of duration and intensity of anesthesia obtained with solutions of 0.5% tetracaine, 0.5% proparacaine, and 0.4% benoxinate. (Modified from Linn, J.G., Jr. Published with permission from The American Journal of Ophthalmology **40:**697-704. Copyright by The Ophthalmic Publishing Company.)

example, during examination and treatment of the throat. Some patients faint in anticipation of ocular surgery; such syncope may be mistaken for anesthetic reaction.

For practical purposes, the onset, intensity, and duration of anesthesia produced by the topical anesthetics are the same for all the commonly used drugs (Fig. 23-5). Within 1 minute of instillation, anesthesia is sufficient for tonometry. For removal of a corneal foreign body, several additional drops may be instilled at 1-minute intervals. Such repeated instillations will enhance and prolong anesthesia beyond that achieved by a single drop.

During the 15- to 20-minute duration of topical anesthesia, the patient will be aware of a peculiar numb sensation of the eye. Commonly, he will rub his eyes in annoyance. Since the anesthetized corneal epithelium can be extensively damaged by self-inflicted abrasions during this painless period, the patient should be instructed to pat away tears from the *closed* lids with a tissue but not to rub the open eye until normal sensation has returned. Such a warning is an important routine precaution; otherwise the patient will almost always rub his eyes.

Commonly used ocular anesthetics are 0.5% proparacaine hydrochloride (Ophthaine), 0.5% tetracaine (Pontocaine), and 0.4% benoxinate hydrochloride (Dorsacaine). Proparacaine instillation causes less initial stinging sensation than does tetracaine. This relative freedom from irritation is helpful in treatment of apprehensive patients or children. Stinging after instillation of an eye drop is considerably reduced by closing the eye for a moment.

Because of the welcome relief from pain, a patient with a corneal abrasion may request that the physician give him some anesthetic drops for home use. Never grant this request! Healing of the corneal epithelium is markedly slowed by topical anesthetics, which inhibit cellular metabolism and growth. Furthermore, if the patient rubs his anesthetized eye, extensive corneal abrasions may result. Severe corneal damage with accompanying iritis can be caused by such unwise use of home anesthetics. Subsequent healing will be delayed for many days.

Local allergy to tetracaine or proparacaine may develop because of repeated use, as in patients with glaucoma. Allergy to medication is recognized by the typical appearance of reddened, swollen eyelids accompanied by the classic symptom of itching. Since most ocular drug allergies are similar in appearance, the specific diagnosis is made by the history of what type of medication was used immediately before the onset of symptoms. A notation on the patient's record will remind the physician to avoid future use of the sensitizing drug. Cold compresses and topical corticosteroid therapy will relieve the symptoms of an acute allergic lid response.

Injection anesthetics. Bupivicaine (Marcaine) and lidocaine (Xylocaine) are the most popular anesthetics for local use in ophthalmic surgical procedures. Not more than 0.5 g of either drug should be given to the average adult during one procedure. This amount represents 50 ml of 1% solution—far more than the 5 to 10 ml usually required for most eye procedures. Either drug is effective in 0.5% to 1% solution. Use of 2% or stronger concentrations does not materially improve anesthesia but does double or quadruple the dosage given, thereby increasing the hazard of the procedure.

Lidocaine diffuses readily through tissue and thereby spreads the anesthetic effect. Its duration permits 30 to 45 minutes of operating time from a single injection. For practical purposes, a large margin of safety exists for the usual eye procedures, which require relatively small amounts of injection anesthetics. During 30 years of eye surgery, I have never personally encountered a single case of serious toxic reaction to the injection of 1% lidocaine. The usual reaction to an anesthetic is a physiologic response to epinephrine. Nevertheless, accidental intravenous injection may greatly reduce the tolerated dose, and the physician should be aware of the hazards of local anesthesia.

Serious reactions to local anesthesia are characterized by respiratory and cardiac arrest and convulsions. Much is written and said about the use of barbiturates to control anesthetic reactions, but the student must clearly understand that barbiturates only worsen respiratory or cardiac arrest and should *not* be used for such reactions. Intravenous administration of barbiturates is of value in controlling convulsions only.

Artificial respiration, a vitally important emergency measure for an anesthetic reaction, must be instituted immediately when arrest of breathing is recognized and must be continued throughout the period of apnea. The physician who uses local anesthesia should have immediately available the facilities for assisting respiration, including an airway, a hand-operated breathing bag capable of delivering positive pressure, and a suction apparatus for clearing the airway of secretions. Assisted respiration should cause visible chest movements. *Be sure the airway is not obstructed.* Extension of the head and elevation of the lower jaw helps clear the airway. The rate of artificially assisted breathing should be ten to fifteen times per minute.

When the heart stops pumping blood, the brain has only 3 or 4 minutes to live. Unless someone present knows what to do, the patient with cardiac arrest from an anesthetic reaction will surely die. Regardless of whether the heart is in asystole or fibrillation, two problems face the physician:

1. Restoration of blood flow (including oxygenation)
2. Restoration of normal heartbeat

Loss of pulse and blood pressure is an emergency that must be met by immediate cardiac massage to achieve restoration of blood flow. There is *no time* to take an electrocardiogram. Because circulation has stopped, medication *cannot* be given by any route, including intravenously. *Do not* simply give artificial respiration and wait hopefully for the heart to start. There is *no time* to experiment or to look up directions; therefore, you must learn *now* the techniques of closed-chest cardiac massage.

The human heart, fixed in the mediastinum, almost completely fills the space between the sternum and the thoracic spine. The chest of the unconscious adult is sufficiently flexible to permit effective cardiac compression when firm pressure is applied on the lower third of the sternum. Such external cardiac massage has maintained effective circulation for as long as 2 hours in human patients. The liver can detoxify a fatal dose of anesthetic in only 20 minutes.

Closed-chest cardiac massage requires that the patient with cardiac arrest be placed supine on a firm surface (such as the operating table or floor). The physician stands or kneels beside the patient; he must be high enough above the patient so that the weight of the physician's body can be used for pressure. The heel of one hand is placed on the lower one third of the sternum, and the second hand is placed on the first. Firm vertical pressure is applied, sufficient to move the sternum 1 to 2 inches toward the vertebral column. Despite the application of considerable pressure, there is little danger of rib fracture when only the heel of the hand is applied to the sternum; however, *no* pressure should be directed on the ribs by the fingers. Finger pressure will fracture the ribs! At the end of each compression, pressure is completely removed from the chest, allowing it to reexpand fully and permitting both ventricles to fill with blood. This cycle is repeated about 60 times a minute, about the rate of a slowly beating heart. Each adequate cardiac compression should produce a palpable pulse and maintain a measurable blood pressure.

Much less force is required in resuscitation of infants. Only moderate fingertip pressure is applied to the middle third of the sternum. Excessive force may cause crushing injury, to which the liver is particularly vulnerable. The pressure of one hand alone is adequate for most children up to 10 years of age.

If the cardiac arrest is caused by asystole rather than fibrillation, intraventricular injection of 1 ml of 1 : 10,000 epinephrine may help restore spontaneous heartbeat. A sharp blow on the chest may stop asystole.

External cardiac massage is a technique that should be familiar to all surgeons, because it is effective and simple and eliminates the problems of infection, hemorrhage, and injury that accompany emergency thoracotomy.

Summary. Remember the following when using anesthetics.

1. Do not use topical anesthetics without warning the patient not to rub his eyes for 15 minutes thereafter.
2. Do not prescribe topical anesthetics for home use.
3. Do not use injection anesthesia unless you know how to perform artificial respiration and closed-chest cardiac massage.

Antibiotics

The first essential of successful antibiotic therapy for a serious ocular disorder is accurate diagnosis of the infectious nature of the disorder. Obviously, the red eye of acute glaucoma or the irritation of a burdock burr imbedded in the upper lid will not respond to antibiotics.

The second essential is choice of a drug effective against the responsible microorganism. Identification of the organism by staining and culture techniques and laboratory measurement of antibiotic sensitivity is required. General knowledge of the appearance of some typical infections (for instance, the hyperacute, purulent conjunctivitis of the newborn caused by gonococcal contamination) and of the spectrum of various antibiotics (for example, colistin is effective against gram-negative bacilli) will permit reasonably accurate antibiotic choice until laboratory reports arrive.

The third essential is knowledge of the toxic effects of antibiotics. Obviously, the surface location of the eye permits topical application of antibiotic preparations in treatment of infections of the conjunctiva, cornea, or lid skin. Intraocular tissues are very delicate and therefore are susceptible to toxic effects of drugs (for example, intraocular injection of as little as 125 μg of amphotericin B will cause irreversible corneal opacification and scarring of the interior of the eye).

The most unique ocular physiologic feature of significance in antibiotic therapy is the blood-aqueous barrier. As its name denotes, this barrier resists the entry of water-soluble ions into the eye. Penicillin, for example, penetrates the eye extremely poorly. The blood-aqueous barrier exists at the walls of the iris and retinal blood vessels, at the epithelial surfaces of the cornea and ciliary body, and at the retinal pigment epithelium. Hence, the cavity of the eye, containing aqueous and vitreous humors and the lens, is a sheltered area within which invading microorganisms may be protected from systemic or topical antibiotic therapy. This barrier is particularly significant in prophylactic antibiotic treatment of an eye after a penetrating wound. The blood-aqueous barrier is permeable to lipid chemicals such as chloramphenicol. For this reason, chloramphenicol is of exceptional value in treatment of intraocular infection.

The extraocular tissues are, of course, entirely outside the blood-aqueous barrier. Hence, the same general principles of antibiotic therapy applicable to any other part of the body would be equally relevant to treatment of an orbital infection.

Choice of antibiotic. For practical reasons, minor eye infections are treated differently from major infections. Such minor diseases as acute conjunctivitis, hordeolum, and

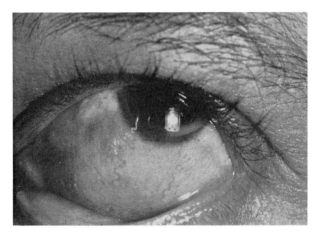

Fig. 23-6. Use of Argyrol as an antibacterial "eyewash" was formerly quite prevalent. The permanent blue-gray staining of this conjunctiva is due to long-continued use of silver salts, which are deposited in the tissues and cause argyria. Modern antibiotics have made the use of Argyrol obsolete.

marginal blepharitis compose the vast majority of eye infections. Cultures, smears, and sensitivity studies are neither economically feasible nor necessary in treatment of these diseases. Excellent results will be obtained with the use of arbitrarily selected topical antibiotics. What antibiotics should be selected (Fig. 23-6)?

The commonly used broad-spectrum antibiotics suitable for systemic administration should be *avoided* for several good reasons:

1. Significantly fewer bacteria will respond to topical use of these systemic drugs, because their widespread use has created many resistant strains.
2. Unnecessary use of these valuable drugs will hasten development of resistant bacterial strains that will later menace community health.
3. The possible sensitization (see Fig. 23-2) of patients to systemic antibiotics is an unwarranted risk when equally good results can otherwise be obtained.

Laboratory studies on bacterial sensitivity of strains isolated from eye patients indicate clearly the superiority of the antibacterial drugs whose use is limited to topical application. Such medications include bacitracin, gramicidin, neomycin, sulfacetamide, and (for gram-negative organisms) polymyxin. Commercially available combinations of these drugs have such broad antibacterial spectra that the great majority of local infections will be adequately treated by this type of prescription.

For the reasons already stated, the drugs whose use is limited to the topical route are best for prophylactic therapy—for example, preoperatively or after corneal abrasion. The prevention of infection suggests that all patients with corneal abrasion be advised to use topical antibacterial drugs until complete epithelial healing occurs. Prevention of secondary infection makes the use of antibiotics worthwhile in many diseases not bacterial in nature. These diseases include erythema multiforme, pemphigus, and other vesicular and ulcerative dermatoses that may encroach on the cornea. Viruses such as herpes zoster or simplex do not themselves respond to antibiotics, but elimination of bacterial invaders will minimize the scarring associated with these diseases.

Most superficial infections cause accumulation of bacteria-laden discharge on the lid margins. Proper management of such infections includes not only topical antibiotic application but also mechanical cleaning techniques. The adherent debris should be thoroughly removed as often as necessary by using moist cotton swabs. Firmly adherent crusts may be softened with warm, moist compresses for several minutes. This material is infectious and should be disposed of in a sanitary fashion. The use of a common washcloth can readily spread bacterial conjunctivitis to the various members of a family.

In treatment of bacterial conjunctivitis, topical antibiotic drops may be prescribed for use three or four times a day. Drops are not greasy, cause less visual blurring than do ointment vehicles, and are less likely to retard epithelial healing. Ointment applications last longer and may therefore be recommended for use at bedtime. They adhere to lid surfaces (desirable in treatment of marginal blepharitis) and have protective and lubricant properties. Ointments are cosmetically greasy, cause annoying blurring of vision for a few minutes, are harder to instill, and may retard epithelial healing (as of abrasions).

Do *not* cover a superficially infected eye with an eye pad. An eye pad interferes with the normal protective blinking and tearing mechanisms and tends to incubate the infection in a warmer environment. As a result, patching the eye enhances the infection. Indeed, simply covering a normal eye will commonly precipitate development of a marginal blepharitis.

The management of minor eye infections, as just outlined, is inadequate for major infections such as the following:

1. Lesions that may threaten life (for example, orbital cellulitis)
2. Lesions that may threaten sight (for example, severe corneal ulcer)
3. Lesions that are potentially disfiguring (for example, destructive cellulitis of the face)

Prompt, vigorous, and intelligent management is required under such circumstances. The expense of sensitivity studies is clearly warranted and will often prove helpful. Therapy must be started immediately, before culture results are available. A Gram stain will help in the initial selection of an antibiotic.

Systemic routes of administration of antibiotics are necessary in treatment of major eye infections, but topical therapy should also be used if the lesion is accessible. Dosage should be generous, in general as high as that which would be used in serious systemic disease. The normal blood-aqueous barrier significantly retards intraocular penetration of most antibiotics but fortunately tends to be broken down by inflammation. Chloramphenicol penetrates the eye more readily than most other antibiotics and should therefore be considered for preferential use. Other indicated therapy (cycloplegic) must not be neglected.

Local toxic effects. Not uncommonly, chronic keratoconjunctivitis will develop after topical antibiotic treatment of a surface ocular infection. Although it is due to the antibiotic, this inflammation is often misinterpreted as being a continuing infection. Such toxic keratoconjunctivitis may gradually become more severe during prolonged treatment. When this diagnosis is suspected, all medications should be discontinued, and treatment should be limited to cold compresses. It will often be difficult to convince these patients that treatment should be stopped, particularly because a latent period of some days may precede improvement. Conjunctival scrapings of toxic keratoconjunctivitis show mononuclear cells with typical basophilic granules.

Allergy to antibiotics is particularly common after topical use of penicillin and neomycin. An allergic response is recognizable by the typical reddened, weeping appearance of the lid skin and by the characteristic itching. The only effective treatment for local drug allergy is recognition of the condition and withdrawal of the offending medication. Subsequent use of the same drug, even years later, will result in prompt return of the allergic changes.

Characteristics of individual antibiotics. *Amphotericin B* is the most effective drug now available against the yeastlike fungi. Unfortunately, this medication is very poisonous and therefore is extremely hazardous for systemic administration. Because intraocular penetration is poor and the drug is highly toxic, the use of amphotericin B for fungus eye infections is of no value.

Bacitracin is a bactericidal antibiotic with a range of activity closely paralleling that of penicillin. It is active chiefly against gram-positive organisms but also destroys spirochetes, gonococci, and actinomycetes. Bacitracin is ineffective against gram-negative bacilli.

Strains of microorganisms resistant to bacitracin are much less frequently encountered than those resistant to penicillin. Bacitracin is not inactivated by pus, blood, necrotic tissue, or bacterial enzymes such as penicillinase. Allergy to bacitracin is far less frequent than it is to penicillin. Topical application of bacitracin in concentrations of 500 to 1000 units/g is nonirritating to the eye and causes no undesirable systemic effects. Most gram-positive organisms are inhibited by 0.001 to 0.5 units/ml. Bacitracin does not penetrate the intact cornea in therapeutic amounts.

In summary, topical bacitracin is an effective treatment for surface ocular infections caused by gram-positive microorganisms. Its use is preferable to that of penicillin.

Chloramphenicol has a broad antimicrobial spectrum, being effective against a wide variety of gram-positive and gram-negative organisms, rickettsiae, and spirochetes. Unfortunately, *Pseudomonas aeruginosa,* an organism particularly likely to destroy the cornea, is usually resistant to chloramphenicol. Since great variations occur in the sensitivity of various strains of organisms, general summaries such as this one are not truly reliable. Rather, the sensitivity of the organism responsible for a given infection must be determined, if possible.

After systemic administration, chloramphenicol penetrates the eye much better than most other antibiotics. Indeed, the intraocular levels of chloramphenicol are approximately half the serum levels. Blood levels of 15 μg/ml are easily achieved by an adult dosage of 3 to 5 g/day, given in divided doses every 4 hours. Oral dosage gives concentrations comparable to the intravenous route; hence, parenteral administration is indicated only if the patient cannot take the drug by mouth (such as preceding general anesthesia).

The superior intraocular penetration of chloramphenicol is due to its lipoid solubility. Chloramphenicol is 10,000 times as fat soluble as penicillin. Since the blood-aqueous barrier is essentially a fatty shield against electrolytes, it is capable of excluding penicillin, tetracyclines, and most other antibiotics, but it does not exclude fat-soluble drugs such as chloramphenicol.

Chloramphenicol is exceptionally well suited to treatment of intraocular infections, which ordinarily follow penetrating trauma or surgery. Unfortunately, in such cases cultures of material from the surface of the eye are usually negative or isolate surface organisms unrelated to the endophthalmitis. For this reason, in most cases of intraocular infection the physician must choose an antibiotic arbitrarily. The drug chosen is selected because of its ability to penetrate the blood-aqueous barrier and because of a reasonably broad antibacterial spectrum. Chloramphenicol meets both these criteria better than other available antibiotics and hence is one of the best medications for treatment or prophylaxis of endophthalmitis. An initial oral dose of 2 or 3 g is advised, followed by 0.5 g every 4 hours.

The toxicity of chloramphenicol has been well publicized—in fact, excessively so. Although it is true that agranulocytosis will kill about 1 of 20,000 to 50,000 patients receiving chloramphenicol, this fact is viewed in better perspective if one realizes that fatal anaphylactic reactions to penicillin have an equal frequency. Stated crudely, the only difference is that the chloramphenicol agranulocytosis causes a lingering death, whereas the penicillin anaphylaxis is immediate.

The LD_{50} dose of chloramphenicol for mice is 245 mg/kg. Hence, although recommended doses are well tolerated without side effects, the clinician must be aware that enormous doses cannot be given with impunity, as is true of penicillin. Very young infants are apparently unable to excrete chloramphenicol *and will die* after frequently repeated large doses.

In summary, because of its lipoid solubility, chloramphenicol penetrates into the intraocular fluids far more readily than do most other antibiotics. Furthermore, it has a broad antibacterial spectrum. For these reasons, it is a drug of choice for treatment of intraocular infections.

Colistin methanesulfonate will effectively inhibit gram-negative organisms such as *Pseudomonas aeruginosa* and *Escherichia coli*. *Pseudomonas* strains are sensitive to colistin in concentrations of 8 to 11 μg/ml. Therapeutically effective aqueous concentrations of colistin may be attained by topical application of 0.12% drops to the surface of an inflamed eye. This concentration does not irritate the conjunctiva or cornea.

Therapeutic vitreous concentrations of colistin are not attainable by topical or systemic routes of administration. This antibiotic causes severe renal and central nervous system toxicity in 30% to 50% of patients receiving therapeutically effective systemic dosages.

Colistin is a drug of choice for topical treatment of gram-negative infections of the cornea and anterior segment of the eye.

Erythromycin has a spectrum of action against gram-positive organisms somewhat comparable to that of penicillin. Staphylococcal resistance to erythromycin develops as readily as to penicillin and is related to the frequency of use. Two percent concentrations of erythromycin are well tolerated by the cornea and produce fair levels of antibiotic in the anterior segment of the eye (for example, 9 μg/ml aqueous). The main indication for ophthalmic use is treatment of organisms shown by sensitivity studies to be vulnerable to erythromycin.

Gentamicin sulfate is another antibiotic effective against gram-negative organisms. At least three fourths of strains of *Pseudomonas* and *E. coli* and almost all staphylococcal strains are sensitive to 4 μg/ml of gentamicin. A high incidence of permanent labyrinthine damage complicates systemic use. Gentamicin is a drug of choice for topical therapy for ocular anterior segment infections caused by gram-negative organisms or by resistant staphylococci.

Neomycin is a broad-spectrum antibiotic effective against a variety of gram-positive and gram-negative microorganisms. Its antibacterial spectrum is broader than that of bacitracin, penicillin, or streptomycin. It is not fungistatic. Neomycin is stable at room temperature and is not inactivated by body fluids. Nephrotoxicity and deafness contraindicate its systemic use. Absorption from topical use is insufficient to cause any toxic systemic effects. Neomycin is a commonly used antibiotic in preparations for topical ophthalmic application.

Novobiocin is effective against a variety of gram-positive and gram-negative microorganisms. It is tolerated topically in concentrations up to 1.2%. Experimental use of 10% solutions causes corneal vascularizaton. Topical applications of tolerable concentrations of novobiocin cause no measurable aqueous penetration. The student may wonder why the blood-aqueous barrier cannot be bypassed by intraocular injections of antibiotics. The reason is that the delicate intraocular cells are easily damaged. For instance, only 25 mg of novobiocin injected intraocularly will destroy sight.

Nystatin is effectively fungistatic against a wide variety of fungi, molds, and yeasts. It has little or no effect on other types of microorganisms. In ophthalmic use, nystatin has been found to be clinically valuable in treatment of surface fungus infections by topical application. Nystatin is reasonably well tolerated by the eye when applied in the form of an ointment containing 100,000 units/g. *Aspergillus* growth is inhibited by 6 to 12 units/ml nystatin; hence, this drug is of value in treatment of corneal mycoses.

Penicillin is a generic term, often used without realization that there exist a number of natural and synthetic derivatives of 6-aminopenicillanic acid. All the clinically useful penicillins effectively inhibit or kill certain bacteria, resist inactivation by human tissues, and are remarkably nontoxic. Considerable variations occur in solubility, stability, and resistance to destruction by penicillinase. In general, penicillins do not penetrate well intraocularly. The resistance of the blood-aqueous barrier may be partially overcome by the use of huge doses of penicillin and is broken down by severe inflammation.

Potassium penicillin G is very water soluble and is ideal for attaining high plasma concentrations rapidly. However, it is also excreted rapidly and therefore must be given intramuscularly every 6 hours to maintain high blood levels. Although penicillin G may be given orally, its absorption is limited because of instability in gastric acid.

Procaine penicillin G is less soluble in water and is therefore absorbed more slowly than is the potassium salt. Intramuscular injections of 600,000 units every 24 hours will maintain demonstrable plasma levels. Higher plasma levels should be attained by the more frequent use of potassium penicillin G rather than by larger doses of procaine penicillin.

Benzathine penicillin G is only slightly water soluble and produces very low blood levels that may last for several weeks. The longer-acting forms of penicillin are troublesome, should the patient happen to be allergic to the drug. Also, they do not penerate the eye effectively.

Phenoxymethyl penicillin (penicillin V) is much more acid stable than penicillin G; hence, it is well suited for oral use. As much as 75% of an oral dose may be recovered in the urine, indicating absorption perhaps five times greater than that of penicillin G. Penicillin V may be given without regard to the time of meals. An oral dose of 250 mg four times daily is adequate for most systemic infections but will give only poor intraocular levels.

The types of penicillin just described differ primarily in solubility and stability. Their antibacterial effect is essentially the same—they are effective against most gram-positive cocci (with the noteworthy exception of penicillinase-producing, and therefore resistant, staphylococci), gonococci, clostridia, and spirochetes. Most gram-negative bacteria (specifically, *Pseudomonas*) are resistant to these types of penicillin.

Sodium methicillin is resistant to destruction by penicillinase and is the agent of choice against resistant staphylococci (unless the patient is allergic to penicillin). Minimal dosage is 1 g intramuscularly every 6 hours. Methicillin is extremely unstable in even slightly acidic solutions and therefore should be dissolved just before injection. When added to infusion fluids, it may be inactivated within several hours. Methicillin is excreted rapidly, half being found in the urine within 2 hours after intramuscular injection.

Sodium oxacillin is pharmacologically comparable to methicillin except that it is more acid stable and so may also be given orally (500 mg every 2 hours).

Ampicillin is an acid-stable, orally absorbed synthetic penicillin with broad-spectrum antibacterial activity. Minimal inhibitory concentrations of ampicillin for the common gram-positive organisms range from 0.01 to 0.05 μg/ml. The majority of gram-negative organisms are considerably more resistant, requiring from 0.5 to 5 μg/ml. Oral administration of ampicillin, 5 mg/kg of body weight, will give aqueous levels of 0.1 to 0.3 μg/ml, lasting for several hours. Intramuscular injection of 100 mg/kg (7 g for a 70 kg adult) will give 1-hour aqueous levels of 40 to 50 μg/ml. Useful levels of ampicillin do not enter the normal vitreous.

For practical purposes, external application and systemic administration of penicillin in any concentration is nontoxic to the eye.

Accidental injection into the sciatic nerve may cause permanent sensory and motor loss. The importance of avoiding sciatic nerve damage is sufficient to warrant cautioning your nurse against injecting into any portion of the buttock except the upper outer quadrant only. The sciatic nerve is particularly vulnerable in infants, who should receive intramuscular injections in the quadriceps muscle.

Allergy to penicillin exists in 5% of the population of the United States. Use penicillin only after ascertaining that the patient has had no previous penicillin reaction. Even a negative history will not exclude allergic reactions. The most common type of penicillin allergy is the delayed response simulating serum sickness. After an incubation period of 1 to 2 weeks, urticaria, fever, and joint pains appear. This response is due to development of antibodies after the injection, and therefore skin testing and the past history will be negative for penicillin sensitivity.

Already-sensitized individuals will manifest allergic reactions more promptly, after periods as brief as a few minutes. Death may occur from acute serum sickness, angioneurotic edema, or anaphylaxis. Despite the relative infrequency of penicillin reactions, an attitude of complacency is unwarranted. Penicillin reactions occur in 2% to 8% of patients receiving the drug. The incidence of death in severe reactions is about 10% and strikes about 1 of 30,000 to 50,000 patients receiving penicillin. Patients found to be allergic to penicillin (or any other medication, for that matter) should be cautioned against its further use and advised to inform their future physicians.

Because of the high incidence of allergic blepharoconjunctivitis, the local ocular use of penicillin is inadvisable.

In summary, penicillin is a first-choice antibiotic for extraocular infections caused by susceptible microorganisms. Because penicillin derivatives have different antimicrobial spectra, laboratory sensitivity studies are essential to the management of severe infections. The intraocular penetration of penicillin is poor; hence, alternate drugs (for example, chloramphenicol) are preferable for treatment of endophthalmitis. The incidence of allergy to penicillin is high and may rarely have a fatal outcome.

Pimaricin is the most effective and least toxic of all the antifungal drugs. Unfortunately, it does not penetrate the eye in adequate concentration to be effective against fungal endophthalmitis. However, application of 5% pimaricin ointment every few hours is the best available treatment for superficial keratomycosis.

Polymyxin B is bactericidal against most gram-negative microorganisms. For example, *Pseudomonas* strains may be sensitive to polymyxin B concentrations ranging from 0.05 to 2 μg/ml. Concentrations of 0.025% are nonirritating to the eye. Hence, polymyxin B can be applied to tissues in concentrations 1000 times greater than that required to destroy sensitive organisms. Topical application achieves effective corneal stromal concentrations if the epithelium is not intact. Adequate intraocular concentrations cannot be produced by topical or parenteral administration because of the toxicity of the drug.

Corneal ulcers resulting from *Pseudomonas* infection are rapidly progressive and highly destructive. Therapy started within 18 hours will usually prevent serious damage. If treatment is delayed for 48 hours, the infection may be controlled, but dense corneal scarring remains. Longer delay permits corneal perforation and loss of the eye. Because of the great importance of early treatment, broad-spectrum antibiotic treatment of serious corneal ulcers should begin immediately. Polymyxin B, 0.2%, should be applied topically at least hourly. The spectrum of polymyxin alone does not include many gram-positive organisms. Hence, the concomitant use of other antibiotics such as bacitracin and neomycin is rational. Atropinization and adequate cleaning of the eye with hot, moist compresses are indicated in treatment of any severe infectious keratitis with associated iritis.

In summary, polymyxin B is one of the most effective antibiotics available for treatment of gram-negative infections of the ocular surface.

Pyrimethamine is a potent folic acid antagonist used in treatment of toxoplasmosis. It is highly synergistic with sulfonamides. Combined therapy requires only one eighth as much sulfonamide and one twenty-fourth as much pyrimethamine as would be necessary if either drug were used alone. Pyrimethamine treatment is so toxic that it should be considered only when the presumed toxoplasmic cause is confirmed by positive laboratory tests and when the retinochoroiditis is sufficiently severe to threaten central visual acuity. The decision to use this drug is difficult because of the uncertainty of the etiologic diagnosis of retinochoroiditis.

Streptomycin is effective against a number of organisms, both gram-negative and gram-positive. Since most gram-positive organisms are much more sensitive to penicillin, its use is preferable for these organisms. Development of the relatively nontoxic broad-spectrum antibiotics has further decreased the usefulness of streptomycin. Contributing greatly to clinical reluctance to use streptomycin is its toxicity to the eighth cranial nerve. Daily use of 2 g of streptomycin for only 2 weeks will permanently destroy vestibular function. The prophylactic use of streptomycin in routine surgery or its prescription for minor or self-limited infections is an unwarranted risk. Perhaps the only clear-cut indication for streptomycin is treatment of tuberculosis.

After intramuscular injection of 10 mg/kg, aqueous concentrations of 8 μg/ml result. Topically applied streptomycin does not penetrate the intact cornea sufficiently well to be of therapeutic value. A 1% concentration is well tolerated by the ocular surface.

In summary, the diagnosis of active systemic and ocular tuberculosis would probably be the only real indication for streptomycin therapy encountered in ophthalmology.

Sulfonamides are bacteriostatic by virtue of their ability to prevent bacterial utilization of *p*-aminobenzoic acid (found in purulent exudate and in local anesthetics, both of which interfere with sulfonamide action). Since the advent of antibiotics, sulfonamides are no longer the drugs of choice for treatment of major infections. However, for topical treatment of ocular infections, sulfacetamide in 10% to 30% concentration is still a valuable drug. Sulfonamides inhibit the growth of most gram-positive microorganisms and a variety of gram-negative organisms, including *Pseudomonas*. Infections such as trachoma may respond somewhat. Corneal infections by some types of fungi may benefit from sulfonamide therapy. With the topical use of 30% sulfacetamide solution, intracorneal concentrations as high as 0.1% can be achieved within 5 minutes.

In summary, sulfacetamide, 30%, still compares favorably with the newer antibiotics for topical use against surface ocular infection.

Tetracyclines are termed broad-spectrum antibiotics because of their ability to inhibit a wide variety of gram-positive and gram-negative organisms—rickettsiae, actinomycetes, spirochetes, large viruses, trichomonads, amebae, and pinworms. Not all strains of these organisms are susceptible; for example, one third or more of the staphylococci may be highly resistant. *Pseudomonas* and *Proteus* are rarely responsive to tetracyclines. Herpetic infections are not benefited by tetracycline therapy.

Concentrations from 1 to 8 μg/ml are usually adequate to inhibit susceptible bacteria. There is little difference in therapeutic effectiveness among the tetracycline derivatives. Hence, if a patient fails to respond to one tetracycline, there is rarely any advantage in changing to another member of this same group of antibiotics.

Surface ocular infections by susceptible microorganisms respond well to topical tetracycline application. The incidence of allergy and irritation is insignificant. Although the intraocular penetration of tetracyclines is poor, large oral doses (6 to 8 g/day) produce demonstrable aqueous concentrations and may be advised for treatment of intraocular infections. If extensive corneal epithelial abrasions are present, topical application of 0.5% solutions will produce aqueous levels as high as 28 μg/ml. The intact corneal epithelium resists tetracycline penetration.

Acute trachoma may be clinically cured by topical application of the tetracyclines. An ointment vehicle is most effective. Treatment must be continued for 2 to 4 weeks.

In summary, the tetracycline derivatives are remarkably nontoxic antibiotics, highly effective against a wide variety of microorganisms. They are useful for treatment of surface ocular infections by topical application, but unfortunately penetrate poorly into the eye.

Vancomycin is a bactericidal antibiotic highly active against gram-positive cocci. Indeed, virtually all strains of staphylococci are sensitive to less than 5 μg/ml. Topical ocular instillation of a 5% solution will produce aqueous levels of vancomycin as high as 8 to 12 μg/ml, lasting for several hours. This concentration is reasonably well tolerated by the eye. The complication of permanent deafness limits the systemic use of vancomycin.

In summary, vancomycin is a drug of choice for treatment of resistant staphylococci.

Antiviral drugs

Clinically useful selective metabolic inhibition of viruses was first achieved against herpes simplex infection of the cornea by the use of idoxuridine. Before this success, no medication had ever been known to cure an established viral infection without destroying the host cells.

The mechanism of action of idoxuridine is that it so closely resembles thymidine that it can substitute for this vital nucleic acid in viral synthesis. Apparently, idoxuridine-containing virus molecules cannot function as infectious agents.

In tissue cultures, an idoxuridine concentration of only 1 μg/ml will inhibit the growth of herpes simplex virus. The cornea will tolerate therapeutic application of 5000 times this concentration (0.5%) without toxicity. Since the continuing presence of idoxuridine is necessary to inhibit viral growth, dosage is 0.5% ointment applied five times daily for several weeks. Premature discontinuance of therapy will result in relapse, with recurrence of the viral corneal ulcer.

Newer antiviral drugs such as triflurothymidine and acycloguanosine are even more effective and less toxic than the original idoxuridine.

The dendritic ulcer, pathognomonic of acute herpetic keratitis, responds well to antiviral treatment. Subjective relief is marked within 24 hours. Conspicuous epithelial healing occurs within 3 days, and residual fluorescein-staining defects usually disappear within 10 days.

Chronic herpetic keratitis penetrates deeply into the corneal stroma, producing large ulcers with ''geographic'' shapes. Such stromal herpes responds poorly to antiviral therapy. Cautious treatment with combinations of antiviral drugs and corticosteroids is currently considered to be the best management of stromal herpes. Since impaired resistance due to poorly advised corticosteroid treatment is a major cause of stromal herpes, the nonspecialist is well advised to avoid use of corticosteroids in the management of any keratitis of possible viral origin.

Autonomic drugs

The autonomic drugs, in which are included the miotic, mydriatic, and cycloplegic agents, represent many of the most important and most commonly used drugs in ophthalmology. The autonomic innervation of the eye and its effector neurochemicals are represented diagrammatically in Fig. 23-7. As indicated in the illustration, adrenergic impulses are transmitted to the muscle cell by norepinephrine. The cholinergic mediator is acetylcholine. Autonomic effects are termed direct when the drug acts on the muscle end-plate in the same manner as norepinephrine or acetylcholine. The effect is termed indirect if the drug either inhibits destruction or induces liberation from nerve endings of the natural effector chemical.

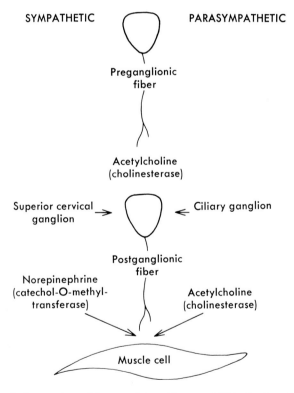

Fig. 23-7. Autonomic innervation of the eye. (From Havener, W.H.: Ocular pharmacology, ed. 5, St. Louis, 1983, The C.V. Mosby Co.)

Since adrenergic and cholinergic actions are mutually antagonistic, a comparable effect results from inhibition of the one (lytic effect) or stimulation of the other (mimetic effect). Hence, autonomic effects may be tabulated as follows:

I. Adrenergic action (mydriasis)
  A. Sympathomimetic (mydriasis)
    1. Direct-acting
      a. Epinephrine
      b. Phenylephrine
    2. Indirect-acting
      a. Cocaine
      b. Hydroxyamphetamine (Paredrine)
  B. Sympatholytic
    1. Timolol (beta blocker)
II. Cholinergic action (miosis and accommodation)
  A. Parasympathomimetic
    1. Direct-acting
      a. Acetylcholine
      b. Carbachol
      c. Pilocarpine
    2. Indirect-acting
      a. Reversible
        (1) Eserine
      b. "Irreversible"
        (1) Isoflurophate (DFP)
        (2) Echothiophate (Phospholine)
  B. Parasympatholytic (cycloplegia)
    1. Atropine
    2. Homatropine
    3. Cyclopentolate
    4. Tropicamide

Mydriatics

Epinephrine. Epinephrine is useful in ophthalmology because of its vasoconstricting effect and because it will lower intraocular pressure in some types of glaucoma.

Topical application of 1:1000 epinephrine to the conjunctival surface will help control bleeding from capillaries and small arterioles but is ineffective against hemorrhage from larger vessels. During most ophthalmic operations it is the oozing from these smaller vessels that is most troublesome in obscuring surgical details; hence, preliminary use of epinephrine is of considerable value in eye surgery. Vasoconstriction occurs almost immediately but lasts for less than an hour.

Inclusion of 1:50,000 concentration of epinephrine in solutions of anesthetics for local injection will cause enough vasoconstriction to delay systemic absorption. Used in this way, epinephrine will prolong the duration of anesthesia and will reduce the likelihood of systemic toxicity of the anesthetic. However, the epinephrine may itself induce tachycardia and apprehension, which may be mistaken for an anesthetic reaction. No local ischemic damage results from injection of epinephrine of this strength about the eye.

Because epinephrine is rapidly inactivated, it is not an effective mydriatic and is rarely used for this purpose. The denervated pupil of Horner's syndrome is sensitized to the effect of epinephrine and will dilate widely in response to 1:1000 epinephrine. However, cocaine (an indirect-acting sympathomimetic) will not dilate such a pupil. Since normally innervated pupils do not dilate with 1:1000 epinephrine and do dilate with cocaine, the use of epinephrine is a clinically helpful pharmacologic test for sympathetic denervation of the pupil.

Although use of a pupil-dilating drug in treatment of glaucoma sounds paradoxical, sound evidence supports such therapy. Sympathomimetic mydriatics reduce intraocular pressure by increasing the facility of aqueous outflow via the uveoscleral (unconventional) pathways. Hence, 1% epinephrine, instilled once or twice daily, is of considerable value in the control of open-angle glaucoma. An additive effect may be achieved by the simultaneous use of epinephrine, miotics, and carbonic anhydrase inhibitors (should the given case of glaucoma be of such severity as to require this amount of therapy).

Gonioscopy is advised before use of sympathomimetic drugs in treatment of glaucoma, in order to avoid closure of the angle in cases of narrow-angle glaucoma. Particular caution is necessary if the anterior chamber is visibly shallow.

Topical use of epinephrine may cause local irritation and discomfort sufficient to preclude use of this medication in some patients. Cardiac extrasystoles are more common in patients receiving epinephrine therapy. Aphakic patients receiving epinephrine therapy sometimes lose vision because of macular edema. This visual loss is reversible if the epinephrine is discontinued. Prolonged epinephrine instillation may cause black oxidation products to accumulate within conjunctival cysts, resulting in the appearance of small black dots in the lower cul-de-sac.

Phenylephrine (Neo-Synephrine). Phenylephrine, a direct-acting sympathomimetic mydriatic, is recommended as a drug of choice for dilating the pupil as an aid to ophthalmoscopy. Instillation of several drops of 2½% phenylephrine about 5 minutes apart will, within 30 minutes, produce good mydriasis lasting for several hours. Phenylephrine does not cause cycloplegia; hence, the patient's ability to perform near work is not impaired.

Phenylephrine is an excellent example of a useful drug whose potential value is not realized by most physicians. Unfounded legends have sprung up concerning the "hazards" of dilating pupils. The patient's inconvenience or discomfort after sympathomimetic dilatation has been exaggerated beyond any resemblance to the truth. Unfamiliarity with the benefits of mydriatic examination promotes an attitude of indifference toward these useful medications.

The primary use for sympathomimetic mydriatics is the improvement of the physician's view of the interior of the eye. It is appropriate to compare the view of the fundus through a small pupil or a dilated pupil with the view of a room as seen through a keyhole or with the door open! Through a dilated pupil, fundus details are observed with ease and can be studied much more accurately. Through a small pupil it is absolutely impossible to see the peripheral portion of the retina or to visualize the most important macular area (because of interference from corneal reflexes at this angle of light incidence). Small details of great diagnostic importance (diabetic microaneurysms, hypertensive arteriolar attenuation, traumatic retinal holes, and so on) are readily overlooked through a small pupil.

Good mydriasis is particularly important in the presence of eye disease. No physician can adequately evaluate complaints pertaining to the eyes through miotic pupils. Symptoms that especially demand thorough fundus examination through a dilated pupil include recent onset of floating opacities in the vision, relatively sudden decrease in visual acuity, visual field loss, ocular pain, and redness of the eye not obviously due to superficial infection or allergy. After contusion, thorough ophthalmoscopy is necessary to rule out internal eye damage. Eye disease often clouds the vitreous or lens and obscures fundus details. Good mydriasis usually reveals such details, which are hidden behind a small pupil.

At this point we should deal with such often-heard comments as the following: ''Drops are unnecessary.'' ''You can see everything you need through the average pupil.'' ''With practice you become expert at seeing fundi without mydriasis.'' I shall meet these comments with the unqualified, authoritarian, flat statement that no other group uses the ophthalmoscope as much or develops such skill in its use as the ophthalmologists. Our use of the ophthalmoscope is under all conditions, including the extreme miosis of treated glaucoma. Without exception, ophthalmologists agree that mydriasis aids fundus examinations, and we use mydriatics routinely in our practices. We are not ashamed to admit that we often cannot see diagnostically important details without the aid of a mydriatic.

Indications. Obviously, all patients do not require mydriatics. If there are no specific eye symptoms, or if the patient has a disease known not to produce eye manifestations (or if he is perfectly healthy), the chances of finding significant fundus disease are not great. Under these circumstances a fair view of the disc and vessels through the undilated pupil will be considered sufficient examination. Many younger patients have spontaneously large pupils that permit relatively thorough fundus examination.

If the patient may have disease known to produce eye manifestations, or if the diagnosis is in doubt, a good view of the fundus may be helpful to the physician. Usually these problems arise in older people, who ordinarily have small pupils. Phenylephrine is useful under these circumstances.

Use of a mydriatic is practically mandatory in evaluation of visual complaints such as floating spots, field loss, and sudden blurring, or if there is unexplained eye pain or redness. A mydriatic is usually necessary for adequate evaluation of ocular contusion.

Cycloplegics, of course, are most helpful in accurate refraction, especially in younger persons.

Precautions. *Before* instilling mydriatics, a minimum physical examination is necessary in view of the following:

1. Intraocular pressure should be evaluated by finger tension to exclude obvious increased pressure.
2. Inspection should rule out the rare case in which the anterior chamber is so shallow that the iris practically touches the cornea. These rare older individuals are predisposed to acute glaucoma and should not have their pupils dilated.
3. The pupil that is miotic due to treated glaucoma can easily be recognized.
4. Findings indicating acute neurologic disease suggest consultation before use of drops.

If these few details are checked early in the physical examination, drops may be instilled and will have dilated the pupil for ophthalmoscopy by the time you have finished examining the patient. Used in this way, mydriatics do not waste your valuable time. The duration of mydriasis is sufficiently short so that there is no benefit in reversing the action with pilocarpine in a normal eye.

As with all other eye drops, sterility is important. Do not contaminate the dropper by touching the patient's lids or your fingers. Holding a tissue below the eye to prevent tears from running down the cheek adds greatly to the patient's comfort.

Contraindications. *Known glaucoma* is a relative contraindication to dilating the pupil. This condition can be determined by asking the patient, by inspecting for the presence of therapeutic miosis, by recognizing scars of previous glaucoma surgery, or by finding obviously elevated intraocular pressure by finger estimation. Under these circumstances dilatation should not be done except by the patient's ophthalmologist. The common type of glaucoma, open-angle glaucoma, which is so likely to exist unknown to the patient and doctor, will *not* become acute with the use of phenylephrine and will probably continue to be undetected. The type of glaucoma that is precipitated by mydriatics is the acute form. It is caused by a mechanical blockage of the angle by the iris and is uncommon. Eyes predisposed to acute glaucoma may often be recognized simply because of the extreme shallowness of the anterior chamber. Statistically, a physician who dilates many eyes in the course of a routine practice might expect to precipitate not more than one case of acute glaucoma during his lifetime. This occurrence can easily be recognized through pain, redness, and hardness of the eye, accompanied by hazy vision and rainbow halos about light. If the condition is recognized, the patient should be referred immediately to an ophthalmologist (after instillation of several drops of pilocarpine).

Unilateral dilatation of the pupil is a sign of grave significance in acute intracranial disease. For this reason, approval of the attending neurosurgeon should be obtained before dilating the pupils in such a patient.

In summary, phenylephrine hydrochloride is a safe and effective aid to ophthalmoscopy. Its use is strongly encouraged for both medical and ophthalmic diagnostic purposes. Known glaucoma and acute neurologic disease are the only real contraindications.

Sympatholytics: timolol

The beta blocker timolol reduces the production of the aqueous humor by approximately 50% and thereby lowers intraocular pressure. Because timolol is applied only twice daily, its use is more convenient than that of pilocarpine, which must be applied four times daily. Pupil size is unchanged by timolol, which eliminates the pilocarpine-induced miosis (causes night blindness and reduced vision in eyes with cataract). No painful and blurring accommodative spasm results from timolol, but this is troublesome with pilocarpine in younger patients.

One drop of 0.25% or 0.5% timolol twice daily is now the most popular initial treatment of glaucoma.

Cholinergics

Acetylcholine. Acetylcholine, an autonomic chemical formed at the parasympathetic nerve endings, is rapidly destroyed by cholinesterase, and hence has little therapeutic value. After delivery of a cataract, some surgeons instill acetylcholine, 1:100, directly on the iris to achieve prompt miosis. Constriction of the pupil lasts for only a few minutes but may help keep the iris away from the limbal incision during completion of the operation.

Carbachol (Carcholin). Carbachol is a synthetic combination of portions of the molecules of acetylcholine and of physostigmine. Because carbachol is not destroyed by cholinesterase, it has a prolonged parasympathomimetic effect. A single instillation of 0.75% carbachol will cause miosis lasting for as long as several days. In clinical use (for glaucoma) the patient usually instills the drops two or three times daily. Of course, the required amount of medication for any given case of glaucoma is determined by clinical trial and depends on the severity of the glaucoma.

In general, 0.75% carbachol will be more effective in control of glaucoma than is 2% pilocarpine. However, it tends to cause more severe accommodative spasm and headache than does pilocarpine. These symptoms often diminish with prolonged use.

Carbachol is usually prescribed as the second miotic used in treatment of glaucoma. It is used when the control of the glaucoma by pilocarpine becomes inadequate, or if the patient becomes allergic to pilocarpine.

Pilocarpine. Pilocarpine has been (prior to timolol) the most popular medication for treatment of primary glaucoma. It is a direct-acting parasympathomimetic alkaloid with the differential solubility characteristics necessary to readily traverse the fat-water-fat corneal barrier.

Although the obvious action of pilocarpine is to constrict the pupil, there is no direct relationship between pupil size and the facility of outflow of aqueous from the anterior chamber. The iris does not itself directly attach to the scleral spur or to the trabecular meshwork; hence, its state of contraction or relaxation does not necessarily affect outflow facility. Rather, it is the ciliary body that primarily affects trabecular patency.

Anatomically, the longitudinal fibers of the ciliary muscle (parasympathomimetic innervation) attach directly to the scleral spur and the trabecular meshwork. By their contraction, these muscle bundles open the trabecular meshwork and thereby enhance aqueous outflow.

Pharmacologically, therefore, parasympathomimetic stimulation of the ciliary muscle (as by pilocarpine) opens the trabecular meshwork and increases aqueous outflow, the pupil being coincidentally miotic. The addition of a sympathomimetic drug (for example, phenylephrine) dilates the pupil but does not alter ciliary innervation and therefore does not diminish aqueous outflow. A parasympatholytic drug (for example, cyclopentolate) blocks contraction of the ciliary muscle, thereby closing the trabecular meshwork and reducing aqueous outflow, the pupil being coincidentally dilated.

The clinical management of glaucoma requires thorough evaluation of the individual case, followed by the trial of one or more of a variety of drugs. Pilocarpine may be used in concentrations of 1% to 4%, in frequency varying from two or three times daily to as often as every 2 hours. If adequate control is not achieved by a reasonable frequency of pilocarpine use in tolerable concentration, the physician should supplement it with other types of medication (for example, epinephrine and/or acetazolamide) or should change to another miotic (for example, carbachol or echothiophate). Timolol is an excellent alternative.

The simultaneous use of two miotics (for example, pilocarpine and eserine) is more likely to result in a competitive than an additive effect. Such combined use was frequently recommended in the past but is no longer considered rational.

As would be expected, parasympathomimetic stimulation results in accommodation for near vision. This drug-induced accommodative spasm causes blurred distance vision and ocular aching, which is more marked in patients younger than the age of presbyopia.

Systemic toxic effects (sweating, nausea) are first noted at a dose of about 5 mg of pilocarpine. One drop of 2% pilocarpine contains more than 1 mg of medication.

Physostigmine (eserine). Physostigmine does not destroy cholinesterase but inactivates it by forming a temporary chemical combination. As physostigmine is gradually destroyed *in vivo*, the cholinesterase is liberated. Hence, physostigmine is classified as a reversible cholinesterase inhibitor and acts by preserving acetylcholine from destruction.

Since some acetylcholine is constantly present in the normally innervated iris and ciliary body, miosis and accommodation result from physostigmine, even when the eye is at rest. In response to accommodative effort, additional acetylcholine is formed. Preservation of this acetylcholine results in the accommodative spasms typical of the indirect-acting parasympathomimetic drugs. These greatly increased muscular responses of the iris and ciliary muscles may be painful and distressing to the glaucomatous patient receiving anticholinesterase therapy.

Within a half hour, 0.25% eserine ointment causes intense miosis lasting from 12 to 36 hours. During this time the facility of outflow of aqueous is increased. Because of its long action, physostigmine ointment has traditionally been prescribed for bedtime use. Alternating use of physostigmine and pilocarpine has been advised for the intensive treatment of acute glaucoma.

Although one might theorize that an additive effect would result from the combined use of a direct-acting parasympathomimetic (pilocarpine) and an indirect-acting parasympathomimetic (physostigmine), these drugs more probably have a competitive effect. Present information indicates that glaucoma responds better to a single miotic than to combinations of miotics. Failure to achieve adequate glaucoma control is met by increasing the concentration or frequency of use of the miotic, by changing to another miotic, or by adding another class of drugs (carbonic anhydrase inhibitor or sympathomimetic drug), but not by the combined use of several different miotics.

Toxicity. Twitching of the eyelids is commonly noted during ocular use of indirect-acting parasympathomimetic agents. This minor but annoying side effect is due to percutaneous drug absorption and inactivation of orbicularis cholinesterase.

Chronic conjunctival irritation is not uncommon after the use of physostigmine. Typical contact allergic dermatitis may develop after prolonged use.

The systemic parasympathomimetic toxicity resulting from physostigmine was the basis for its use as an ordeal poison in ancient Africa.

Black patients sometimes develop depigmentation of the lid skin, which appears after many months of physostigmine use. The depigmentation may gradually disappear when drug use is discontinued, but recognizable changes persist for years.

Isoflurophate (DFP). The synthesis of war gases and insecticides has resulted in the development of long-lasting, indirect-acting parasympathomimetic drugs. Although these medications were originally believed to form an irreversible bond with cholinesterase, the development of pralidoxime chloride disproved this concept, for such oximes can reactivate inhibited cholinesterase.

A single drop of 0.05% isoflurophate will cause intense miosis, with onset within 10 to 15 minutes and a duration of 2 to 4 weeks. Isoflurophate-induced ciliary spasm induces myopia lasting for as long as a week. The pain accompanying such spasm is worse during close work because of the greater production of acetylcholine during accommodation.

Isoflurophate reduces intraocular pressure, the maximal depression occurring during the first day. Return to the preexisting intraocular pressure requires about 1 week. Control of glaucoma may be achieved by instillation of a drop once daily or even less frequently. Because of systemic toxicity and local ocular side effects, more frequent use of isoflurophate is rarely advisable.

In general, any case of glaucoma (except narrow-angle glaucoma) that can be controlled with weaker miotic therapy (for example, pilocarpine, carbachol, physostigmine) will be controlled by isoflurophate. Cases uncontrolled by the weaker miotics will often achieve substantially better control through use of isoflurophate, thereby sparing the patient from surgery.

In practice, the use of isoflurophate is reserved for cases of open-angle glaucoma that have not responded well to weaker miotics and for aphakic glaucoma. The reason for this restriction is the expectation of severe side effects when a strong miotic is used, especially in younger persons.

The use of isoflurophate is contraindicated in narrow-angle glaucoma because it is likely to precipitate a medically uncontrollable acute attack that will require immediate surgery. Prevention of such an attack requires gonioscopic confirmation of the presence of an open angle before prescription of isoflurophate. The mechanism of isoflurophate-induced angle closure may be that the extreme miosis increases physiologic iris bombé, with consequent deepening of the posterior chamber and closure of the chamber angle.

The accommodative component of esotropia may be eliminated by nightly instillation of 0.025% isoflurophate. Dosage is adjusted to the smallest effective amount. Instillation every second or third night only, or even less often, may maintain straightness of the eyes. Perhaps a third of children with esotropia have a sufficient accommodative component to permit effective straightening of the eyes by miotic therapy.

The mechanism whereby esotropia is corrected is, of course, unrelated to the miosis. Because a fixed relationship exists between accommodation and convergence, the hyperopic child must also converge when he accommodates to obtain clear vision. This excessive accommodation and convergence may cause esotropia in a hyperopic child—hence the name "accommodative" esotropia. Inhibition of cholinesterase enhances the response of the ciliary muscle to a minimal accommodative innervation. Since less accommodative innervation is used, less convergence will occur.

Children are likely to develop pigment cysts of the pupil margin after use of isoflurophate. Rarely, these cysts reach such a size as to occlude the miotic pupil. Isoflurophate cyst formation is prevented by simultaneous use of 2.5% phenylephrine.

Toxicity. Generalized parasympathomimetic poisoning is much less likely to occur with isoflurophate than with echothiophate and hence is discussed in the next section, which deals with echothiophate. Nevertheless, isoflurophate is a highly poisonous drug, and the contents of a patient's bottle of eye drops could easily kill a child.

Systemic absorption of anticholinesterase drugs applied topically to the eye is rapid and of surprising magnitude. Systemic anticholinesterase activity is detectable within a few minutes of ocular instillation and approaches the levels produced by intravenous administration of the same dose.

Echothiophate (Phospholine). The clinical characteristics and indications for use of echothiophate are almost identical to those of isoflurophate. Because of greater stability, echothiophate is clinically more popular than isoflurophate. Both drugs are extremely poisonous, and toxic side effects are commonly associated with their use.

The systemic side effects of the potent cholinesterase inhibitors include diarrhea, weakness, abdominal cramps, and general fatigue and weakness. These toxic manifestations may simulate an acute gastrointestinal upset or upper respiratory tract infection. If such symptoms arise in a patient receiving anticholinesterase therapy, determination of the cholinesterase values in red blood cells may indicate whether the symptoms are iatrogenic. Red blood cell cholinesterase values may be reduced for as long as 4 months by potent drugs such as echothiophate.

Because echothiophate poisoning is cumulative, toxic systemic symptoms do not appear for weeks or months after the start of therapy. For this reason, the relationship of symptoms and the ocular therapy may not be recognized. Frequently symptoms are discovered only by direct questioning. Paresthesia and circulatory collapse may be among the symptoms of echothiophate toxicity.

Since plasma cholinesterase hydrolyzes succinycholine and procaine, patients with low blood levels of cholinesterase due to anticholinesterase therapy for glaucoma or esotropia are more susceptible to the toxic effects of these anesthetic drugs. Death has been reported from use of succinylcholine during anesthesia in a patient with low blood levels of cholinesterase.

The most serious ocular complication of anticholinesterase therapy is cataract formation. The typical anticholinesterase cataract begins in the form of anterior subcapsular vacuoles. It is dose related, being more frequent with prolonged and frequent use. A year or more is required before recognizable lens changes occur.

Anticholinesterase antidote. Pralidoxime chloride is capable of separating the cholinesterase molecule from its phosphoryl bond to anticholinesterase drugs such as echothiophate or isofluorphate. Pralidoxime does not have a parasympatholytic action as does atropine, but simply frees and reactivates cholinesterase. The neutralizing action of pralidoxime does not permit recurrent cholinesterase inactivation from the original dose of isoflurophate.

Since accidental swallowing of eye drops (as by children) could easily be lethal, a brief outline of treatment is appropriate:

1. Gastric lavage will prevent further absorption of any chemical remaining in the stomach. Since anticholinesterase drugs may be absorbed percutaneously, contaminated skin should be washed with water.
2. In severe poisoning, artificial respiration and maintenance of an open airway are essential. Nasopharyngeal and bronchial secretions are increased by parasympathomimetic stimulation and may require removal by suction.
3. Atropine should be given intravenously in a dosage of 2 mg every 5 minutes until the symptoms of parasympathomimetic overdosage disappear; atropine should be repeated whenever such symptoms recur.
4. Pralidoxime chloride, 1000 mg, should be given slowly intravenously in not less than 2 to 5 minutes. An additional 500 mg may be given in 30 minutes if weakness is not relieved. Pralidoxime is effective orally, but this route is usually not feasible because of vomiting.
5. Diazepam (Valium) (10 mg) will effectively combat central nervous system toxicity such as convulsions.

Parasympatholytics (cycloplegics)

Atropine. Atropine acts directly on the smooth muscles and secretory glands innervated by postganglionic cholinergic nerves. At these nerve endings, it blocks the response to acetylcholine. This blockage is relative and can be overcome by parasympathomimetic drugs such as pilocarpine if they are applied in sufficient concentration and frequency relative to the amount of atropine used.

Atropine produces both mydriasis and cycloplegia, as is true of all parasympatholytic drugs. Additional mydriasis occurs with simultaneous use of sympathomimetic drugs such as phenylephrine. In clinical use, such additive medications are commonly prescribed to achieve maximal dilatation of the pupil.

The response of individual eyes to atropine varies with pigmentation. Darkly pigmented patients are more resistant to atropinization. Usually atropine cycloplegia is attained within a few hours and will last for a week or more. In contrast, homatropine cycloplegia lasts only several days.

Clinical use. Atropine is one of the best medications for treatment of iridocyclitis. By relaxing the inflamed musculature of the ciliary body, atropinization reduces the pain characteristic of iridocyclitis. If started early enough, atropine will break adhesions of the iris to the lens. Untreated, such adhesions may cause glaucoma, occlude the pupil, or induce cataract formation. Perhaps most important, atropine restores to normal the permeability of inflamed iris vessels, thereby decreasing the leakage of protein and cellular debris into the aqueous chamber.

The eye suffering from iridocyclitis is unusually resistant to atropinization. Repeated instillation of 1% atropine, perhaps three times daily, supplemented by 10% phenylephrine, may be necessary to break iris adhesions to the lens.

The red-eyed patient without iridocyclitis will not benefit from atropinization. A common mistake of emergency room interns is to atropinize an eye with a minor corneal abrasion. Such treatment does not benefit the patient and disables him from performing near work for a week or more.

Toxicity. Only 10 mg of atropine may be a fatal dose to a child. Since one drop of 1% atropine contains about 0.5 mg of drug (the usual preoperative dose for drying nasopharyngeal secretions), simple calculation will reveal that an insignificant-looking 5 ml ophthalmic bottle of atropine contains enough alkaloid to kill several children. Patients should be warned to keep all drugs out of reach of children, and especially such poisonous medications as atropine or pilocarpine.

Parasympatholytic drugs such as atropine will increase intraocular pressure in eyes with glaucoma. Eyes predisposed to acute glaucoma because of an anatomically shallow angle are especially intolerant of atropinization.

Will preoperative atropinization (as for general anesthesia) harm open-angle glaucoma? This question frequently arises. The answer is no. The sensitivity of the eye to the relatively small systemic dose is low. If miotic therapy is being used, the local effects of pilocarpine are far greater than can be overcome by systemic atropinization. Of course, the usual frequency of miotic therapy should be continued through the hospital stay, just as at home. Actually, even if a small elevation of intraocular pressure should occur, no significant damage would occur during a period of a few days.

Contact dermatitis confined to the lids of the treated eye is not uncommonly caused by atropine. This allergy is recognized by the characteristic itching and by the reddened and swollen, weeping texture of the skin. No treatment is satisfactory except discontinuance of the offending allergen. Even years later, reuse of atropine usually causes prompt return of the allergy.

Homatropine. Homatropine is a parasympatholytic drug similar to atropine except that it has a much shorter duration of action, its effect lasting less than 24 hours. Because of the shorter duration of homatropine cycloplegia, its use was formerly popular for refraction. Cyclopentolate and tropicamide have replaced homatropine because of their more rapid onset of cycloplegia.

Scopolamine. Except for a much shorter duration of action, the effects of scopolamine are, for practical purposes, the same as those of atropine. Half the cycloplegic effect of scopolamine is lost within 3 to 4 hours, and accommodation returns to normal in about 1 day.

Scopolamine may be used as a substitute for atropine in cases of atropine allergy.

Cyclopentolate (Cyclogyl). Cyclopentolate is a potent parasympatholytic drug of great value for inducing cycloplegia and wide mydriasis. Its cycloplegic effect is superior to that of homatropine or scopolamine; it has a more rapid onset, greater intensity, and shorter duration. One drop of 0.5% cyclopentolate, repeated in 10 minutes, will produce maximum cycloplegia in 40% of white patients within 15 minutes. This cycloplegic effect is usually dissipated within 24 hours.

The physician should be aware of the frequency of individual variations in drug response. A dosage of two drops of cyclopentolate requires 45 minutes to achieve maximum cycloplegic effect in 20% of white patients. The eyes of black patients are resistant to cyclopentolate, just as to other cycloplegics, and may require repeated instillation of 2% solution and a longer time than usual for dilatation.

Excellent mydriasis is produced by cyclopentolate. Pupils dilated with this drug do not constrict, even with the prolonged, intense light of the indirect ophthalmoscope or during fundus photography. This maximal mydriasis is of great value during the examination of patients with retinal detachment, for instance.

Patients with atropine allergy do not have a cross sensitivity to cyclopentolate. This drug is an effective medication in treatment of iridocyclitis complicated by atropine allergy. Because of its shorter duration of action, cyclopentolate must be instilled as often as every 3 or 4 hours in the management of a severe case of iridocyclitis, whereas atropine could be used once or twice daily.

As is true of all parasympatholytic drugs, cyclopentolate will increase the intraocular pressure of most patients with chronic simple glaucoma. Dilatation with any drug, including cyclopentolate, may precipitate an attack of acute glaucoma in patients predisposed to this disorder because of a narrow anterior chamber angle.

Ocular instillation of cyclopentolate may cause disturbances of the central nevous system in children. Symptoms develop about 30 to 45 minutes after instillation of the drops and include restlessness, aimless wandering, ataxia, irrelevant talking, incoherent

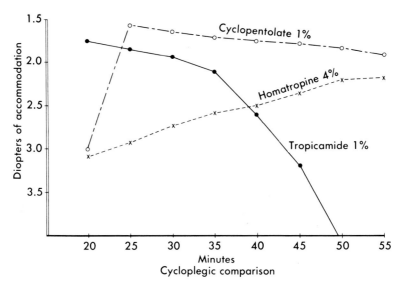

Fig. 23-8. Duration and effectiveness of cycloplegia induced by two instillations of 1% tropicamide, one instillation of 1% cyclopentolate, and two instillations of 4% homatropine. (Modified from Gettes, B.C., and Belmont, O.: Arch. Ophthalmol. **66:**336, 1961. Copyright 1961, American Medical Association.)

speech, hallucinations, memory loss, and faulty orientation as to time and place. Ten percent of children may develop such symptoms after use of 2% cyclopentolate (this concentration is unnecessarily strong—0.5% solution is adequate).

Tropicamide (Mydriacyl). Tropicamide is a rapid-acting parasympatholytic drug suitable for producing cycloplegia and mydriasis of very short duration. As shown in Fig. 23-8, the duration of tropicamide cycloplegia is less than an hour. This extremely short action has obvious value to the patient in sparing him the nuisance of prolonged cycloplegia. However, if used for cycloplegic refraction, tropicamide instillation must be repeated, lest the effect wear off too soon.

Corticosteroids

Corticosteroids decrease cellular and fibrinous exudation and tissue infiltration, inhibit fibroblastic and collagen-forming activity, retard epithelial and endothelial regeneration, diminish postinflammatory neovascularization, and restore toward normal the excessively permeable inflamed capillaries. These anti-inflammatory effects are nonspecific, occurring whether the etiology is allergic, traumatic, or infectious. The degree of response is dose related, and corticosteroid therapy must therefore be titrated against the individual disease. Subject to the limitations of toxic side effects, enough corticosteroid is given to obtain a therapeutic response. It must be emphasized that an infectious or allergic cause of inflammation is *not* eliminated by corticosteroid therapy but continues to be present even though the inflammatory response of the body is inhibited. The clinical implication of this fact is that treatment must be continued after apparent cure and that dosage must be tapered off gradually to avoid relapse.

The anti-inflammatory effects of corticosteroids are useful in ophthalmology because the delicate and transparent ocular structures are particularly susceptible to functional damage by inflammation and scarring. Properly used, corticosteroids will markedly reduce the amount of permanent scarring and may make the difference between useful vision and its loss. In general, therapeutic responses are obtained in clinically nonpyogenic inflammations such as uveitis and scleritis and in all forms of ocular allergy. Although pyogenic inflammations are initially reduced in severity, the ultimate tissue destruction will be more severe because of the loss of body defense mechanisms. Corticosteroids reduce resistance to almost all types of invading microorganisms—bacteria, viruses, and fungi—and should *not* be used in the presence of such infections except simultaneously with an *effective* antibiotic. Degenerative diseases are completely refractory to corticosteroid therapy.

These facts indicate the great practical importance of accurate differential diagnosis. As an illustration, the similar-appearing lesions of idiopathic paramacular chorioretinitis, tuberculous choroiditis, and senile macular degeneration will, respectively, be improved, be made considerably worse, and be unaffected despite great expense to the patient through corticosteroid therapy.

Administration. The route of administration of corticosteroids depends primarily on the site of involvement. Topical therapy is effective in anterior segment disease, including disorders of the lids, conjunctiva, cornea, iris, and ciliary body. Ease of application, relatively low cost, and absence of systemic complications strongly favor local routes whenever they are effective. Unusually stubborn anterior segment disease rarely requires supplementary systemic or subconjunctival routes of administration.

The course of posterior segment disease (chorioretinitis, optic neuritis, posterior scleritis) is not appreciably affected by topical medication and requires systemic therapy. Patients prefer oral corticosteroids to injections. Since the peak concentration of plasma corticosteroids occurs within an hour after oral administration, it is unnecessary to resort to intravenous injections for faster or better results. Four to eight hours after an oral dose, plasma corticosteroid levels have returned to normal.

Dosage will vary with the severity of disease. For most topical purposes, 0.5% suspensions of cortisone, hydrocortisone, prednisone, or prednisolone are adequate. Usually, increased frequency of instillation is at least as effective as a stronger concentration. The danger of relapse exists if therapy is prematurely discontinued in a disease such as iritis; hence, the frequency of use should be tapered off gradually over a week or more, depending on the response of the given eye. Usually little difference is noted clinically in the response to the various available corticosteroid derivatives.

The minimum acceptable response is arrest of further progress of the disease. When improvement is noted, the physician may choose to reduce corticosteroid dosage to the

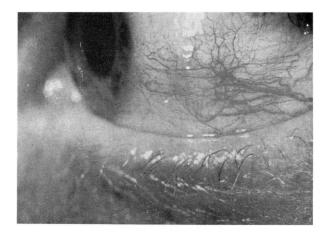

Fig. 23-9. A localized patch of dilated superficial and deep vessels, without purulent discharge or ulceration, without a history or evidence of trauma, and surrounded by normally white conjunctiva, is characteristic of episcleritis. Topical corticosteroids rapidly cure episcleritis.

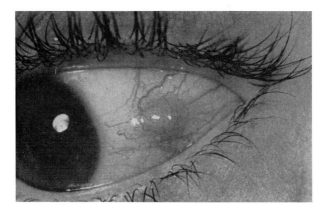

Fig. 23-10. A phlyctenule is similar to episcleritis except that it contains a yellowish, elevated nodule in its center. Therapy is the same as for episcleritis.

minimum level necessary to produce steady regression of a lesion, or he may prefer to maintain high dosage in an attempt to restore a vital area, such as the macula, to normal as quickly as possible. Less critical inflammations will tend to be treated by the first choice and more critical ones by the second choice.

Indications. In general, corticosteroid therapy is indicated for many nonpyogenic inflammations (episcleritis [Fig. 23-9], scleritis, uveitis, phlyctenulosis [Fig. 23-10], interstitial keratitis, sclerokeratitis, rosacea keratoconjunctivitis, optic neuritis, and so on), and for the reduction of scarring from certain types of severe injury (chemical or thermal corneal burns). Corticosteroid therapy is of no benefit whatever in degenerative diseases (senile macular degeneration, cataract, corneal dystrophies, glaucoma, keratoconjunctivitis sicca, and so on). Old scars (inactive chorioretinitis, band keratopathy, traumatic corneal scars and so on) are not altered by cortisone. Some rare diseases responsive to corticosteroid therapy include Boeck's sarcoid, malignant thyroid exophthalmos, temporal arteritis, and herpes zoster ophthalmicus.

Contraindications. A common mistake is the routine use of corticosteroids in the management of minor corneal abrasions. This practice must be strongly condemned, for no benefit results and the susceptibility to infection is increased. For some illogical reason, corticosteroid-antibiotic ointments are popular in the management of marginal blepharitis. Almost all marginal blepharitis is infectious and responds well to mechanical cleaning and topical antibiotic ointment. Corticosteroids do not benefit such cases, may reduce resistance to infection, and are inevitably more expensive.

The systemic complications of cortisone use are well known and do not require repeating here. Topical ocular use does not cause these systemic complications. The main ocular complications of corticosteroid use are activation of infection, worsening of glaucoma, and cataract development.

General agreement exists that cortisone treatment of the typical dendritic keratitis caused by herpes simplex infection leads to much more severe corneal scarring than would otherwise be expected. This disease is a not uncommon cause of red eye and is perhaps the most outstanding reason why the physician should be wary of ''shotgun'' use of corticosteroids for red eyes. Unless you are absolutely certain the diagnosis is not herpetic infection, you should not prescribe corticosteroids for a red eye with corneal involvement. Do not be misled by the fact that a knowledgeable ophthalmologist will use corticosteroids cautiously in combination with antivirals for treatment of some stages of chronic herpetic keratitis. Your patient can have serious trouble from such treatment unless you know what you are doing. Dense corneal scarring, corneal perforation, uveitis, and even encephalitis can result.

Under certain circumstances of chronic corneal ulceration, the epithelial cells adjacent to the ulcer will produce collagenase, an enzyme capable of dissolving the exposed corneal stroma. Corticosteroid therapy enhances such stromal dissolution. In fact, stromal loss may occur so rapidly (only a few days) that the cornea is said to ''melt.'' Ocular perforation may result.

Vaccinia and trachoma viruses are also activated by corticosteroids. Almost all fungi grow better with the aid of corticosteroid inhibition of host defenses. Since the advent of corticosteroids and their widespread use, severe fungus eye infections are more commonly encountered. Bacterial infections are also enhanced by corticosteroid therapy. *Pseudomonas* and tuberculosis ocular infections particularly contraindicate corticosteroid therapy.

The effect on intraocular pressure of topical corticosteroids applied three or four times daily for a month is of special clinical significance. In two thirds of the population, the intraocular pressure does not change. However, in one third a moderate rise in intraocular pressure—to the level of 20 to 30 mm Hg—occurs. Perhaps 5% of the population will respond to such corticosteroid use with a marked pressure elevation—to 40 mm Hg and higher. Genetic research has established that open-angle glaucoma is due to a recessive gene present in one third of the population—the group responding to corticosteroids with a moderate pressure elevation. The 5% with a marked pressure have a double gene for glaucoma and hence have the potential to develop clinical glaucoma spontaneously. Obviously, a substantial proportion of the population will develop abnormally high intra-ocular pressure if treated with topical corticosteroids for a month or more. This hazard *must* be considered whenever prolonged corticosteroid use is prescribed.

Long-term systemic corticosteroid therapy (1 year or more) is capable of causing posterior subcapsular cataract. This complication is dose related and may occur in as many as 80% of patients receiving 15 mg of prednisone daily for 4 years or more. These cataracts are not usually sufficiently dense to require surgery, but they do not regress when the drug is stopped. In time, some of these patients will require cataract surgery.

Fluorescein

Fluorescein does not actually stain tissues but is useful as an indicator dye by virtue of its visibility in very high dilutions. The intact corneal epithelium, having a high lipid content, resists penetration by any water-soluble molecule such as fluorescein and hence is not colored by it. Any break in the epithelium permits fluorescein penetration into Bowman's membrane and the corneal stroma. Whether due to trauma, infection, or any other cause, such epithelial defects appear bright green with fluorescein and are thereby easily visualized. When the epithelial surface regenerates, the characteristic green coloration disappears, regardless of whether the underlying stroma is normal or scarred. Bright oblique illumination and some method of magnification help identify the minute staining defects characteristic of many types of disease. Grossly visible defects occur only with extensive trauma or large ulcers. Be aware that the typical dendritic ulcer of herpetic keratitis, a particularly serious problem, is small and inconspicuous, even with the aid of fluorescein.

The safest, most convenient method of using fluorescein is to use sterile fluorescein-impregnated filter paper. The strip of fluorescein paper is touched to the lower conjunctival sac for a moment, until the tears dissolve out the desired amount of fluorescein. The tear film will now appear to be a uniform faint green or yellow color. The excess fluorescein should be irrigated away with saline solution to enhance the contrast between the colored lesion and the adjacent normal areas. Fluorescein staining of the eye is transient, disappearing within minutes, and is therefore not cosmetically objectionable to the patient. Stain of the skin are easily removed with a tissue moistened with water.

Fluorescein solutions are notoriously susceptible to contamination. Since the purpose of fluorescein is to identify epithelial defects, the patients for whom this drug is used are particularly vulnerable to infection. Hence, the practice of keeping a bottle of fluorescein solution in the office is unsafe.

Fluorescein may also be used to test the patency of the lacrimal drainage system in patients with epiphora. A generous amount of dye is placed in the suspected eye. Five minutes later the patient blows his nose and clears his throat into paper tissues. Traces of fluorescein will be visible in these oral and nasal secretions in patients with normal tear passages.

Given intravenously, 10 ml of 5% fluorescein will circulate from an arm vein to the eye. The dye appears in the retinal arterioles after about 13 seconds and persists in the fundus circulation for about 20 seconds. Study of the fundus by fluorescein photography will provide three types of information:

1. The presence or absence of abnormally opaque or transparent areas, as demonstrated by exceptionally poor or good retroillumination
2. The presence or absence of areas of abnormal capillary permeability
3. The time relationships of retinal flow

By providing this specialized information, fluorescein photography may be helpful in the differential diagnosis of fundus lesions.

Osmotic agents

The blood-aqueous barrier behaves as a semipermeable membrane between the plasma and the ocular fluids. Osmotically active molecules such as urea, mannitol, or glycerol

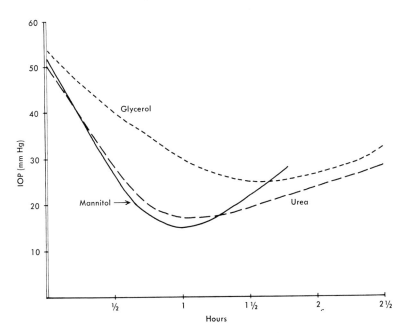

Fig. 23-11. Pressure-lowering effect of oral glycerol (1.5 mg/kg), urea (1 g/kg intravenously), and mannitol (3 g/kg intravenously). All drugs used in each one of 30 glaucoma patients. (Modified from Galin, M.A., Davidson, R., and Schachter, N. Published with permission from The American Journal of Ophthalmology **62:**629-634, 1966. Copyright by The Ophthalmic Publishing Company.)

cannot readily cross the blood-aqueous barrier; hence, they create an osmotic differential between plasma and the aqueous and vitreous. This osmotic differential withdraws fluid from the eye and will effectively reduce intraocular pressure in any type of glaucoma.

Osmotherapy acts rapidly, reducing pressure within minutes to an hour (Fig. 23-11). As shown, the drop in pressure is capable of bringing an eye from 50 mm Hg to normal levels in 30 to 60 minutes. The duration of osmotic pressure reduction is only 5 or 6 hours; hence, this method of treatment is not of value in management of chronic glaucoma. However, it is the most effective method available for control of acute glaucoma.

Mannitol is the most satisfactory osmotherapeutic drug. Its dosage is 2 g/kg of 20% solution given intravenously during a 30-minute period. The patient may not drink fluid during the period of osmotic dehydration, or the therapeutic effect will be lost. He must be specifically instructed against drinking, for mannitol dehydration causes intense thirst. Provision must be made for the intense diuresis that results. Since mannitol is soluble only to a 15% solution in cold water, the 20% solution must be warmed before administration to eliminate the crystals present in cold solutions. Mannitol is stable in solution and therefore can be sterilized by heat and stored without deterioration, thus avoiding the bothersome preparation of a fresh solution that is necessary with urea.

Since mannitol is not absorbed from the gastrointestinal tract, it does not reduce intraocular pressure when given orally. Mannitol is not significantly metabolized and thus can be used in a diabetic patient without creating metabolic problems. Mannitol does not cause tissue necrosis if it extravasates into the tissues. (Urea causes destructive sloughing of the tissue if it extravasates.)

Glycerol is given orally in a dosage of 1 to 1.5 g/kg in 50% solution. Refrigeration and flavoring with lemon juice makes this unpleasant medication more palatable. Because glycerol is the most easily used osmotic agent, it is the most suitable for office use in the initial treatment of acute glaucoma.

Glycerol is utilized as a carbohydrate and can cause hyperglycemia and glycosuria. If given intravenously, it causes hematuria because of damage to the afferent glomerular arterioles.

Headache due to increased intracranial pressure is the most unpleasant common side effect of all osmotic drugs. It affects more than 90% of patients and is comparable to a lumbar puncture headache. Such headaches are easily relieved simply by lying down. Nausea affects one third of patients and may preclude the use of oral glycerol. About 20% of patients are confused and perhaps disoriented during the period of cerebral dehydration; osmotherapy should therefore be given only when the patient is under continuing observation.

Although pure water does not have therapeutic value, its effect on the eye is of great importance. Part of the dehydrating mechanism that maintains corneal clarity depends on the hypertonicity of the tear film. Irrigation of the corneal surface with a hypotonic solution, such as pure distilled water, interferes with corneal dehydration and results in corneal edema. This condition is transient, leaving promptly when irrigation ceases.

A more serious problem follows accidental irrigation of the anterior chamber with distilled water during eye surgery. The single layer of endothelial cells lining the posterior cornea is absolutely vital to corneal dehydration. Just as red blood cells hemolyze in distilled water, so also the corneal endothelial cells hydrate and burst in distilled water. They do not regenerate, and the cornea remains permanently opaque after death of the endothelial cells. For this reason, distilled water is not permitted in the eye surgical room.

Secretory inhibitors

When the increased outflow of aqueous resulting from miotic therapy is insufficient to control glaucoma, the ophthalmologist usually resorts to medications that reduce aqueous secretion. The most effective of such medications inhibit the carbonic anhydrase enzyme, which is essential in maintaining the normal rate of aqueous secretion. When carbonic anhydrase is maximally inhibited, the rate of aqueous secretion drops to about 40% of normal. Obviously, if the damaged outflow mechanism responsible for the given case of glaucoma is capable of handling 40% of the normal flow, carbonic anhydrase inhibitors will control the intraocular pressure. If greater damage to the outflow mechanism exists, control will be inadequate.

The most commonly used secretory inhibitor is acetazolamide (Diamox). Its dosage is 250 mg every 6 hours. The effect of acetazolamide may be prolonged by dispensing it in coated granule form (Diamox Sequels). A 500-mg Sequel is given every 12 hours.

The hypotensive effect of acetazolamide is not due to its diuretic action. Particular confusion has arisen because of the similarity of the brand names of two diuretics: Diamox and Diuril. Although a potent diuretic, Diuril has no effect on intraocular pressure.

Only rarely is chronic glaucoma treated with a carbonic anhydrase inhibitor alone. Ordinarily, carbonic anhydrase inhibitors are added to miotic therapy when the latter has been inadequate to control a difficult case of open-angle glaucoma. Angle-closure glaucoma should *not* be treated with carbonic anhydrase inhibitors, for such management gives the illusion of pressure control while the narrow angle progressively occludes, and the opportunity for surgical cure by iridectomy is irrevocably lost. Perhaps half the open-angle glaucoma patients in whom the condition is poorly controlled by miotics alone will respond to the addition of secretory inhibitors.

Gastrointestinal upsets are the most frequent cause of acetazolamide intolerance so severe as to force discontinuance of treatment. Symptoms may range from vague abdominal discomfort and a peculiar metallic taste to severe nausea and diarrhea. Paresthesias commonly affect hands and feet and the circumoral region. Drowsiness and malaise affect some patients. These side effects are less annoying with the sustained-release form of medication.

Tolerance to the various carbonic anhydrase inhibitors may vary considerably from one patient to another. The individual with acetazolamide intolerance may do well with another carbonic anhydrase inhibitor. Dosage of the other commonly used carbonic anhydrase inhibitors is methazolamide, 100 mg three times daily; dichlorphenamide, 50 mg three times daily; and ethoxzolamide, 125 mg three times daily.

Timolol, levo-epinephrine, and carbonic anhydrase inhibitors have a similar mechanism of action, all three decreasing aqueous secretion. In practice, timolol is usually the first choice for open-angle glaucoma therapy. Miotics or levo-epinephrine may be added if control is inadequate. When all else fails, acetazolamide may be used before resorting to surgery.

RECOMMENDED READING

Havener, W.H.: Ocular pharmacology, ed. 5, St. Louis, 1983, The C.V. Mosby Co.

chapter 24 Metaphysical Therapy (Reassurance Therapy)

One important method of treatment a physician can offer his patients has nothing to do with pills and knives. The treatment itself can neither be seen nor weighed, and yet its effects are indisputably evident and beneficial. Obviously, I am referring to what has been called the "art of medicine." In ivory tower circles this modality is often in disrepute, being equated with the hocus-pocus of the charlatan. True, the charlatan has nothing to offer but a form of "art," but his severest critics must concede that an accomplished quack is able to influence profoundly the attitudes of his patients. I submit to your consideration the proposition that a comparable ability on the part of an ethical physician is of benefit to all his patients and may even be of greater value to most patients than are the pills and knives. Furthermore, the intent of this writing is to define precisely the great power of metaphysical forms of therapy and to explain clearly the rules that govern the application of such treatment.

Historically, the broad tapestry of human activity contains a constant thread of healing power. This healing power has been known by many different names, all of which refer to the same entity. I prefer one of the current names, "life force." Life force is supposed to flow from the touch of the healer. And it does.

Accept for the moment that "life force" will be a name by which we designate whatever is the common denominator of metaphysical therapy. And accept that there is a common denominator in these therapies—that each method is simply a different outside wrapping for the same life force. To what do I refer? To the primitive medicine man; to the grandmother who is an expert in using potent herbs; to the frontier salesman of snake oil; to the modern promoter of krebiozen, laetrile, and other comparable past, present, and future cancer remedies; to the Christian Scientist, the yoga disciple, the exorcist, and the shrines of religious healing; to the legalized cults that flourish in the United States today and would sue me if I named them; to the current fair-haired child of metaphysics— acupuncture. And let us also include as a life force practitioner every single ethical physician who is beloved by his patients.

A valid method of treatment, whether it is penicillin or life force, requires a basis for effectiveness. The basis for life force is the genuine need of a human being for being comforted, supported, reassured, and loved. Whether sick or well, a person has such needs, and in sickness these needs are greatly intensified. Perhaps I can explain my point by comparing the sick patient to a lost puppy.

A lost puppy cries loud and long and with great intensity. Why? Because he knows he will die if his mother does not find him. Barring human intervention, every lost puppy from the beginning of time has been eaten up or has perished from starvation, freezing, drowning, or other unpleasant difficulties. There is nothing imaginary about the value of having your mother beside you in the dark, especially if you are out in the primitive woods and your mother is an 85-pound Doberman pinscher with teeth an inch long. Maybe such a comparison does not seem relevant to present human civilized existence, but our bodies, minds, and emotions were designed for survival under circumstances more closely resembling the lost puppy's environment than a modern hospital environment. In short, life force works because it evokes a response from the basic primitive instincts for survival.

As the current vogue in life force therapy, acupuncture deserves mention. The Orientals have perfected a format that maximizes the placebo component of therapy. A complex nonsense ritual endowed with mystery is virtually guaranteed to work under placebo rules (which I will shortly explain). Within a few years these words will seem inexplicable, but at the time of this writing, almost every layman will concede that he believes there is probably value in acupuncture. More surprisingly, in January 1974, I asked a class of 150 intermediate medical students whether they did not believe acupuncture had specific curative value. Only *three* of the entire group were willing to indicate they did not believe acupuncture had such value. Even *Today's Health,* the lay journal of the American Medical Association, has presented a favorable attitude toward acupuncture. Neurophysiologists seek explanations for acupuncture effects and propose the "gate theory," a concept of competitive cancellation of neural effects. Legislators authorize research on acupuncture. And, as always, desperate patients travel in endless search of the miracle.

PLACEBO THERAPY

Is medical science unaware of the nature of metaphysical therapy? Not at all. Many physicians, however, grossly underestimate its value. The accepted medical name for life force is placebo therapy. "Just a placebo" is the common deprecatory classification of a worthless remedy. However, let us be clear as to what is worthless—it is not the placebo that is worthless, but the specific medication selected for use.

A placebo may be defined as any therapy (or component of a therapy) that has no specific value in treatment of the given medical condition. For example, if we treat the common cold with sugar pills or with penicillin, both are placebos. If we similarly treat a streptococcal pharyngitis, the penicillin has both definitive value and placebo effectiveness, whereas the sugar pill has only a placebo effect.

At least one third of patients suffering from almost any disease will be completely cured or greatly benefited after use of a placebo. Placebo response is not a property of the disease but a characteristic of the patient and of the amount of suggestion employed in the therapy. The attitudes and efforts of the physician determine the magnitude of placebo response. The composition and amount of the placebo do not matter in the least, so long as it is not detected by the patient as being a placebo. A placebo is *not* worthless—it is one of the most powerful medications we use.

The self-limited nature of most disorders results in credit for the cure being given to any treatment, whether of value or not. Even inexorably progressive disorders have objectively measurable remissions, so that striking but transitory improvements occur in the course of multiple sclerosis, cancer, and many other major diseases. Placebo therapy instituted before such a remission will, of course, produce a ''cure''—at least for a short time.

Note that I am classifying the giving of a placebo as simply another ritual method of transmitting life force. The placebo is no more valuable than are the acupuncture needles—the value accrues from the amount of life force transmitted.

REASSURANCE THERAPY

All the preceding material is preamble to my advocacy of reassurance therapy, which is the way in which the ethical physician transmits life force.

Each patient should be confident he is receiving good care. From his standpoint, this confidence is much more an emotional state than an intellectual evaluation. You can and should contribute to this confidence by the deliberate use of what may be termed reassurance therapy.

You may dismiss this concept with lofty scientific disdain; nevertheless, reassurance therapy is required to a greater or lesser degree by every patient and is the sole treatment required in the management in about half of our patient visits. The patient's satisfaction with you as his physician will usually be determined more by your skillful use of reassurance therapy than by your pills. If you are a surgeon, bear in mind that any sensible patient requires a great deal of confidence in a man whom he will permit to cut into his body. I am discussing reassurance therapy in detail because of its inherent importance and because its characteristics are not usually stressed in traditional medical education.

Reassurance therapy begins with the history taking, which is the patient's introduction to you. The patient's first impressions of you will be good or bad, depending on your skill in taking a history. Note that from the patient's standpoint the history represents more than half of his verbal communication with you and therefore assumes proportionate importance in his assessment of you. I have already told you this in Chapter 4, but I am repeating it here because these are the important steps you must follow with each patient for the rest of your professional life.

Step one of reassurance therapy is simply a *standard medical history*. Do *not* attempt to reassure the patient while taking a history—such attempts are counterproductive by inhibiting the patient from giving you further information and by betraying your anxiety or impatience. In fact, permitting the patient to experience some anxiety during the history preconditions him to accept reassurance therapy more effectively at the appropriate later time. (Remember that reassurance therapy requires six steps—it will not work otherwise.)

Step two is *evaluation of affect*. This evaluation is to be performed during the same time that you are taking the history. Affect is evaluated nonverbally, by interpretation of "body language." The tone of voice, the ease or apprehension of the patient, and his mannerisms convey affect more than do his words. When you realize that you feel uneasy with a patient, he has successfully conveyed to you his concern about his problems.

Evaluation of affect is important because it shows you the significance of the symptoms to the patient and guides you as to how much reassurance therapy will be needed.

Step three is *examination of the affected part*. It is not only a necessity of physical diagnosis, but it also "talks" to the patient. The gentleness and assurance of your physical contact contributes significantly to the patient's evaluation of your ability. Touch carefully—remember your touch "talks" nonverbally to the patient.

Step four is *medical diagnosis*. You must accurately assess the nature of the patient's problem. Note that the patient cannot judge your accuracy or your knowledge. This step will, of course, determine the definitive medical care you render to the patient.

Step five is *explanation*. You may misunderstand this step. Although an explanation of the problem is a necessary part of reassurance therapy, is basic to the legal doctrine of informed consent, and is essential to the cooperation of your patient in therapy, the patient does *not* need to understand your explanation to be reassured. The explanation must, however, convey three beliefs to the patient:

1. Belief that the physician understands the symptoms
2. Belief that the physician is not uncertain about the management of the symptoms (Do not undermine yourself by spontaneous small talk that shakes the patient's confidence; keep your mouth *shut* during the indecisive period of your thinking about the evaluation and management.)
3. Belief that the physician is sympathetic (that is, not antiseptic in manner) and wishes to be helpful.

Only as the sixth and final step is *reassurance* appropriate. What is reassurance? Is it saying, "Oh, don't worry?" Did you ever see anyone worry less after such an admonition?

Reassurance may be defined as a *credible and acceptable prognosis*. Predict the patient's future appropriately. Be as specific as possible with respect to the patient's particular situation. What can he do and what can he not do? Seek out and stress all positive aspects. Do not volunteer negative and threatening facts unless he must know them (for example, informed consent to surgery requires general knowledge that not every operation is successful). Do not be unrealistic—future problems arise if the patient's expectations exceed the physician's ability to deliver. Banish unwarranted fears—patients usually imagine worse problems than actually exist.

Your verbal communication with the patient includes the history, explanation, and reassurance. They merge inextricably into the total emotional and factual impact the physician makes on the patient. So be aware that history taking is also part of your therapy—for good or ill.

SUMMARY

I do not advocate that you relax in any way your efforts to deliver traditional high-quality medical care. Such care is essential, and no compromise with quality is acceptable.

However, the delivery of antiseptic care is an incomplete form of patient management. I do advocate that you should integrate the principles of reassurance therapy into your medical practice. You will be rewarded by the gratitude of your patients and will find that the patients actually get well faster (as measured by return to normal activity).

chapter 25 Evaluation of Therapeutic Response

PROBLEMS DUE TO OBSERVATION

Controlled observation. Once, long ago, a physician prescribed cabbage for the relief of certain symptoms suffered by a blacksmith. Recovery followed. In time, a clergyman developed similar symptoms; he was also treated with cabbage, but he died. The physician concluded that, for these symptoms, cabbages would cure blacksmiths but kill clergymen.

Do such clinical coincidences still influence our treatment of patients? Certainly! The emotional impact of a single dramatic clinical experience creates lasting but invalid impressions as to the effect of a given medication or procedure. Such a trap can be avoided only by study of a carefully controlled and adequately large series of cases.

The basic question in a controlled study is: With what patients should the treated patients be compared? Ideally, the control and treated patients should be identical in all respects except for the factor under evaluation. "Controls" cannot be the same number of patients seen 10 years ago, or a group of patients failing to respond to treatment.

Inaccurate observation. Our enthusiasms and prejudices distort our evaluation of circumstances to an unbelievable degree. Our ability to perceive detail is far more limited and unreliable than we think it is. One need only discuss a series of previously observed patients with a group of competent physicians to realize the amazing differences of opinion as to the history and physical findings.

Many reports have documented that a 25% variability commonly exists in the accuracy of clinical and laboratory observations. Indeed, recognition of the probability of faulty determinations and observations is part of the skill of an astute physician.

Double-blind controlled observation. The intent of double-blind studies is to eliminate observer bias. Supposedly, errors are neutralized by the comparable control. In practice, this technique works well, but monumental bloopers still occur in experimental design. Even the most careful scientific study must be regarded with caution if its results conflict with other sources of information, or if it is not subsequently confirmed by other studies.

418

PROBLEMS DUE TO STATISTICS AND PATIENTS

Statistical significance. ''Significance'' is often accepted as a seal of approval verifying the conclusions of the author. Actually, a ''statistically significant difference'' simply establishes that the control and experimental groups do differ in some respect. However, this difference is not necessarily the treatment administered but often will be another factor in selection of the two groups. The relevant factor may be apparent to the critic or may be subtly concealed by inadequate description of the experiment.

For example, a statistically significant correlation exists between the number of marriages performed by the Church of England and the incidence of venereal disease. However, this correlation does not mean that the ceremony causes disease; rather, both marriage and disease rates are related to the number of individuals in the marriageable age group at any given time.

Patient (un)reliability. At least 30% to 40% of patients do not follow instructions at all, and everyone fails to obey prolonged and detailed recommendations with 100% accuracy. Failure to cooperate cannot reliably be correlated with environment, education, socioeconomic status, age, sex, or any other variable. Reliability of clinic attendance and of obtaining the drug does not correlate with cooperation in actually taking the medication. Failure to cooperate cannot be detected by inquiry because the patients lie—even honest patients lie!

Duration of therapy is one consistent factor. Patients become progressively less cooperative in taking medication during prolonged treatment (of glaucoma, for instance). Also, multiple medications are less likely to be used according to instructions.

Hence, in the evaluation of therapeutic response (either good or bad), we cannot fail to consider the *probability* that the patient is not using his medication properly.

Pharmacogenetics. Even if we are positive the proper medication has been given as directed, constitutionally determined individual differences in response occur. Allergy, idiosyncrasy, and hypersensitivity are common examples of pharmacogenetic differences.

Placebo effect. The words and attitudes of a physician cause measurable positive or negative patient responses. We recognize this placebo effect when it occurs with the giving of a sugar pill. Actually, of course, the placebo effect will also account for part of the patient response to a potent drug. It can be a trap for the unwary physician who may confuse the placebo response with specific therapeutic benefit. Such confusion has resulted in many enthusiastic but subsequently unconfirmed reports in the literature.

About 35% of patients show a significant response to placebo therapy. Stated differently, almost any treatment will cause subjective improvement in one of every three patients suffering from almost anything. Objective improvement will occur in the psychosomatic parameters (pulse, respiration, gastric acid, and so on). The placebo effect is greatest in situations where the stress and psychologic reactions of the patient are greatest. It does not matter in the least of what the placebo is made or how large the dose—only that the patient does not detect that it is intended as a placebo.

PROBLEMS DUE TO DRUGS

Generic nonequivalence. Chemical identity is not the same as biologic availability. Differences in vehicle, freedom from contamination, and a host of other variables, even including the type of container, do cause variations in response. For example, an allergic response to a particular preservative used by one manufacturer may be entirely absent in a generic "equivalent."

Counterfeit drugs represent a problem of unknown magnitude. Penalties are token, and potential profits are great. Detection of a spurious medication would be beyond my capability except that a puzzling failure of therapeutic response might be recognized.

Drug stability. Prolonged storage of medications commonly results in loss of potency and occasionally in toxic degradation products. Many dry medications break down rapidly when placed in solution. Exposure to warmth, light, and oxygen causes deterioration of epinephrine, for instance.

Medication errors. Tribute to the faithfulness of nurses and pharmacists in appropriate. Nevertheless, human errors routinely occur. Do not exclude the possibility of error in medication if the therapeutic response is greatly different from what was expected— and double-check the accuracy of your own written orders.

Toxic effects. The evaluation of therapeutic response must take into account the possibility of adverse side effects. Such complications are commonplace. Perhaps 10% of hospitalized patients are there for the management of complications of treatment. Sometimes one cannot readily distinguish the course of the disease from iatrogenic problems.

SUMMARY

The evaluation of therapy requires that we apply the scientific method to each patient as follows:

1. Gather all available facts (history and physical).
2. Formulate a hypothesis (preliminary diagnosis).
3. On the basis of the hypothesis, seek corroborating or conflicting facts (look at the patient again, seeking pertinent findings).
4. Formulate a theory (presume that the diagnosis is correct).
5. Finally, use the theory to predict (prescribe appropriate medication and observe whether the expected therapeutic response occurs).

Most faults in patient management result from insufficient fact gathering. The most overlooked step is the second check of the patient, intended to elicit subtle corroborative or conflicting facts. Such details require intellectually guided seeking, rather than hopeful looking. Such intellectually guided analysis is mandatory in evaluation of therapeutic response. Otherwise, at the end of a self-limited disease, the unwary physician will attribute the "cure" to the final treatment prescribed—but it will not work the next time (just as the cabbages at the beginning of this chapter failed to cure the clergyman).

chapter 26 Surgery
of the Eye

The indications for and techniques of ophthalmic surgery are not of general interest. However, many physicians will wish to undertake the surgical care of small lid lesions and the repair of superficial trauma.

SURGERY OF THE LID

Repair of lid lacerations. Careful examination of the underlying eyeball is the most important step in the treatment of any patient with lid injury. Care of an injured eye enjoys a high priority over lid repair. Please note the criteria for diagnosis of penetrating trauma presented in Chapter 13.

Simple surface lacerations that do not penetrate the full lid thickness require only accurate suturing. As in the case of any other wound, all foreign matter and dirt should be meticulously removed. Enthusiastic debridement is *not* desirable. Lost lid tissue is not easily replaced and creates a cosmetic defect. Furthermore, the rich vascular supply is ample to ensure survival of even a free full-thickness graft; therefore, pedicles of tissue will be entirely viable and should not be sacrificed. Fine sutures (6-0 or smaller) and needles and delicate forceps will give best results. Excess sutures are undesirable, and only the number required to give good apposition should be used.

Full thickness lacerations should be closed in three layers (see Fig. 13-4). The deepest layer of tarsus with firmly adherent conjunctiva should be accurately and snugly apposed with absorbable sutures that do not penetrate through to rub the cornea and that are knotted anteriorly. Apposition of the orbicularis layer will minimize tension and prevent a thin, depressed scar. The surface layer of skin should be closed separately. If gut sutures are used for closure of skin lacerations in children, the difficult problem of suture removal from a frightened child is solved. Fine gut sutures cause little or no undesirable skin reaction.

If the lid margin is involved, apposition must be meticulous to avoid an unsightly irregularity. Full-thickness lacerations nasal to the lower punctum require canaliculus anastomosis if permanent tearing is to be avoided. Unrepaired ruptures of lateral or medial palpebral ligaments result in poor lid apposition to the globe. Ptosis occurs if a severed levator tendon is not reattached. If the lid is extensively lacerated, the initial surgical repair requires tedious and careful anatomic restoration for an acceptable result. The

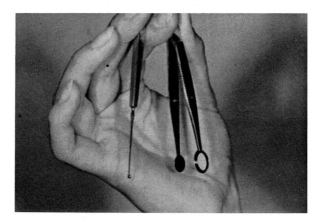

Fig. 26-1. The open ring of the chalazion clamp is applied on the conjunctival surface, and through its opening the chalazion may be incised. The small chalazion curet is used to remove the tenacious contents, which tend to form pockets of material and do not flow out readily.

surgeon undertaking repair of a major lid injury should be entirely familiar with the anatomy of this specialized area; otherwise, great cosmetic, functional, and financial distress will ensue.

Lid tumors. Small papillomas, basal cell carcinomas, nevi, and so on, are easily removed with elliptic incisions running parallel to the lid margin. The skin edges should *never* be closed under tension, because such closure will result in late development of ectropion. If the defect is too large to close readily, a complicated plastic sliding of the lid or a full-thickness skin graft will be necessary. Removal of extensive plaques of xanthelasma will cause trouble and should be avoided. Unsightly bulging of the relaxed lids of older people is *not* reparable by simple skin excision.

Chalazion. The most common lid operation is incision and curettage of a chalazion. A chalazion is a retention cyst of the meibomian glands in the tarsal plate, lies deep in the lid, and must be differentiated from a hordeolum (see Figs. 20-6 and 20-7). A hordeolum (sty) is an inflammation of the glands about the hair follicles in the anterior lid margin and is almost never helped by surgery. About one half of acute chalazia will spontaneously disappear after the application of hot compresses for 5 to 10 minutes three times a day. Surgery should be avoided if the chalazion is less than 2 weeks old or if it is inflamed and painful.

Infiltration anesthesia deep to the orbicularis muscle and surrounding the chalazion (about 2 ml of 1% xylocaine is ample), supplemented by 0.5% topical tetracaine, should permit a completely painless procedure. The lid is everted and fixed with a chalazion clamp (Fig. 26-1), which also provides hemostasis. The incision is made from the conjunctival surface perpendicular to the lid margin, should extend the full length of the meibomian gland, should penetrate no deeper than the lumen of the chalazion, and should

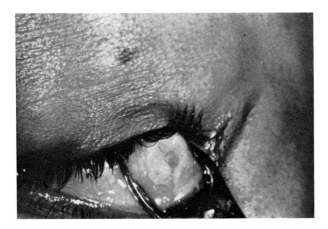

Fig. 26-2. The lower lid is everted in the firm grip of a chalazion clamp. A vertical incision has been made into the chalazion (but not through the tarsal plate into the orbicularis muscle), and its contents have been evacuated by curettage. The average chalazion has a surprisingly large cavity.

never continue anterior to the gray line of the lid margin. If the incision is made with a disposable cautery instead of a knife, it will not bleed. If no gelatinous material is encountered, the chalazion has not been found and another incision will be necessary. Chalazia are filled with tenacious material and therefore require curettage to remove their contents. At the close of the procedure the gray, glistening clean cyst walls should be visible throughout their extent (Fig. 26-2). Antibiotic ointment and an eye pad are then applied. Minimal pain will be experienced for several hours. Hot, moist compresses are helpful after several hours. Healing requires only a few days.

Unless a physician has observed a number of chalazion operations, he is advised not to undertake his first such procedure without supervision. I have observed total occlusion of the central retinal artery resulting from excessive pressure on the eye during chalazion surgery.

LACRIMAL IRRIGATION

Chronic tearing of an eye, often associated with crusting and purulent discharge, suggests blockage of the nasolacrimal duct. Pressure on the lacrimal sac in the lower nasal orbit (see Fig. 5-7) will cause regurgitation of purulent fluid (see Fig. 20-9) in many such patients but not in all of them. A certain test for patency of the lacrimal drainage system is irrigation—if the irrigating fluid flows freely into the nose, the duct must be open. Inability to irrigate or probe through the ducts usually means that surgery will be required to stop the tearing. Often epiphora will be relieved by successful irrigation or probing.

Irrigation is done with the patient under anesthesia with 0.5% topical tetracaine or 0.5% proparacaine. Drops are instilled into the lower conjunctival sac and flow into the

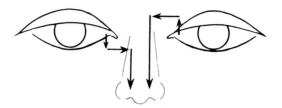

Fig. 26-3. The direction in which a probe traverses the lacrimal passages is first at right angles to the lid margin, then directly toward the midline, and finally straight down. These changes in direction are abrupt, and failure to turn properly will tear the delicate tissues, causing serious and possibly permanent damage.

punctum and canaliculus by capillary action. Usually the punctum will be too small to admit the lacrimal cannula and must be dilated. The best dilator is the blunt point of a large safety pin, of the size commonly used for baby diapers. The canaliculus runs exactly perpendicular to the lid margin for about 1 mm and then makes a right-angle turn to extend toward the nose (Fig. 26-3). The dilating pin is therefore introduced straight into the punctum for 1 mm and then turned 90 degrees toward the nose. Because the shaft of the pin is considerably larger than the point, only about 2 mm can be introduced into the usual canaliculus; it will suffice, however, for dilatation of the punctum. A finger placed on the lateral part of the lid to pull it down and temporal (for the lower lid, and up and temporal for the upper lid) will steady the lid and facilitate manipulation.

The blunt-tipped lacrimal irrigation cannula is usually easily introduced into the dilated punctum. After entering the vertical portion for about 1 mm, the cannula is turned 90 degrees toward the nose and passed deeper into the canaliculus. Usually a depth of 4 or 5 mm will suffice to hold the cannula securely in the canaliculus and prevent fluid regurgitation around the cannula. A 2 ml glass syringe filled with saline solution has been attached to the cannula throughout the entire procedure and is now used to deliver fluid into the lacrimal sac. Excessive force should never be used for irrigation or for passage of the cannula, lest the delicate passages be torn. Flow into the nose and throat will be evident because of the patient's coughing or swallowing, as well as because the fluid disappears somewhere and must therefore be passing internally.

Lacrimal probing starts in the same way, except that 0.5 ml of tetracaine is irrigated into the sac and left there for a few minutes. (Probing is unnecessary and undesirable if irrigation fluid freely enters the nose.) The probe is introduced perpendicularly 1 mm and then turned at right angles and slid through the canaliculus until it meets the absolutely solid obstacle of nasal bone. Pulling the lid laterally is helpful during the procedure of threading the probe through the canaliculus. If soft, resilient tissue can still be felt before the tip of the probe, it is not yet in position to tip into the sac. The tip *must* be solidly against bone to avoid tearing the canaliculus. When the probe tip is definitely against the nasal bone, the shaft is tilted upward 90 degrees so as to point directly down to the chin. The shaft should press firmly against the brow in order to be aligned to pass into the lacrimal sac and nasolacrimal duct. If the brow is prominent, the probe may have to be

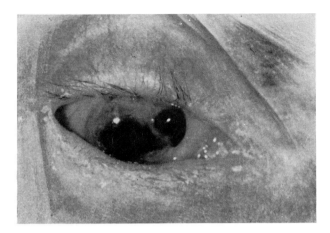

Fig. 26-4. This iris prolapse has occurred at a site of rupture of a cataract incision. Wound rupture is a serious complication and may result in infection, uveitis, glaucoma, corneal opacity, and other unpleasant conditions. Pressure exerted on the eye by the patient or his attendants is the usual cause of wound rupture.

curved slightly (concave forward) to achieve the proper angle of the tip. As soon as the probe is tipped upward, if the tip is properly positioned, it will easily be advanced into the sac and will progress downward freely for about 1 cm. A constricted passageway will be evident at the beginning of the nasolacrimal duct. Many solid obstructions are present at this point and may either be impassable or require considerable skillfully directed force. *Do not* exert force at this point or anywhere else unless you know from experience what you are doing. Irreparable lacerations of the lacrimal passage will result. Passage of a too-large probe is also damaging; choose a size that will slide easily into the canaliculus.

POSTOPERATIVE HOSPITAL CARE

Considerable variation exists in the postoperative orders for different procedures and as prescribed by individual physicians. In general, few if any restrictions will be placed on the activity of a patient who has not had an intraocular procedure. Should an intraocular operation have been performed (cataract, glaucoma, detachment, and so on), the eye will be in an extremely delicate condition for weeks or months (Fig. 26-4), and it is entirely possible to cause serious and disastrous damage through slight external pressure. For this reason, the ophthalmologist is understandably reluctant to have anyone else change dressings for his patients after intraocular surgery. If an eye bandage falls off, it should be gently replaced, including the shield that guards against accidental bumps. If a patient complains of eye pain or discomfort after intraocular surgery, the ophthalmologist should be notified. *Under no circumstances* should the bandage be removed by anyone other than the ophthalmologist in order to inspect the eye during the immediate postoperative period. I have seen several instances in which the patient destroyed his own eye by reaching up to rub it after the shield was removed.

chapter 27   Ophthalmic Terminology

Words are the tools with which you think. In our heritage of language, thoughtful minds have assembled these words from Greek and Latin roots, with lesser contributions from other languages. The derivation of the word is, therefore, descriptive of the concept it expresses. You can remember and understand a word better if you know its derivation; also, you can figure out the meaning of a brand new word you have never seen before if you know the roots of which it is composed.

The purpose of this presentation is to introduce you to some of the common roots used in eye words and to provide examples of their usage.

Blepharo means eyelid.
> *-itis* means inflammation; *blepharitis* is inflammation of the eyelids.
> *-spasmos* means spasm; *blepharospasm* is spasmodic contraction of the orbicularis muscle of the eyelid.

Chorio means choroid.
> *-itis* means inflammation; *chorioretinitis* is inflammation of the choroid and retina.
> *-pathy* means disease; *chorioretinopathy* is disease of the choroid and retina.

Cor means pupil.
> *aniso-* means unequal; *anisocoria* is inequality of the pupils, a readily observed sign of ocular or neurologic disease.
> *-ek* means out; *-topos* means place; *corectopia* is a displaced pupil, usually referring to a congenital malformation.
> *leuko-* means white; *leukocoria* is a white pupil, due to inflammatory or neoplastic cells within the vitreous cavity.

Cyclo means circle. It refers to the ciliary body, which encircles the eye.
> *-cryo* means cold; *cyclocryotherapy* is freezing the ciliary body to reduce aqueous secretion in treatment of glaucoma.
> *-dialysis* means dissolution; *cyclodialysis* is separation of the ciliary body from the choroid, performed surgically in treatment of glaucoma.
> *-itis* means inflammation; *cyclitis* is inflammation of the ciliary body.
> *-plegia* means paralysis; *cycloplegia* is paralysis of accommodation, as results from use of eye drops to block contraction of the ciliary muscle.

Dacryo means tear.
> *-aden* means gland; *dacryoadenitis* is inflammation of the lacrimal gland.
> *-cyst* means cavity; *dacryocystitis* is inflammation of the lacrimal sac.
> *-rhino* means nose; *-stoma* means opening; *dacryocystorhinostomy* is surgical creation of an opening between the lacrimal sac and the nose for the correction of a blockage of the tear flow.

426

Duction means to lead.

ab- means away from, and is used in reference to the midline; *abduction* is turning the eye laterally (away from the midline). The lateral rectus muscle abducts the eye; hence, its cranial nerve (VI) is called the *abducens* nerve.

ad- means toward, and is also used in reference to the midline; *adduction* is turning the eye nasally (toward the midline).

supra- means above; *supraduction* means upward turning of the eye.

infra- means below; *infraduction* means downward turning of the eye.

Irid means iris.

-ectomy means surgical removal of; *iridectomy* is surgical removal of part of the iris to enhance aqueous flow, and is used in treatment of glaucoma.

Kerato means cornea.

-itis means inflammation; *keratitis* is inflammation of the cornea.

-conus means cone; *keratoconus* is a conical distortion of the cornea, usually occurring as a spontaneous bilateral degenerative change in young adults.

-tome means cut; *keratome* is a triangular knife used to make a corneal incision, as in cataract surgery.

-meter means measure; a *keratometer* measures the curvature of the cornea.

-mycosis means fungus; *keratomycosis* is fungus infection of the cornea.

-pathy means disease; *keratopathy* is a noninflammatory corneal disease; for example, exposure keratopathy.

-plasty means repair; *keratoplasty* refers to a corneal transplant.

Ocul means eye.

intra- means within; *intraocular* means within the eye.

OD stands for oculus dexter; *dexter* means right; *OD* means right eye.

OS stands for oculus sinister; *sinister* means left; *OS* means left eye.

OU stands for oculus uterque; *uterque* means each; *OU* means both eyes.

Ophthalm means eye.

-ologist means specialist in the study of; an *ophthalmologist* is a specialist in the study of eyes.

-scope means an instrument for examining; an *ophthalmoscope* is an instrument used to examine the eyes.

Opia, Opsia means vision.

an- or *al-* means without; *anopia* or *alopia* means without sight.

ambly- means dull; *amblyopia* is reduced vision in an eye appearing apparently normal on examination. This is most commonly used as "suppression amblyopia," which refers to loss of vision resulting from strabismus or monocular refractive error.

ametros- means disproportionate; *ametropia* is the faulty combination of the optical components of an eye, resulting in refractive error. Ametropia is a general term including any type of refractive error.

aniso- means unequal; *anisometropia* is a difference in the refractive error of the two eyes.

asthenic- means weak; *asthenopia* is rapid fatigue with use of the eyes.

deuter- means second; *deuteranopia* is inability to see the second primary color (green), a form of red-green color blindness.

diplo- means double; *diplopia* is double vision, the simultaneous seeing of two images of a single object (like a photographic double exposure).

emmetros- means in proper measure; *emmetropia* is the refractive condition of an eye that is perfectly focused for distance vision without the aid of accommodation.

hemer- means day; *hemeralopia* is inability to see in daylight.

hemi means half; *hemianopia* is half sight (loss of half the visual field). For instance, bitemporal hemianopia is loss of the temporal half of the visual field in each eye.

hyper- means beyond; *hyperopia* is the refractive error in which parallel light is focused beyond (behind) the retina (synonym, farsighted).

meta- means change; *morph-* means shape or form; *metamorphopsia* is distorted vision, a symptom characteristic of displacement of the cones of the central retina.

micro- means small; *micropsia* is a minification of vision resulting from retinal edema.

myein- means to shut; *myopia* (nearsightedness) is the refractive error in which parallel light focuses in front of the retina, a condition that cannot be helped by accommodation. However, partially shutting the eyelids eliminates the poorly focused peripheral light rays, allowing the myope to improve his distance vision.

nyct- means night; *nyctalopia* is inability to see in relative darkness.

presby- means old; *presbyopia* is the sight of old age, the inability to accommodate the lens to focus on near objects.

prot- means first; *protanopia* is inability to see the first primary color (red), a form of red-green color blindness.

Phakos means lentil, or lentil-shaped; hence the lens.

a- means without; *aphakia* is absence of the lens, as following cataract extraction.

-emulsio means suspension of small globules; *phacoemulsification* is a technique of cataract extraction in which the lens is broken into tiny fragments by ultrasonic vibrations.

-lysis means solution; *phacolytic* glaucoma is the result of spontaneous breakdown of the lens, including a macrophage response that clogs the trabecular meshwork.

erysis- means drawing; *erysiphake* is a small suction cup designed to grasp the lens for withdrawal during cataract extraction.

Tarsos means broad, flat surface and refers to the eyelid framework.

-orrhaphy means suture; *tarsorrhaphy* is suturing together of the eyelids.

-malacia means softening; *tarsomalacia* is softening of the edges of the eyelids.

Trope means turn.

eso- means in; *esotropia* is inward turning of the eyes (convergent strabismus).

exo- means out; *exotropia* is outward turning of the eyes (divergent strabismus).

hyper- means above; *hypertropia* is upward turning of one eye, which is higher than the other eye.

TERMINOLOGY TEST

1. Blepharoplasty refers to plastic surgery on the
   - ☐ Eyebrow
   - ☐ Eyelid
   - ☐ Cornea
2. Polycoria means multiple
   - ☐ Choroidal vessels
   - ☐ Corneas
   - ☐ Pupil openings

3. Cyclectomy is removal of part of the
   - ☐ Ciliary body
   - ☐ Sclera
   - ☐ Vitreous
4. Dacryocystectomy is removal of
   - ☐ The tear sac
   - ☐ A malignant tumor
   - ☐ The ethmoid bone
5. Iridodonesis is
   - ☐ Scleral collapse
   - ☐ Choroidal hemorrhage
   - ☐ Movement of the iris, seen in aphakia
6. A superficial keratectomy would be performed to remove
   - ☐ The abnormal fluid in retinal detachment
   - ☐ A scar resulting from corneal injury
   - ☐ A papilloma of the eyelid
7. Metamorphopsia means change in the shape of
   - ☐ The eyeball
   - ☐ Details seen in the central visual field
   - ☐ The pupil
8. Entropion is
   - ☐ Accumulation of pus within the eyeball
   - ☐ The seeing of false or imaginary images
   - ☐ Turning in of the eyelid against the eye
9. Phakic refers to the presence of
   - ☐ The crystalline lens
   - ☐ An intact vitreous face
   - ☐ Excessive softness of the eye
10. Symblepharon means adhesion of
    - ☐ The iris to the lens
    - ☐ Both sides of a detached retina together
    - ☐ The eyelid to the eyeball

Glossary

Throughout the text the majority of common ophthalmologic terms have been described in more detail than is possible in a list of definitions. Reference to the index will locate these terms. This glossary is a supplement to the text and is not intended as a complete dictionary.

abducens nerve Sixth cranial nerve, which innervates the lateral rectus muscle.

abduct To move the eye laterally (away from the midline).

abduction Rotation of an eye temporarily.

abductor Muscle, such as the lateral rectus, that rotates the eye temporally.

aberration Imperfect passage of light rays through an optical system.

    chromatic aberration Separation of colors due to the refractive differences between the various wavelengths of light.

    spherical aberration Axial focusing defect resulting from the greater refractive strength of a lens periphery as compared with its axial portion.

abiotrophy Synonym for degenerative change.

ablatio retinae Retinal detachment.

AC/A ratio Proportion between accommodative convergence and accommodation; of clinical importance in ocular alignment, because it determines the amount of convergence automatically resulting from the dioptric focusing of the eyes at a given distance.

accommodation Near focusing of the eye, accomplished by an increase in strength of the lens achieved by contraction of the ciliary muscle.

accommodation-convergence ratio Relationship between accommodation and convergence of the two eyes that determines (in part) whether they will be straight.

acetylcholine Chemical that transmits parasympathetic impulses to the muscle fiber (for example, sphincter of iris) and that transmits impulses across most nerve synapses.

achromatic Corrected for chromatic aberration.

achromatope Person afflicted with achromatopia.

achromatopia Color blindness for all colors.

acne rosacea Chronic dermatosis of unknown cause that may result in corneal scarring.

acuity Ability of the eye to see fine detail.

acyanopsia (acyanoblepsia) Faulty ability to perceive blue wavelengths of light.

adaptometer Device to measure the rate and amount of increased sensitivity of the retina to light, as occurs when the light-adapted eye is placed in darkness.

add Additional lens strength of the bifocal part of an eyeglass.

adduct To rotate an eye medially.

adduction Turning of an eye toward the nose.

adductor Muscle, such as the medial rectus, that turns the eye toward the nose.

adherent leukoma Adhesion of the iris to a white corneal scar.

Adie's syndrome Slowness of the reflexes, including a tendency for one or both pupils to respond only slowly to light or dark.

430

adnexa oculi Adjacent structures of the eye; for example, lids or extraocular muscles.

adrenaline Chemical that transmits sympathetic impulses to the muscle fiber; for example, dilator of iris.

advancement Moving forward of an extraocular muscle for surgical correction of strabismus with the intent of increasing its function.

aftercataract Opacity remaining subsequent to incomplete removal of the crystalline lens of the eye.

afterimage Visual sensation remaining, even though the eye no longer looks at the object producing the afterimage; for example, the bright sensation seen when the eyes are closed after looking at a light.

agnosia Cerebral inability to recognize the meaning of details seen or otherwise perceived.

agonist One of several muscles acting together to rotate the eye in the same direction. For example, the inferior rectus muscle and the superior oblique muscle each have action components for downward rotation of the eye and are agonists in accomplishing this particular movement.

akinesia Blocking of muscle movement; for example, paralysis of orbicularis muscle by anesthesia of the seventh nerve to prevent squeezing of eyelids during surgery.

albinism Genetically determined deficiency of pigment, either localized or general throughout the body; if the retina is involved, vision is reduced.

alexia Inability to read because of damage to the reading centers of the cerebral cortex.

Allen gonioprism Four-sided contact lens used for microscopic viewing of the internal aspect of the peripheral circumference of the anterior chamber of the eye.

alpha angle Angle between the visual axis (the line of sight) and the optic axis (the anatomic centerline of direction of the eyeball).

amaurosis Little-used synonym for blindness; frequently used to designate visual loss in a structurally normal eye (as from pituitary tumor).

amblyope Person suffering from amblyopia.

amblyopia Reduced vision in an eye appearing normal to examination; this term is most commonly used as "suppression amblyopia," which refers to cerebral blocking of vision in an eye that is deviated or suffers from a refractive error more marked than that of the good eye.

amblyoscope Stereoscope-like instrument that can present different pictures to the two eyes at various angles of ocular deviation; such instruments are useful in orthoptic evaluation and treatment of patients with strabismus.

ametropia General term meaning the presence of refractive error of any type.

ametropic Pertaining to refractive error.

amplitude (of accommodation) Amount in diopters by which accommodation of the crystalline lens can increase the optical strength of the eye.

ampulla (lacrimal) Enlargement of the lacrimal canaliculus located at the right-angled bend about 2 mm from the punctum. This is a component of the lacrimal pump mechanism that propels tears toward the nose.

Amsler grid Checkerboard-like pattern of lines used as a background for the subjective drawing of visual field defects.

angioid streaks Linear retinal changes resembling a blood vessel but representing a rupture of Bruch's membrane; appear in pseudoxanthoma elasticum, sickle cell anemia, Paget's disease, and senile elastosis.

angioscotoma Extension of the normal blind spot due to local blocking of vision by a large retinal vessel.

angle kappa Difference between the direction of gaze and the apparent direction in which the eye points; this normal structural feature may cause errors in measurement of strabismus.

anirida Absence of the iris.

aniseikonia Difference in size of the images received by the two eyes.

anisocoria Difference in size of the two pupils.

anisometropia Difference in refractive error of the two eyes.

ankyloblepharon Abnormal adhesion between the margins of the upper and lower eyelids.

annulus of Zinn Circular fibrous origin of the extraocular muscles in the back of the orbit.

anomaloscope Research instrument for measuring color vision.

anomalous retinal correspondence (ARC) Adaptation to strabismus, whereby the deviating eye relearns direction orientation in terms of its abnormal position; for example, the brain no longer interprets the macula as looking straight ahead.

anomaly angle Angle between the visual axis (the normal line of sight) and the abnormal direction of alignment of an eye with macular suppression and selective use of a nonmacular portion of the retina for fixation.

anophthalmia Total failure of the eye to develop.

anopsia Loss of vision; usually used in a combining form, as hemianopsia.

antagonist Extraocular muscle exerting opposing pull; for example, the medial rectus muscle is the antagonist of the lateral rectus muscle of the same eye.

anterior chamber Aqueous-containing space between the cornea and the iris.

aphakia Absence of the lens.

applanation tonometry Measurement of intraocular pressure by an instrument that flattens a predetermined area of the cornea.

aqueous Clear fluid that is secreted by the ciliary processes and fills the anterior and posterior chambers.

arcus juvenilis Corneal ring comparable in appearance to an arcus senilis but often associated with lipoidal degenerations of the blood vessel walls.

arcus senilis Gray ring commonly observed in the peripheral cornea of older persons; represents a benign lipoid infiltration of no local or general significance.

Argyll-Robertson pupil Miotic pupil reacting to the accommodation reflex but not to the light reflex; caused by neurologic lesions between the lateral geniculate body and the third-nerve nucleus; frequently caused by syphilis.

argyria Dirty blue discoloration of conjunctiva due to deposition of silver, usually after prolonged use of Argyrol.

Arlt's line. Horizontal scar of the upper palpebral conjunctiva that is almost pathognomonic of chronic trachoma.

aspheric lens Special lens corrected for peripheral distortions; such lenses give improved vision after cataract extraction.

asteroid hyalosis Deterioration of the vitreous body, in which degenerative vitreous change causes numerous tiny white nodules to develop within the vitreous framework; rarely impairs vision.

asthenopia Inability to use the eyes for a reasonable length of time without discomfort or fatigue.

astigmatism Optical distortion, usually caused by irregular corneal curvature, which prevents a clear focus of light at any point.

atropine Drug that blocks parasympathetic innervation (causes dilatation of the pupil and paralysis of accommodation); used in treatment of intraocular inflammation and in refraction of children.

aura (visual) Subjective visual sensations originating from the cerebral cortex, as in association with the vasoconstriction of migraine.

autokeratoplasty Corneal transplantation with tissue from the patient himself (from the other eye, or by rotation from a peripheral portion of the same cornea).

Axenfeld's nerve loop. Intrascleral nerve commonly associated with a small cuff of uveal pigment, usually occurring several millimeters above the upper limbus in heavily pigmented persons. Its clinical significance is that it may be mistaken for an imbedded foreign body.

axis Meridian in which astigmatism is oriented.

band keratopathy Horizontal exposure scar of central cornea, often associated with degenerative diseases of the eye.

bar reading Method of training and diagnosis of binocular vision in which a barrier blocks part of the vision of each eye, thereby resulting in alternating monocular and binocular vision.

Barany's nystagmus Vestibular nystagmus resulting from rotation of the body in the planes of the semicircular canals.

bedewing Delicate edema of the corneal epithelium, recognizable by biomicroscopy.

belladonna Herbal name for the alkaloid or plant source of parasympatholytic drugs such as atropine; the "beautiful lady" meaning originates from its supposed cosmetic use to dilate the pupils and enhance attractiveness.

Bell's palsy Paralysis of seventh cranial nerve, resulting from a specific cause—swelling of the nerve within its bony canal, which causes inadequate closure of the lids (orbicularis oculi paralysis), as well as paralysis of the other facial muscles.

Bell's phenomenon Reflex upward rotation of the eye associated with closure of the eyelids.

Bergmeister's papilla Embryologically, the connective tissue base surrounding the hyaloid artery just anterior to the optic nerve.

Berlin's edema Reversible edema of the central retina resulting from ocular contusion.

Best's disease Vitelliruptive degeneration of the macula, a dominantly inherited juvenile degeneration affecting primarily the pigment epithelium of the retina.

Bielschowsky's test Method of identifying superior oblique paralysis as a cause of head tilt. When the head is tilted in the opposite direction from the normal posture, the affected eye (on the side toward which the head spontaneously tilts) rotates upward.

bifocal Double lens, usually prescribed for older persons who can no longer accommodate; lower portion focuses for near vision.

binocular vision Normal simultaneous use of both eyes (which results in depth perception).

biomicroscope Clinical examining instrument (slit-lamp microscope) that combines a microscope with a very thin beam of light and permits observation of minute details within the transparent eye.

Bitot's spots Small foamy deposits on the conjunctiva on either side of the cornea, within the interpalpebral space, commonly containing *Bacillus xerosis*. Although they are traditionally associated with vitamin A deficiency, this clinical association is not usually present.

Bjerrum scotoma Nerve fiber bundle visual field defect on the nasal side, characteristically associated with glaucomatous optic atrophy.

blackout Loss of vision before loss of consciousness; caused by inadequate cerebral perfusion, which can result from postural hypotension or positive G forces encountered in aerial maneuvers.

blennorrhea Conjunctival inflammation resulting in mucoid discharge.

  inclusion blennorrhea Chlamydial infection transmitted from the genital area to the eye, as during the birth process, in poorly chlorinated swimming pools, or by finger transmission.

blephar- Prefix signifying the eyelid.

blepharitis Inflammation of the eyelid.

blepharochalasis Redundancy of the upper lid skin.

blepharoconjunctivitis Associated inflammation of both the eyelid margins and the conjunctiva.

blepharospasm Involuntary contraction of the orbicularis muscle.

Blessig's cysts Benign microscopic cystic degeneration of the peripheral retina, almost universally present, even in children.

blind spot Normal visual field defect corresponding to the location of the optic disc.

blindness Although the ophthalmologist usually considers blindness to mean inability to see, legal blindness is defined as vision (corrected by eyeglasses) of 20/200 or less, or less than 20 degrees of visual field in the better eye.

blink Regularly repeated reflex closure of the eyelids necessary to maintain the tear film lubrication and protection of the cornea.

bombé (of iris) Forward displacement of the iris caused by block of the pupil, which prevents forward flow of aqueous.

Bowman's membrane Thin layer between the corneal epithelium and the stroma.

Bruch's membrane Hyaline membrane between the choroid and the retinal pigment epithelium; same as lamina vitrea.

Brushfield's spots Pale spots of the peripheral iris, occurring more frequently in mongolism (Down's syndrome).

bullous keratopathy Blisterlike elevations of the corneal epithelium resulting from decompensation of the dehydrating mechanism.

buphthalmos Enlargement of the eye due to secondary glaucoma at an early age.

Butyn (butacaine) Topical anesthetic; little used because it causes discomfort and frequently allergy.

campimeter Synonym for tangent screen; a surface used for evaluation of the central part of the visual field.

canal of Schlemm Important aqueous drainage channel encircling the periphery of the anterior chamber.

caniculitis Inflammation of the lacrimal canaliculus.

caniculus Portion of the lacrimal drainage apparatus between the punctum and the sac.

canthotomy Horizontal cut extending the palpebral aperture, most frequently used to aid the exposure of the eye during cataract surgery.

canthus Outer or inner angle between the eyelids.

capsule (of lens) Elastic membrane surrounding the crystalline lens. It has sufficient inherent elasticity to induce the change of lens contour that causes accommodation.

capsulotomy Surgical incision of the lens capsule as part of a cataract operation.

carbachol Synthetic parasympathomimetic drug frequently used in treatment of glaucoma.

caruncle Nodular elevated structure at the inner corner of the eye.

cataract Any defect in transparency of the lens.

chalazion Cystic dilatation of a meibomian gland, usually due to postinflammatory blockage of its duct.

chalcosis oculi Copper deposits within the eye, usually due to a retained intraocular copper foreign body. An almost pathognomonic feature is the "sunflower" cataract—a central disc of opacity of the anterior lens capsule corresponding to the pupil area, with surrounding petal-like opacities extending into the peripheral capsule.

chemosis Severe edema of conjunctiva and underlying connective tissue.

chiasm, optic Junction of the two optic nerves, within which a semidecussation of the visual fibers occurs.

choked disc Synonym for papilledema.

choriocapillaris Capillary layer of the choroid, which lies on its inner aspect and serves to nourish the external layers of the retina.

chorioretinitis Inflammation involving both the choroid and the retina. Because of their thinness and proximity, almost any inflammation will involve both layers; however, the primary site may be in one or the other tissue. For example, *Toxoplasma* organisms are found exclusively within the retina, whereas *Histoplasma* organisms affect the choroid.

choroid Vascular layer responsible for the nutrition of the outer portion of the retina. It is the posterior portion of the uveal tract (composed anteriorly of the ciliary body and iris).

choroideremia Abiotrophy of the choroid.

choroiditis Inflammation of the choroid. Older usage included a variety of degenerative changes more properly referred to as choroidopathy.

choroidopathy Degenerative or traumatic changes of the choroid, as distinguished from choroiditis; at times this clinical distinction may be difficult.

chromatopsia Abnormal subjective perception of color, as may occur following cataract extraction or in digitalis poisoning.

chrysiasis Deposition of gold within tissues, as may visibly occur in the cornea and conjunctiva following gold therapy for arthritis.

cilia Eyelashes; each hair grows to a fixed length, lives for about 3 months, and then is replaced by a new cilium.

ciliary body Portion of the uveal tract between the iris and the choroid that contains the muscles of accommodation and secretes aqueous.

cilioretinal Referring to an artery entering the temporal retina from the posterior ciliary circulation rather than from the central retinal artery. This minor anomaly occurs in at least 5% of all eyes.

cilium Eyelash.

Cloquet's canal Axial space in the vitreous that contained the hyaloid artery during early development.

Coats's disease Retinal telangiectasis of childhood.

cocaine Narcotic that was the first anesthetic used topically in the eye; because of its corneal toxicity, cocaine is rarely used except as a diagnostic aid in Horner's syndrome.

collarette Circular inner edge of the anterior mesodermal leaf of the iris, which is visible as a zigzag circular elevated edge several millimeters peripheral to the pupil edge.

collector channels Communicating vessels joining the canal of Schlemm to the intrascleral veins, functioning to permit escape of aqueous humor from the eye into the bloodstream.

collyrium Synonym for eye drops.

coloboma Any notchlike defect in the eye or lids.

color blindness Inability to differentiate normally between colors; the most common type causes confusion between red and green.

comitance Characteristic of strabismus in which the angle of deviation between the two eyes remains constant regardless of the direction of gaze. This indicates a supranuclear origin of the strabismus, rather than an infranuclear or nuclear muscle paresis.

commotio retinae Edema of the retina after ocular contusion.

concave lens Incurved (center thinner than edges) lens that corrects nearsightedness by diverging light rays.

concomitant strabismus Nonparalytic strabismus that does not change in amount with different positions of the eye.

cone Retinal cell used for daylight vision.

conformer Oval shell fitted in the eye socket immediately after surgical removal of the eye in order to minimize contraction before fitting of the artificial eye (usually done 1 month postoperatively).

conjunctiva Mucous membrane lining the back of the lids (palpebral) and the front of the eye (bulbar) except for the cornea.

conjunctivitis Inflammation of the conjunctiva. Also refers to a variety of degenerative changes, such as keratoconjunctivitis sicca, the consequence of dryness.

consensual reflex Contraction of the opposite, not illuminated, pupil in response to a light stimulus to its fellow eye.

contact lens Thin lens that fits directly on the cornea under the eyelids.

conus Crescent-shaped degenerative area adjacent to the optic nerve; myopia is a common cause.

convergence Turning of the two eyes toward each other.

convergent Condition in which both eyes are rotated toward each other.

convex lens Outcurved (center thicker than edges) lens that corrects farsightedness by converging light rays.

corectopia Eccentric position of the pupil; normal in small amount.

cornea Normally transparent structure forming the surface of the eye.

couching Primitive surgical practice of dislocating a cataract into the vitreous; visual improvement obtained in this way is transient, because lens-induced inflammation usually destroys the eye.

craniostenosis Inherited defect of the skull suture lines; of ophthalmologic interest because of the frequency with which an abnormally shallow orbit develops and because bony constriction may damage the cranial nerves.

cross cylinder Lens made up of two astigmatic lenses at right angles to each other; used in refraction to measure astigmatism.

cross-eyes Lay term for convergent strabismus.

crystalline lens Lens of the eye, situated just behind the pupil. Its function is to contribute to the optical power of the eye and to accommodate the eye for near vision.

cul-de-sac Upper or lower conjunctival recess.

cup Excavation in the surface of the optic disc.

cyclectomy Surgical removal of part of the ciliary body, as in treatment of a neoplasm.

cyclitic membrane Sheet of inflammatory scar tissue behind the lens.

cyclitis Inflammation of the ciliary body.

cyclocryotherapy Freezing of the ciliary body, performed to reduce the secretion of aqueous in glaucoma.

cyclodeviation Torsional fault of eye position, due to rotation on the anteroposterior axis.

cyclodialysis Antiglaucoma operation that separates the ciliary body from the sclera, thereby creating a new exit for the aqueous.

cyclodiathermy Antiglaucoma operation that partially destroys the ciliary body, thereby reducing aqueous formation.

cyclophoria Tendency of the eye to become misaligned by rotating on an anteroposterior axis.

cyclopia Developmental anomaly in which both eyes are joined together to form a single partially duplicated eye located in the central forehead.

cycloplegia Paralysis of accommodation.

cycloplegic Parasympatholytic drug that blocks the innervation of the ciliary body.

cyclops Abnormal fetus with cyclopia.

cyclotropia Form of strabismus in which the deviation consists of rotation around an anteroposterior axis.

cylinder Lens used for the correction of astigmatism.

cytoid body Retinal microinfarction synonymous with soft exudate.

dacryoadenitis Inflammation of a lacrimal gland

dacryocystectomy Surgical removal of the tear sac.

dacryocystitis Inflammation of a tear sac, usually due to faulty drainage.

dacryocystography Evaluation of the status of the lacrimal drainage system by means of radiopaque dyes.

dacryocystorhinostomy Surgical communication between a blocked tear sac and the nose.

dacryolith Calcific deposit within the lacrimal drainage system, usually a consequence of fungus infection.

Dalen-Fuchs nodule Aggregation of epithelioid cells in the choroid, characteristic of sympathetic ophthalmia.

decentration Eccentric positioning of a lens to produce a prism effect.

deorsumvergence Turning of both eyes downward.

dermoid Developmental inclusion of aberrant ectoderm and mesoderm.

descemetocele Protrusion of Descemet's membrane; occurs after loss of corneal stroma from disease or injury.

Descemet's membrane Elastic layer on the posterior corneal surface.

detachment Separation of one layer of the eye from the adjacent one; a choroidal detachment is separated from the sclera, a retinal detachment is separated from the pigment layer, and a vitreous detachment is separated from the retina.

deuteranomaly Mild form of red-green color blindness, with reduced sensitivity for green.

deuteranopia Severe form of red-green color blindness, with greatest loss of sensitivity for green.

deviating eye Eye that is not straight in strabismus, as distinguished from the "fixing eye."

dextroversion Simultaneous turning of both eyes to the right.

DFP Diisopropyl flurophosphate; isoflurophate; a long-acting cholinesterase inhibitor used in therapy for glaucoma and accommodative esotropia.

dialysis of retina Tearing of the retina almost at the ora serrata, leaving only a narrow fringe of the peripheral retinal attached.

dichromat Individual unable to utilize one of the primary colors in color matching—he requires only two colors to match the entire spectrum.

diktyoma Neoplasm originating from the neuroepithelium of the pars plana.

dionin Irritant causing vasodilation after topical application, used without success to "slow the growth" of cataract; ethylmorphine hydrochloride.

diopter Unit in which the refracting strength of a lens is designated; diopters are calculated as the reciprocal of the focal length of a lens measured in meters.

diplopia Double vision; usually due to faulty alignment of the two eyes.

diploscope Device used for the evaluation and treatment of ocular misalignment.

disc Portion of the optic nerve visible with an ophthalmoscope.

discission Technique of incising a cataract with a knife-needle in order to create an optical opening; this method is applicable to cataracts in children or to thin secondary membranes in adults but will not remove the nucleus of an adult cataract.

disinsertion of retina Large circumferential tear of the retina in its far periphery, leaving only a narrow rim still attached at the ora serrata.

dislocation of lens Abnormal positioning of the crystalline lens, as may result from trauma, Marfan's syndrome, homocystinuria, or syphilis. Dislocation usually refers to a position entirely away from the normal site, in contrast to a subluxation, in which the lens is at least partly within its original location.

dispersion of light Separation of the wavelengths of visible light, as may occur with a prism or from the fault of chromatic aberration.

distichiasis Reduplication of the eyelashes; the inner lashes originate behind the gray line and usually irritate the cornea.

divergence Movement of the two eyes apart from each other.

drusen Hyaline nodules of the lamina vitrea of the choroid; commonly present but rarely disturbing vision.

duction Movement of one eye. For example, adduction refers to movement of an eye toward the midline. Distinguish from vergence, which refers to movement of both eyes; convergence is the movement of both eyes toward the midline.

dyschromatopsia Faulty color discrimination resulting in incomplete color blindness.

dyscoria Distorted pupil shape.

dystrophy Inherited degenerative change; for example, the cornea may be affected by a number of different types of dystrophy.

Eales' disease Focal proliferation of new-formed blood vessels on the retinal surface and invading the vitreous cavity. The cause is unknown, and the diagnosis does not include somewhat similar neovascularization associated with sickle cell retinopathy, diabetic retinopathy, or retinopathy of prematurity. All of these disorders are variants of retinal vasoocclusive disease.

ectasia Bulging forward of a weakened cornea; differentiate ectasia from staphyloma, which is a bulging area lined with uveal tissue.

ectopia Faulty position of a structure, such as the pupil or crystalline lens.

ectropion Abnormal outward displacement of the lid away from the eye.

ectropion uveae Eversion of iris pigment epithelium around the pupil margin.

Egger's line Circular attachment of the hyaloideocapsular ligament to the posterior periphery of the crystalline lens.

eikonometer Instrument that measures the relative size of images seen by the two eyes.

electrooculogram Recording of the electrical potential of the whole eye.

electroretinogram Recording of the electrical potential of the retina.

elevator Extraocular muscle that rotates the eye upward.

Elschnig's pearls Globular abortive lens fibers occurring in secondary cataracts after injury or extracapsular extraction.

embryotoxon Developmental opacity of the posterior surface of the peripheral cornea.

emmetropia Refractive condition of an eye that is perfectly focused for distance without the aid of accommodation.

emmetropic Referring to an eye without refractive error.

endophthalmitis Suppurative inflammation of the interior of the eye.

enophthalmos Abnormal displacement of the eye backward into the orbit due to atrophy of orbital contents or their loss through a fracture.

entoptic phenomena Sensations perceived for mechanical reasons within the eye; for example, the floaters and flashes caused by retinal detachment.

entropion Abnormal inward displacement of the lid margin toward the eye.

enucleation Surgical removal of the entire eye, including the sclera.

epiblepharon Congenital redundant skin fold overlying the inner portion of the lower lid.

epibulbar Located on the surface of the eye.

epicanthus Congenital skin fold overling the inner portion of the upper lid and the inner canthus; simulates the appearance of esotropia.

epilation Permanent removal of a hair, such as a misdirected cilium, including destruction of its bulb.

epinephrine Chemical mediator at sympathetic nerve endings; useful as a vasoconstrictor in ophthalmic surgery and may be used in glaucoma therapy to reduce aqueous secretion.

epiphora Tearing due to blockage of the lacrimal drainage apparatus or overproduction of tears.

episclera Loose connective tissue on the scleral surface.

episcleritis Inflammation that is an allergic response of the episclera; differentiated from other causes of red eye.

epithelial ingrowth Invasion of the interior of the eye by surface epithelium entering a penetrating wound.

equator Midportion of the eye; of significance in surgical or retinal localization.

erysiphake Small vacuum cup designed to hold a cataract during its removal.

erythropsia Visual sensation of excessive red coloration.

eserine Indirect-acting parasympathomimetic drug used in treatment of glaucoma.

esodeviation Misalignment of one eye into an abnormally convergent position.

esophoria Latent convergent deviation of the two eyes.

esotropia Convergent strabismus.

euthyscope Instrument designed to treat eccentric fixation by dazzling the retina adjacent to the macula, thereby relatively enhancing macular vision.

eversion (of eyelid) Outward turning of an eyelid, so that the tarsal plate is reversed.

evisceration Removal of the contents of the eye with retention of the sclera.

exenteration Removal of all soft tissues within the bony orbit.

exodeviation Misalignment of the eye into an abnormally divergent position.

exophoria Latent divergent deviation of the two eyes.

exophthalmometer Instrument that measures the anteroposterior position of the eye within the orbit.

exophthalmos Abnormal displacement of the eye forward out of the orbit due to an increase in volume of orbital contents or to an abnormally shallow orbital bony structure.

exotropia Divergent strabismus.

extorsion Rotation of an eye on its anteroposterior axis so that its upper portion moves away from the midline.

extraocular Pertaining to structures outside the sclerocorneal covering of the eye.

eye Visual apparatus. Medical terminology usually refers to the eyeball alone, whereas most laymen refer to the general area of the eye, including the lids.

eyecup Container with an oval opening that can be fitted snugly against the skin around the eye. In use, it is filled with liquid and the eye placed against it. When the head is turned upward and the eyelids opened, the medication bathes the eye. This is an unsanitary device, the use of which should be discouraged.

eyeground Ophthalmoscopically visible ocular fundus.

eyelash Protective cilium located along the anterior portion of the eyelid margin.

eyelid Entire structure covering and protecting the eye, including the skin and conjunctiva and the intervening tarsal plate, connective tissue, and muscles.

eyestrain Lay term describing poorly defined discomfort associated with use of the eyes and localized in the general area of the eyes.

farsightedness Refractive error in which parallel light is focused behind the retina; accommodation is required in order to see clearly in the distance. Hyperopia.

Fick's axes Theoretical concept that all rotations of the eye can be described by rotation on three axes. The X axis is anteroposterior; the Y axis is horizontal; the Z axis is vertical.

field of vision Entire area that can be seen by an eye.

fixation Act of directing vision at a given point.

fixing eye Nondeviating eye in strabismus.

flare Visible reflection of light from the aqueous or vitreous humors when they become turbid because of a pathologic amount of protein, present because of breakdown of the blood-aqueous barrier. It is recognized by biomicroscopic observation of the path of a sharply focused light beam.

fleck syndromes Group of fundus abnormalities that have the appearance of multiple light-colored spots. These conditions affect the pigment epithelium of the retina.

floaters Opacities within the vitreous space that cast moving shadows on the retina.

fluorescein Harmless indicator stain useful in recognizing corneal epithelial abrasions and in verifying the fit of contact lenses.

flush, limbal Circumcorneal hyperemia, of importance because it usually indicates the presence of a severe inflammation of the anterior portion of the eye.

focus To adjust a lens system to produce a sharp, clear picture.

fogging Technique of refraction in which distance vision is blurred by an excess of plus lens strength. The intent is to reduce the tendency of the eye to accommodate during the examination.

folliculosis Chronic conjunctivitis that causes multiple tiny lymphatic nodules to become visible, especially in the inferior cul-de-sac.

foot-candle Unit of illumination; 1 foot-candle is generated by 1 lumen on 1 square foot of surface.

fornix Conjunctival recess, cul-de-sac.

fovea centralis Central portion of the retina with the highest visual acuity; ophthalmoscopically visible as a bright light reflection seen in healthy eyes.

Fuchs's dystrophy Abiotrophy of the corneal endothelium resulting in corneal edema.

fundus Internal surface of the eye, including the optic disc, the retina, and the choroidal or scleral details visible through the retina.

fusion Cerebral synthesis of the two ocular pictures into a single mental picture.

gerontoxon Arcus senilis.

glare Irregularly scattered light that interferes with the focused retinal picture and reduces visual acuity.

glaucoma Abnormally increased intraocular pressure that causes irreversible death of the optic nerve fibers.

glioma Tumors of the optic nerve or retina.

gliosis Astrocytic scar proliferation on or within the retina.

gonioprism (gonioscope) Special type of contact lens that permits examination of the periphery of the anterior chamber; study of this portion of the eye is important in patients with glaucoma.

goniopuncture Antiglaucoma operation in which a tiny slit is made through the trabeculum and anterior sclera to permit aqueous to flow into sub-Tenon's space.

gonioscopy Study of the angle of the anterior chamber with the aid of a special contact lens (gonioscope).

goniosynechiae Tiny adhesions between the peripheral iris and the trabecular meshwork.

goniotomy Antiglaucoma operation in which the abnormal tissue present in the anterior chamber angle of an eye with congenital glaucoma is excised.

granulomatous uveitis Inflammation of the iris, ciliary body, or choroid characterized by a chronic, destructive course and supposedly due to active bacterial infection (for example, tuberculosis).

Gunn's dots Minute punctate reflections from the inner surface of the retina, occurring physiologically in healthy young eyes, perhaps due to dimpling of the surface by traction from Müller's fibers.

gyrate atrophy Atrophy of the choroid and retina affecting the midperipheral to posterior portions of the fundus; may be associated with hyperornithemia.

Haidinger's brushes Radiating entopic lines extending to either side of fixation, induced by viewing polarized light. Rotation of the plane of polarization causes a corresponding rotation of the brushes.

haploscope Stereoscope-like instrument used in orthoptic training and diagnosis.

Hasner's valve Mucosal folds within the nasolacrimal duct, resulting in unidirectional lacrimal flow.

Hassall-Henle bodies Nodular thickenings of Descemet's membrane.

hemeralopia Inability to see well in daylight illumination, with preservation of good night vision.

hemianopia (hemianopsia) Loss of vision in approximately one half of the visual field.

heterochromia Difference in color of the two irides or in parts of the same iris.

heteronymous Indicates involvement of the temporal visual field in both eye or of both nasal fields (distinguish from homonymous).

heterophoria Tendency of the eyes to deviate from straightness.

heterotropia Strabismus.

hippus Rapidly alternating increase and decrease in pupil size associated with neurologic disturbances or occurring to a lesser degree physiologically.

homatropine Parasympatholytic drug with shorter action than atropine; useful in refraction.

homonymous Indicates involvement of the same side of the two visual fields (for example, right homonymous hemianopia).

hordeolum (sty) Infection of a gland near the eyelid margin.

horopter Curved plane in space seen simultaneously by corresponding portions of the two retinas at a given position of the eyes; this concept is of value in theoretical considerations of binocular vision.

Hruby lens Strong concave lens that may be positioned in front of the cornea (not in contact with it) to neutralize the corneal refraction and thereby permit biomicroscopic observation of the fundus.

hue Color.

hyalitis Vitreous inflammation or degeneration.

hyaloid artery Artery present during the embryologic period, running from the optic disc to the posterior lens.

hyalosis Degenerative change of the vitreous body.

hydrophthalmos Congenital glaucoma resulting in enlargement of the eye.

hydrops of cornea Gross entry of aqueous humor into the cornea as a result of rupture of endothelium and Descemet's membrane, as may occur in keratoconus.

hypermetropia Refractive error in which a convex lens is required for correction of distance vision; farsightedness.

hyperopia Farsightedness; the refractive error in which light rays focus behind the retina.

hyperphoria Latent upward deviation of an eye.

hypertelorism Lateral displacement of the eyes due to an orbital anomaly.

hypertropia Vertical strabismus.

hyphema Blood in the anterior chamber.

hypopyon Purulent discharge in the anterior chamber.

hypotony Abnormal softness of the eye.

implant Rounded prosthesis buried in the orbit to replace partially the volume of an enucleated or eviscerated eye.

incomitance Characteristic of strabismus whereby the amount of ocular misalignment changes with different positions of gaze.

incomitant Referring to incomitance.

infraduction Rotation of one eye downward.

infraorbital Located below the orbit.

infraversion Rotation downward of both eyes.

interpalpebral Between the upper and lower eyelids.

interpupillary distance Distance between the two pupils centers.

intorsion Rotation of the eye on an anteroposterior axis so that the upper portion of the eye moves toward the nose.

intraocular Within the eye.

intraretinal Within the retina.

intrasclera Within the sclera.

intravitreal Within the vitreous cavity.

iodopsin Photopic (day vision) photopigment within the cones.

iridectomy Prophylactic antiglaucoma procedure in which a small portion of peripheral iris is excised.

iridencleisis Antiglaucoma operation in which a wick of iris is used to maintain a scleral opening through which aqueous drains to sub-Tenon's space.

iridocyclitis Inflammation of the iris and ciliary body.

iridodialysis Tearing of the iris from the ciliary body, either traumatic or as part of an antiglaucoma procedure.

iridodonesis Trembling of the iris with eye movement, indicating loss of lens support, as in aphakia or a dislocated lens.

iridoplegia Paralysis of the iris.

iridoschisis Frontal plane splitting of the mesodermal layers of the iris, usually as a spontaneous degenerative change.

iridotomy Cut into the iris without removal of tissue. Performed during cataract extraction as a prophylactic measure against possible pupillary blockage by the vitreous humor.

iris Colored portion of the eye surrounding the pupil.

iris bombé Forward displacement of the iris, resulting when the aqueous flow is obstructed at the pupil.

iritis Inflammation of the iris.

iseikonia Equality of image size of the two eyes.

Ishihara test Series of plates for the detection of deficiencies of color vision.

isopter Outer limit of the visual field as measured with a specific test object.

Jaeger's type Print of varying size used for measurement of near visual acuity.

jaw-winking Congenital anomalous connection between innervation to the levator and the pterygoid muscles of the jaw, resulting in elevation of the upper lid when the mandible is moved.

Jensen's choroiditis Severe juxtapapillary chorioretinitis resulting in a nerve fiber bundle visual field defect.

kappa angle Angle between the visual axis (the line of sight) and the axis imagined to exit the eye from the center of the pupil.

Kayser-Fleischer ring Copper deposit occurring in the peripheral Descemet's membrane in hepatolenticular degeneration (Wilson's disease or syndrome).

keratectomy Excision of a superficial portion of the cornea.

keratic precipitates (KP) Inflammatory deposits on the back surface of the cornea.

keratitis Corneal inflammation.

keratoconjunctivitis Inflammation of both the cornea and the conjunctiva.

keratoconus Cone-shaped distortion of the central cornea due to degeneration of the stromal lamellae.

keratomalacia Corneal breakdown due to vitamin A deficiency.

keratometer Instrument for measuring corneal curvature; useful in fitting contact lenses and in refraction.

keratomycosis Fungus infection of the cornea.

keratopathy Noninflammatory corneal disease.

keratoplasty Corneal transplantation.

Krukenberg's spindle Vertical pigment line on the posterior cornea resulting from breakdown of the iris pigment.

Kuhnt-Junius disciform macular degeneration Senile degenerative loss of macular function due to fibrovascular invasion through a break in the lamina vitrea (Bruch's membrane).

lacrimal Pertaining to the structures that produce or drain the tears.

lacrimation Excessive tearing.

lagophthalmos Failure of the eyelids to close completely.

lamina vitrea Inner layer of the choroid; synonymous with Bruch's membrane.

Landolt ring Visual acuity chart for illiterate patients, consisting of broken rings (resembling the letter C) with the break oriented in different directions.

Leber's optic atrophy Hereditary, bilateral optic atrophy usually affecting young males.

lens Focusing structure immediately behind the iris with which accommodation is accomplished.

lensometer Instrument that measures the strength of an eyeglass.

lenticonus Inherited abnormal curvature of the posterior or anterior lens surface.

leukocoria White pupil caused by opaque tissue within the eye.

leukoma Dense scar of the cornea.

levator palpebrae Muscle raising the upper lid.

levoversion Simultaneous rotation of both eyes to the left.

limbus Transition zone between the cornea and the sclera.

loupe Binocular magnifier; useful in ophthalmic surgery.

lumen Unit of light energy.

lysozyme Enzyme present in tears that can destroy some types of bacteria.

macropsia Visual fault that causes objects to appear magnified in size.

macula lutea Central portion of the retina; several disc diameters in area.

madarosis Loss of eyelashes.

Maddox rod Lens composed of a parallel series of very strong cylinders; when viewed through a Maddox rod, a point of light appears as a line; used to measure extraocular muscle balance (phoria).

magnification Increase in size achieved by a lens system.

Mariotte's blind spot Physiologic blind spot corresponding to the location of the optic disc projected into the visual field.

megalocornea Inherited abnormally large cornea; must be differentiated from the enlarged cornea due to congenital glaucoma.

meibomian glands Sebaceous glands within the tarsal plates, discharging just behind the gray line of the lid margin.

melanin Uveal pigment.

melanocytoma Heavily pigmented benign tumor of the optic disc.

melanoma Neoplasm arising from the uveal tract.

melanosis bulbi Congenital hyperpigmentation of an eye.

metamorphopsia Distortion of vision due to retinal edema or damage.

microcornea Abnormally small cornea on an otherwise normal-sized eyeball.

micronystagmus Very fine movements of the eyes normally present at all times.

microphthalmos Abnormal smallness of the entire eyeball.

micropsia Minification of vision due to retinal edema.

migraine Unilateral headache associated with premonitory visual disturbances; attributed to cerebral vasospasm.

minus lens Concave lens.

miosis Marked constriction of the pupil.

miotic Medication causing the pupil to become constricted.

Mittendorf dot Congenital remnant of the hyaloid artery just behind the lens.

monochromatism Total color blindness.

monocular Pertaining to one eye.

morgagnian cataract Hypermature, partially liquefied cataract, with a freely movable central nucleus.

mucocele Mucus-filled distention of a sinus or of the lacrimal sac.

muscae volitantes Small floaters due to minute opacities contained within the vitreous humor.

mydriasis Enlargement of pupil size.

mydriatic Medication causing the pupil to become dilated.

myectomy Surgical removal of part of a muscle; most often done to correct overaction of the inferior oblique muscle.

myokymia Twitching of the orbicularis oculi; usually due to fatigue.

myope Nearsighted individual.

myopia Nearsightedness; the refractive error in which parallel light rays focus in front of the retina.

myotomy Surgical transection of a muscle; most often done to correct overaction of the inferior oblique muscle.

nanophthalmos Congenital smallness of the eyeball without other abnormalities of the eye.

nasolacrimal duct Channel between the lacrimal sac and the nasal cavity.

nearsightedness Myopia.

nebula Very small corneal opacity.

needling Incision of the lens capsule with a tiny knife intended to remove a secondary membrane or to permit absorption of a cataract in a young person.

neuroepithelium Rods and cones.

nevus Localized hyperpigmentation of the choroid, iris, or conjunctiva.

nicking Compression of a vein by an arteriosclerotic arteriole at an arteriovenous crossing.

nictitation Blinking of the lids.

noncomitant Describes a strabismus varying in amount with the position of the eyes, thereby indicating the presence of a paralyzed muscle.

nuclear sclerosis Form of senile cataract affecting the central lens.

nyctalopia Night blindness with preservation of normal daylight vision.

nystagmus Rhythmic involuntary oscillation of the eye due to abnormal innervation or to lifelong reduced vision.

occluder Cover for the eye; used in therapy for suppression amblyopia, to eliminate diplopia, for examination purposes, or to conceal a deformity.

oculi uterque Both eyes, basis for the abbreviation OU.

oculist Medically trained eye specialist.

oculoglandular conjunctivitis (Parinaud's syndrome) Severe granulomatous conjunctivitis associated with enlarged preauricular nodes.

oculogyric Producing movements of the eyes, as may occur in parkinsonism.

oculomotor nerve Third cranial nerve.

oculus Synonym for eye.

OD Oculus dexter; right eye.

ophthalmia Ocular inflammation.

ophthalmic Referring to the eye.

ophthalmodynamometer Instrument for clinical measurement of the blood pressure of the ophthalmic artery.

ophthalmologist Medically trained eye specialist.

ophthalmology Medical and surgical specialty of eye care.

ophthalmoplegia Paralysis of ocular muscles.

ophthalmoscope Instrument for clinical examination of the posterior portion of the eye.
ophthalmoscopy Clinical examination of the interior of the eye.
opsin Protein constituent of the visual pigment rhodopsin.
optic nerve Second cranial nerve.
optician Technician who prepares and dispenses eyeglasses.
optometrist Nonmedically trained refractionist.
optometry Practice of nonmedical eye care, primarily refraction.
ora serrata Anterior boundary of the retina.
orbicularis oculi Muscle that closes the eyelids.
orbit Bony eye socket.
orbitonometry Measurement of the ease of displacement of the eye into the orbital tissues; of value in the study of exophthalmos.
orthophoria Freedom from a latent tendency to ocular deviation.
orthoptics Techniques used in diagnosis and treatment of strabismus or heterophoria.
OS Oculus sinister; left eye.
OU Oculus uterque; both eyes.

palpebral Referring to the eyelids.
pannus Vascular corneal scar.
panophthalmitis Generalized suppurative inflammation of the eye.
Panum's area Extent of receptor field in a retina capable of contributing to binocular vision in cooperation with a corresponding point in the opposite retina.
papilla, optic Optic disc.
papilledema Ophthalmoscopically visible swelling of the optic disc due to increased intracranial pressure.
papillitis (optic neuritis) Inflammatory swelling of the optic disc.
papilloma Benign ectodermal tumor that may arise from any surface part of the eye and its appendages (except the cornea).
papillomacular bundle Ganglion cell axons extending from the macula to the optic disc.
paracentesis Surgical drainage of the aqueous; very rarely indicated since the development of modern medical therapy.
parafoveal area Retinal area adjacent to the fovea; usually the site of eccentric fixation in suppression amblyopia.
parallax Apparent displacement of the background some distance behind an object when the observer changes his position of view. Parallactic displacement observed during ophthalmoscopy establishes the fact that the object under examination is elevated above the fundus background.
parallelepiped Corneal section illuminated by a slit lamp.
paresis Incomplete paralysis.
pars plana Smooth posterior part of the ciliary body.
pars plicata Part of the ciliary body having the ciliary processes.
PCB Punctum convergens basalis; near point of convergence plus the distance to the center of ocular rotation.
PD Interpupillary distance.
perimeter Instrument for clinical measurement of the visual field.
perimetry Examination and measurement of the visual field, of value in documenting and diagnosing lesions of the visual pathways.
periorbita Periosteum lining the inside of the orbit.

peripapillary Surrounding the optic disc.

peritomy Surgical separation of the conjunctiva from the limbus; performed as a preliminary step in various procedures.

phaco- Signifying the lens.

phacoanaphylaxis Intraocular reaction resulting from sensitivity to lens material.

phacoemulsification Technique of cataract extraction by ultrasonic fragmentation and subsequent aspiration.

phacolytic Referring to liquefaction of the lens cortex.

phacolytic glaucoma Increased intraocular pressure due to the toxic effect of liquefied lens cortex.

phakomatosis One of several inherited tumorous states, all of which frequently affect the eye and the skin; they include neurofibromatosis, encephalotrigeminal angiomatosis, tuberous sclerosis, and cerebellar-retinal angiomatosis.

phlyctenule Localized conjunctival or corneal inflammatory nodule, supposedly due to tuberculous hypersensitivity.

phoria Latent tendency to ocular deviation.

phorometer Instrument for clinical measurement of ocular muscle balance.

phoropter Instrument for clinical measurement of refractive error and ocular muscle balance.

phosphene Sensation of light caused by mechanical or electrical stimulation of the retina or optic nerve.

photochemical visual pigment Light-sensitive visual pigment.

photocoagulation Use of an intense, precisely focused light beam for sealing of retinal tears or for destruction of intraocular vascular anomalies or neoplasms.

photophobia Abnormal intolerance of light, usually due to inflammation of the iris and ciliary body.

photopic vision Vision at daylight illumination.

photopsia Flashing light sensations due to retinal disease.

photoreceptor Rod or cone cell.

phthiriasis palpebrarum Body louse infestation of the lids.

phthisis bulbi Mushy soft atrophic destruction of the eye due to very severe infection or injury.

physostigmine (eserine) Indirect-acting parasympathomimetic drug used in therapy for glaucoma.

pilocarpine Direct-acting parasympathomimetic drug used in therapy for glaucoma.

pinguecula Inherited benign nodule situated in the interpalpebral space several millimeters nasal or temporal to the cornea; long-continued irritation may cause transformation into a pterygium.

pinkeye Acute bacterial conjunctivitis.

Placido's disc Illuminated disc marked with concentric rings that reveals abnormalities of corneal curvature when its reflection is observed on the corneal surface.

plano- Lens having no refractive strength.

pleoptics Orthoptic method of treating eccentric fixation.

plica semilunaris Remnant of the third eyelid situated in the inner canthus.

plus lens Convex lens.

poliosis Loss of pigment in the eyelashes or other hairs, as may occur in the Vogt-Koyanagi syndrome of poliosis, uveitis, and dysacousia (all these manifestations involve pigmented cells).

polycoria Congenital anomaly in which an eye has more than one pupil.

Pontocaine Topical anesthetic used for minor ocular surgery and tonometry; trade name for tetracaine.

preretinal Located in the space between the retina and the vitreous humor.

presbyopia Loss of accommodation due to age.

prism Wedge-shaped lens that displaces the position of objects viewed through it.

proptosis Forward protrusion of the eye.

protanomaly Mild form of red-green color blindness, with reduced sensitivity for red.

protanopia Type of red-green color blindness, with greatest loss of sensitivity for red.

pseudoglaucoma Optic atrophy and cupping resembling glaucoma but due to vascular damage rather than increased intraocular pressure.

pseudoglioma Condition simulating a retinoblastoma, in which the interior of the eye is filled with inflammatory or fibrovascular material.

pseudoisochromatic Pertaining to a testing method for color blindness in which numbers or figures are formed with hues chosen so that they appear alike (isochromatic) to the color-blind individual, yet may be differentiated by the normal eye. As a result, the color-blind person cannot distinguish any numbers, although they are obvious to the normal person.

pseudoneuritis Physiologic variation in appearance of the optic disc that may be confused with the appearance of papillitis.

pseudopterygium Superficial, vascularized corneal scar.

pseudotumor of orbit Increase in orbital volume due to a low-grade inflammatory reaction.

pterygium Elastic degenerative change that slowly proliferates from the conjunctiva on the cornea; originates from a pinguecula in response to irritation.

ptosis Drooping of the upper eyelid due to deficient innervation or muscular strength.

punctum, lacrimal Tiny tear drainage opening in the medial aspect of the margin of each eyelid.

pupil Central opening of the eye encircled by the iris.

pupillometer Device for measuring pupil diameter.

Purtscher's retinopathy Edema and hemorrhage of the retina secondary to severe crushing injury.

quadrantanopia (quadrantopsia) Loss of approximately one fourth of the visual field.

range of accommodation Linear distance between the far point and the near point of clear vision.

recession Operation for strabismus in which the effect of a muscle is decreased by moving its insertion backward.

rectus muscle One of the four extraocular muscles originating from the apex of the orbit and inserting on the sclera less than a centimeter from the limbus. Designated as superior, inferior, medial, or lateral, depending on the location on the eye.

reflex Reflection of light from a curved smooth surface, such as the cornea, fovea centralis, or retinal arterioles.

refraction Clinical measurement of the error of focus in an eye.

refractor Device containing lenses and prisms, used in determining the dioptric status of the eye.

relucence Property of partially reflecting light, as occurs in any imperfectly transparent structure, such as the cornea or lens. Relucency of these structures is the basis for their visibility when illuminated by a sharply focused beam of light, as with the biomicroscope.

resection Operation for strabismus in which the effect of a muscle is increased by shortening its tendon.

retina Innermost, light-sensitive layer of the eye.

retinene Intermediate pigment in the photochemical visual cycle. It is a combination of the *cis*-isomer of vitamin A with a protein, opsin.

retinitis pigmentosa Retinal abiotrophy characterized by migration of pigment to form linear sheathing of retinal vessels.

retinoblastoma Malignant tumor of childhood originating from the retina.

retinochoroiditis Inflammation of both the retina and the choroid, with the primary disease within the retina.

retinopathy Noninflammatory disease of the retina.

retinopexy Operation for correction of a detached retina.

retinoschisis Retinal abiotrophy characterized by splitting of the retina into anterior and posterior layers.

retinoscope Instrument for the objective determination of refractive error.

retinoscopy Objective measurement of the refractive status of an eye by observation with a retinoscope of the direction of movement of light reflected from the ocular fundus.

retrobulbar Behind the eye; the site of injection anesthesia for ocular surgery.

retroillumination Valuable technique of examination of translucent tissues by light reflected from behind; useful in biomicroscopy and ophthalmoscopy.

retrolental Located immediately behind the crystalline lens.

retrolental fibroplasia Destructive vascular and fibrous overgrowth of the retina occurring in premature infants placed in high concentrations of oxygen.

rhodopsin Light-sensitive pigment contained in the rods.

Riolan's muscle Portion of the orbicularis oculi muscle nearest the eyelid margin.

rivalry, retinal Normal spontaneous alteration of perception of the visual field between the two eyes. It is as if the occipital cortex scans portions of the visual field by alternating use of the messages from the two eyes. This is clinically recognizable by presenting to the eyes dissimilar images that cannot be fused and forcing recognition of their alternation.

rod Visual cell used when the eye is dark adapted.

rubeosis iridis Neovascularization of the iris resulting from diabetes, occlusion of the central retinal vein, or some chronic inflammatory conditions.

sac, lacrimal Dilated portion of the lacrimal drainage apparatus situated between the canaliculi and the nasolacrimal duct.

Sattler's veil Corneal haze resulting from the anoxia induced by prolonged wearing of a contact lens.

scatter Irregular diffusion of light through translucent structures such as the sclera, or through corneal scar tissue. Of importance in ocular biomicroscopy, because it discloses imperfections in optical structure.

Schiøtz tonometer Device to measure intraocular pressure by the degree of indentation of the cornea resulting from application of a standard weight.

Schlemm's canal Aqueous outflow channel located just external to the trabecular meshwork of the anterior chamber angle of the eye.

Schnabel's cavernous atrophy Vascular atrophy of the anterior portion of the optic nerve, resulting in a deep, atrophic cupping of the optic disc, resembling the cupping of glaucomatous atrophy.

Schwalbe's line Peripheral border of Descemet's membrane.

sclera Tough, white outer layer of the eye.

scleral spur (spur of sclera) In gonioscopic view, the white scleral edge immediately behind the trabecular meshwork.

sclerectomy Antiglaucoma operation permitting aqueous to escape through a notch cut from the sclera.

scleritis Inflammation of the sclera.

sclerokeratitis Inflammation of both the sclera and the cornea.

scleromalacia perforans Extreme thinning of the sclera usually associated with rheumatic uveitis.

scotoma Area of loss of vision within the visual field.

scotopic vision Night vision; mediated by the rods.

seclusio pupillae Total blocking of the pupillary opening by a 360-degree posterior synechia (complete adherence of the pupil margin to the lens).

Seidel's scotoma Small nerve fiber bundle field defect adjacent to the physiologic blind spot, usually caused by glaucoma.

siderosis bulbi Iron deposits resulting from a retained intraocular foreign body; iron is toxic and causes extensive degenerative changes within the eye.

situs inversus Mirror reversal of the appearance of the optic disc in which the large vessels run predominantly nasalward from the disc; associated with myopia and uncorrectable visual loss; usually affects only one eye.

skew deviation Vertical nonparalytic deviation of the eyes due to cerebellar disease.

skiascope Synonym for retinoscope.

slit-lamp microscope (biomicroscope) Instrument for examining the eye under high magnification and in optical section obtained by a finely focused slit of light.

socket Conjunctival sac remaining after enucleation into which an artificial eye fits.

Soemmering's ring Peripheral ring of lens capsule and cortex remaining after injury to the lens.

spasmus nutans Syndrome including nystagmus and head nodding occurring transiently in infants.

spectrum Various wavelengths of light in orderly sequence.

spherocylinder Spectacle lens correcting both a spherical error (hyperopia or myopia) and astigmatism.

spherophakia Small round lens found in patients with certain mesodermal anomalies (Marchesani's syndrome).

sphincter iridis Constrictor muscle of the iris.

squint Synonym for strabismus.

staphyloma Bulging defect of cornea or sclera that is lined with uveal tissue.

stenopeic slit Narrow aperture that excludes stray light and thereby enhances the focus of the retinal image.

stereocampimeter Instrument for measurement of the central visual field of each eye separately, although both eyes are used for fixation.

stereopsis Binocular depth perception.

stereoscope Instrument that permits different pictures to be positioned before each of the two eyes.

strabismus Failure of straightness of the eyes; one eye (the fixing eye) looks directly at the object of attention, whereas the other eye (the deviating eye) does not.

stroma of cornea Central framework of the cornea, situated between Bowman's and Descemet's membranes.

stroma of iris Mesodermal portion of the iris and also its ectodermal muscles (sphincter and dilator). This includes all of the iris except its posterior pigment epithelium.

sty (hordeolum) Infection of a gland of the eyelid margin.

subcapsular Located just internal to the capsule of the crystalline lens.

subconjunctival Located just beneath the bulbar conjunctiva.

subluxation of lens Partial displacement of the lens from its normal position.

subretinal Located between the retinal rods and cones and the retinal pigment epithelium. Note that this customary terminology is a misnomer—the location is within the retina, in the original cavity of the embryonic optic vesicle, not underneath the retina.

suppression Cortical inhibition of the vision of one eye under conditions of binocular vision.

suppression amblyopia Relatively irreversible cortical inhibition of the central vision of one eye, persisting when the amblyopic eye is used by itself.

suprachoroid Outer layer of the choroid.

supraduction Upward rotation of one eye.

supraversion Simultaneous rotation of the eyes upward.

suture Junction of the ends of the lens fibers, which results in the formation of Y and stellate figures within the lens.

symblepharon Adhesion of the lid to the eyeball.

sympathetic ophthalmia Sensitization to the uveal pigment of an injured eye that results in severe uveitis in the uninjured fellow eye.

synchysis scintillans Degenerative vitreous condition in which cholesterol crystals float freely within the liquefied vitreous cavity.

synechia Adhesion of the iris to the lens (posterior) or cornea (anterior).

syneresis of vitreous Liquefaction of vitreous humor.

synergists (yoke muscles) Two muscles, one in each eye, that move the eyes in the same direction (for example, right lateral and left medial recti).

synoptophore Stereoscope-like instrument used in orthoptic diagnosis and treatment.

tachistoscope Instrument that projects a slide for only a fraction of a second; helpful in measuring speed of perception and possibly in some types of visual training.

tangent screen Instrument for clinical measurement of the central visual field.

tarsorrhaphy Partial fusion of the lids for the purpose of protecting the cornea from exposure.

tarsus Fibrous plate that forms the lid contour and provides its strength.

tears Lacrimal secretion.

Tenon's capsule Connective tissue sheath encircling the eyeball posteriorly.

Tenon's space Location behind the eye, within the cone contained within the rectus muscles and their intermuscular membranes.

tenotomy Severing of all or part of a tendon; performed to decrease the function of a muscle in the surgical correction of strabismus.

tetartanopia Type of blue-yellow color blindness.

timolol A beta sympathetic blocker that reduces aqueous formation; therapy reduces intraocular pressure. This is now the most popular medical therapy for glaucoma.

tonography Measurement of the rate of aqueous outflow; clinically feasible and a valuable method of evaluation of glaucoma.

tonometer Instrument for measuring intraocular pressure; vitally important for the early detection of glaucoma.

trabeculum Meshwork in the anterior chamber angle through which the aqueous flows to leave the eye.

trachoma Blinding chlamydial infection of the cornea and conjunctiva; widely prevalent throughout the world and probably the most common cause of blindness.

transillumination Method of determining with transmitted light whether a lesion is solid or cystic.

translucency Incomplete transparency, so that light is scattered as it passes through.

transposition Conversion of a spherocylindrical notation from one form to another (may be written as either a positive or a negative cylinder, which is added to a smaller spherical power or subtracted from a larger spherical power).

trephination Antiglaucoma operation in which a small circular scleral opening is made to permit aqueous to escape to sub-Tenon's space.

trichiasis Aberrant lashes that turn against the cornea.

trigeminal nerve Fifth cranial nerve.

triplopia Abnormal perception of three images corresponding to only one object.

tritanopia Type of blue-yellow color blindness.

trochlea Fibrous pulley of the superior oblique tendon.

trochlear nerve Fourth cranial nerve, which innervates the superior oblique muscle.

tropia Manifest misalignment of the eyes, present without interruption of fusion, as by covering one eye; strabismus.

tucking Folding of an extraocular muscle tendon in order to shorten it and increase its action to correct strabismus.

tunica vasculosa lentis Vascular network surrounding the fetal lens.

uvea Vascular and pigmented layer of the eye, including the choroid, ciliary body, and iris.

uveitis Inflammation of all or any part of the uveal tract.

vergence Movement together (convergence) or apart (divergence) of the two eyes.

version Similar movement of the two eyes in the same direction (for example, dextroversion).

vertex distance Distance of a spectacle lens from the cornea. This is of significance in the fitting of a strong lens, as in correction of aphakia, because the effective strength of a plus lens increases with distance, whereas the effective strength of a minus lens diminishes.

visuscope Modified ophthalmoscope used to identify the fixation characteristics of an amblyopic eye.

vitreous Gel that fills the eye behind the lens.

xanthelasma Form of xanthoma characterized by yellowish lipoid plaques in the eyelids of patients with excessive cholesterol.

xerophthalmia Dryness of the eyes.

xerosis Corneal drying in vitamin A deficiency.

zonule System of fibers that suspend the lens.

zonulysis Dissolving of the zonule by a solution of alpha-chymortrypsin in order to facilitate cataract extraction.

Index

A

Accommodation, 353
  reaction, 50
Accommodative esotropia, 306, 400
Acetazolamide, 411
Acetylcholine, 393, 397
Acne rosacea, 344
Acupuncture, 414
Acute bacterial conjunctivitis, 258, 259
Acute glaucoma, 258, 266, 283
Acute iritis, 258
Affect, 32
Agranulocytosis, 386
Albinism, 209
Albinotic fundus, Plate 2
Allergy, lid, 344
Alternate cover test, 54
Amblyopia, 309, 310
Amphotericin B, 384
Ampicillin, 388
Amsler grid, 59
Anatomy, 7
Anesthesia, corneal, 246
Anesthetics, 378
Angioid streaks, 178, 182
Angioma, 288
  retinal, 177
Anisocoria, 50
Anisometropia, 356
Anterior chamber depth, 279
Antibiotic, 381
Anticholinesterase antidote, 401
Antiviral drugs, 391
Aphakia, 322
Applanation tonometer, Goldmann, 293
Aqueous flow, 282
Argyll Robertson pupil, 50
Argyrol, 382
Arteriolar attenuation, Plate 23
Arteriolar constriction, 104
Arteriolar light reflex, 78, 106

Arteriolar occlusion, 130, 132, 170
  findings, 151
Arteriolar sclerosis, 108, 199, 201
  findings, 150
Artificial respiration, 380
Ascarid, 331
Astigmatism, 356
Atropine, 393, 401
  with glaucoma, 281
Autonomic drugs, 392

B

Bacitracin, 385
Bacterial conjunctivitis, acute, 258, 259
Bacterial endocarditis, subacute, 209
Basal cell, 346
Bayes theorum, 70
Beading, 77
Benoxinate, 378
Berlin's edema, 168
Biomicroscopy, 59
Birth injury, 241
Bjerrum's scotoma, 218, 225
Black diagnostic sequence, 165
Blepharitis, 336
Blepharochalasis, 345
Blind adult
  examination, 68
  guidance, 67
Blind spot, enlarged, 218
Blond periphery, Plate 8
Blood dyscrasia, 203
Blood-eye barrier, 11, 382
Bloom's taxonomy, 22
Body language, 32, 416
Bone corpuscle, 147; Plate 16
Bowman's membrane, 11
Bupivacaine, 379
Burn(s)
  chemical, therapy, 374
  corneal, 242

Burn(s)—cont'd
  thermal, 244
  ultraviolet, 244

C
Carbachol, 393, 397
Carbonic anhydrase, 411
Cardiac massage, 380
Cardinal gaze, 53
Cardinal position, 296
Carotid artery ulcerations, 209
Carotid cavernous fistula, 75, 207
Caruncle, 43
Cataract
  congenital, 323
  coronary, 325
  developmental, 324
  endocrine, 325
  senile, 320
  traumatic, 325
  zonular, 324
Cellulitis, 240, 339
Central nervous system, 209
Central serous choroidopathy, 176
Cerebromacular degenerations, 208
Chalazion, 338, 422
Chalazion clamp, 422
Chemical burn, therapy, 374
Cherry red spot, 76
Chief complaint, 17
Child, examination, 66
Chloramphenicol, 385
Cholinesterase, 392
Choriocapillaris atrophy, 183
Chorioretinitis, 82, 131, 136, 164, 185
  findings, 151
  histoplasmosis, Plate 12
  juxtapapillary, Plate 3
  macular, Plate 13
  old, 165; Plate 15
  toxoplasmosis, Plate 27
Choroid, 15
Choroidal nevus, 83, 165; Plate 17
Choroideremia, 184
Choroidopathy, central serous, 176
Chronic vitamin A intoxication, 208
Ciliary artery, 96
Ciliary body, 12
Ciliary retinal artery, 78, 218; Plate 2
Circulation of fundus, 98, 99
Circumpapillary atrophy, 73
Coats' disease, 178
Cocaine, 393
Colistin, 386

Collagen diseases, 208
Coloboma of disc, 73; Plate 5
Color of hemorrhage, 122
Color line, 164
Color testing, 57
Communication by touch, 46
Complaint, chief, 17
Concentric constriction, 227
Cones, 7
Confrontation fields, 57
Confrontation perimetry, 216
Congenital tortuosity, 77
Conjunctiva, 41
  bulbar, 11
Conjunctival cysts, 247
Conjunctivitis
  allergic, 262, 376
  bacterial, acute, 258, 259
    therapy, 371
  vernal, 262
Consensual reaction, 48
Constriction
  arteriolar, 104
  concentric, 227
Contact lenses, 274, 360
  aphakic, 322
Contusion, 179
  findings, 152
Convergence, 306
Corectopia, 302
Cornea, 7
  examination, 46
Corneal anesthesia, 246
Corneal burns, 242
Corneal epithelium, 11
Corneal foreign body, 245
Corneal light reflex, 55
  strabismus measurement, 302
Corneal pump, 11
Corneal sensitivity, 48
Corneal ulcer, 264
  or trauma, 258
Corticosteroids, 404
  contraindications, 247
Counting fingers, 36
Cover test, 54, 300
Credé prophylaxis, 271
Crepitus, 241
Crescent, myopic, 355
Cup/disc ratio, 64, 280; Plate 29
Cyclogyl, 403
Cyclopentolate, 393, 403
Cycloplegia, 359, 401

Cysticercus, 208
Cysts
  conjunctival, 247
  macular, 171

D

Dacryocystitis, 338
Dandruff, 337
Degenerative fundus lesions, 164, 165
Degenerative myopia, 355; Plate 28
Demyelinating diseases, 209, 213
Dendritic ulcer, 261, 342
Depth of hemorrhage, 121
Detachment
  pigment epithelial, 181
  retinal; *see* Retinal detachment
  rhegmatogenous, 328
Diabetes, 194, 287
  findings, 149
Diabetic retinopathy, 327; Plates 10, 21
Diagnosis
  etiologic, 29
  differential, 21
Diagnostic sequence(s), 160
  black, 165
  red, 161
  white, 163
Diagnostic significance of fundus findings, 149
Diamox, 411
Diazepam, 401
Differential diagnosis, 21
Dilatation, contraindications, 396
Dioptric focusing, 157, 327
Diplopia, 300
  monocular, 29, 320
  physiologic, 302
Direct illumination, 153
Disc
  coloboma, 73; Plate 5
  details, 73
  enlarged, 94
  pallor, 100
  physiologic blurring, 74
  schematic, 92
Disc diameter, 101
Disciform degeneration, 178
Disciform keratitis, 342
Disciform macular degeneration, Plate 20
Double-blind observation, 418
Drusen, 82, 142, 164, 181
  of macula, Plate 11
Drugs
  antiviral, 391
  autonomic, 392
Dry eye, therapy, 377

E

E charts for measurement of visual acuity, 37, 310
Echothiophate, 393, 400
  for convergence, 306
Eclipse, 219
Ectropion, 39, 349
Edema
  Berlin's, 168
  of fundus, 80
  retinal, 168
Elevation measurement, 157, 158
Emboli, 76, 109
Emmetropia, 354
Endocarditis, subacute bacterial, 209
Endothelium, 11
Enlarged blind spot, 218
Enophthalmos, 56
Entropion, 41, 269, 350
Epicanthus, 316
Epinephrine, 393
Epiphora, 12, 260
Episcleritis, 258, 263, 406
Epithelium, corneal, 11
Erythromycin, 386
Eserine, 393, 398
Esotropia, 294
  accommodative, 306, 400
Etiologic diagnosis, 29
Examination, 35
  of blind adult, 68
  of child, 66
  of eyelid, 39
  of optic disc, 63
Exophthalmometer, 56
Exophthalmos, 56, 203
  thyrotrophic, 295
Exposure keratopathy, 268, 376
Exudates, 200
  hard, 81, 117, 140, 141, 164, 196; Plates 7, 10, 23
  soft, 81, 139, 164, 196; Plate 23
  subretinal, 177
Eye drop instillation, 373
Eye pad, 384
Eye symptoms, 25
Eye wash, 377
Eyelid, examination, 39

F

Family history, 20
Finger tension measurement, 51
Fistula, carotid cavernous, 75, 207
Fixation, eccentric, 79
Fixation behavior, 310
Flashlight illumination, 72

Flashlight inspection, 367
Flashlight test, swinging, 49
Floaters, 326
Fluorescein, 408
    staining, 44
    use, 232
Focusing, dioptric, 157, 327
Foreign body
    corneal, 245
    intraocular, Plate 25
    removal, 246
    therapy, 371
Fovea, 112
Fovea centralis, 65
Fuchs' spot, Plate 28
Fundus
    background, 66
    circulation, 162
    diagrammatic anatomy, 88
    edema, 80
    examination routine, 63
    exudates; *see* Exudates
    findings, diagnostic significance, 149
    folds, 186
    myopic, Plate 4
    potential spaces within, 119
Fundus flavimaculata, 179
Fusion, 307

G

Gaze, cardinal, 53
Gentamicin, 386
German measles, 209
Giant cell arteritis, 214
Glare, 319
Glaucoma
    acute (closed angle), 258, 266, 283
    atropine with, 393, 401
    congenital, 285
    hereditary, 277
    open-angle, 276
    secondary, 286
    therapy, 281
Glaucomatous cup(ping), 97; Plates 5, 26
Glial veil, 74
Glycerol, 409
Goldmann applanation tonometer, 293
Gonococcal conjunctivitis, 260
Gravity and retinal detachment, 328
Gyrate atrophy, 184

H

Hard exudates, 81, 117, 140, 141, 164, 196; Plates 7,
    10, 23

Hemangioma, 346
Hematologic dyscrasia, findings, 150
Hemorrhage, 128
    choroidal, 162
    color, 122
    deep intraretinal, 162
    depth, 121
    diagram, 118
    flat top, Plate 9
    fundus, 81
    intraretinal, 125
    nerve fiber layer, 162
    preretinal, 126, 162; Plate 9
    size, 120
    subconjunctival, 235
    subretinal, 162
    venous, 110
    vitreous, 127, 239
Hemianopia, 224
Henle's fibers, 172
Hereditary afflictions, 208
Hereditary glaucoma, 277
Herpes conjunctivitis, 261
Herpes simplex, 342
Herpes zoster, 332, 343
Histoplasmosis, 330; Plates 3, 12
History, 16
    as therapy, 30
Homatropine, 393, 403
Hordeolum, 39, 338
Hyaloid artery, 74
Hydroxyamphetamine, 393
Hyperopia, 356
Hypertelorism, 318
Hypertension, 198
    findings, 150
Hypertensive retinopathy, Plate 23
Hypertropia, 309
Hypopyon, 264
Hysteria, 217, 365

I

Idoxuridine, 391
Illumination
    direct, 153
    flashlight, 72
    oblique, 47, 231, 279
    proximal, 154, 156
Implant, lens, 322
Injury, 229
    birth, 241
    penetrating; *see* Penetrating injury
Interstitial keratitis, 271
Intraocular foreign body, Plate 25

Intraocular pressure measurement, 50
Iridectomy, peripheral, 284
Iridocyclitis, 286, 334
Iris, 12
Iritis, acute, 258, 267
    therapy, 377
Ischemic optic neuritis, 213
Isoflurophate, 393, 399

K

Keratitis
    disciform, 342
    interstitial, 271
Keratoconus, 357
Keratomalacia, 273
Keratopathy, exposure, 268, 376

L

Lacrimal apparatus, 12
    examination, 41
Lacrimal cannula, 341
Lacrimal drainage fault, 260
Lacrimal fossa, 42
Lacrimal irrigation, 423
Lacrimal passages, 424
Lacrimal probing, 424
Lacrimal pump, 12
Lamina cribrosa, 7
Laser
    for diabetes, 198
    for glaucoma, 282
Lateral geniculate body, 89
Lead poisoning, 208
Lens, dislocation, 288
Lens implant, 322
Lid(s)
    allergy, 344
    eversion, 43
    laceration, 233
    separation, 41
Lid lag, 205
Lid retraction, 205
Lidocaine, 379
Light
    perception, 37
    projection, 36
Light reflex
    arteriolar, 78, 106
    corneal; see Corneal light reflex
    pupillary, 48
Limbal flush, 12
Limbus, 7
Lipemia retinalis, 78, 197

M

Macula, 65, 79, 112, 167
    detached, 328
Macular cysts, 171
Macular degeneration
    disciform, Plate 20
    senile; see Senile macular degeneration
Malingering, 217, 365
Mannitol, 409
Marcaine, 379
Marcus Gunn pupil, 50
Marfan's syndrome, 288
Marginal blepharitis, therapy, 375
Media, 66, 72, 87, 364
Medical allergy, 19
Medical ophthalmology, 194
Meibomian gland, 40
Melanoma, 84, 146, 165, 184, 250, 347; Plate 18
Metastatic neoplasms, 208
Methacillin, 388
Microaneurysms, 77, 110, 128, 129, 173, 195; Plate
        10
Migraine, 364
Miosis, 50, 398
Mucocele, 207
Multiple sclerosis, 57
Muscle star, 53
Mydriacyl, 404
Mydriasis, 50
Mydriatics, 394
Myelin sheath, 143
Myelinated nerve fibers, 83, 164; Plate 14
Myopia, 354
    adult, 320
    degenerative, 355; Plate 28
Myopic crescent, 73
Myopic fundus, Plate 4

N

Neomycin, 386
Neoplasm, 287
Neovascularization, 76, 110, 111, 195
Neuroophthalmology, 210
Nevus, 146
    choroidal, 83, 165; Plate 17
Nicking, 76, 108
Nonparalytic strabismus, 302
Novobiocin, 387
Nystagmus, 54
Nystatin, 387

O

Oblique illumination, 47, 231, 279
Occluded arteriole, 164

Occlusion, 310, 315
 arteriolar; *see* Arteriolar occlusion
Oculoglandular syndrome, 270
Ointment vehicle, 383
Old chorioretinitis, 165; Plate 15
Ophthaine, 379
Ophthalmoscope, details of use, 188
Ophthalmoscopy, 59
 teaching, 188
Optic atrophy, 73, 97, 98, 100, 215
Optic disc, examination, 63
Optic neuritis, 98, 212
 ischemic, 213
Optical strength, 11
Orbit
 contusion, 232
 neoplasm, 186
Orthoptics, 313
Osmotherapy, 285, 409
Oxacillin, 388

P

Paget's disease, 178
Panophthalmitis, 265
Papilledema, 73, 98, 99, 210; Plate 24
 findings, 150
Papilloma, 346
Parallax, 159
Paralytic strabismus, 295
Past history, 19
Penetrating injury, 230, 237
 therapy, 375
Penicillin, 387
 allergy, 372
Perimetry, 216, 366
Peripheral iridectomy, 284
Phakomatoses, 208, 348
Pharmacogenetics, 419
Phenylephrine, 393, 394
Phlyctenule, 406
Phoria, 307
Phospholine, 400
Physiologic depression, 74, 95
Physiologic disc variance, 215
Physiology, 7
Physostigmine, 398
Pigment
 abnormalities, 83
 crescent, Plate 2
 detachment, 181
 location, 91
 rupture, 179
Pilocarpine, 393, 397
Pimaricin, 389

Pinguecula, 251
Pityrosporon, 336
Placebo, 414
Plica semilunaris, 43
Poison ivy, 344
Polycythemia, 75
Polymyxin B, 389
Pontocaine, 379
Potential spaces within fundus, 119
Pralidoxime, 399, 401
Presbyopia, 357
Present illness, 18
Prevalence, 70
Prism diopter, 305
Prism measurement, 305
Probing, lacrimal, 424
Proparacaine, 378
Proximal illumination, 154, 156
Pseudostrabismus, 316
Pseudoxanthoma elasticum, 178; Plate 20
Ptosis, 349
Ptyergium, 251
Pulsation
 venous, Plate 24
 of vessels, 79
Pupil
 Argyll Robertson, 50
 dilatation, 394
 examination, 48
 Marcus Gunn, 50
Pupillary light reflex, 48
Pyrimethamine, 389

Q

Quinine poisoning, 208

R

Reassurance therapy, 31, 413
Red diagnostic sequence, 161
Red eye, 255
Red glass, 300
Red reflex, 62, 72, 87, 238; Plate 1
 for study of cataract, 321
Red spot, cherry, 76
Reflections, 114, 144, 168
Refractive error, 351
Regurgitation, 41
Reliability, 419
Resuscitation, 380
Retinal angioma, 177
Retinal artery
 ciliary, 78, 218; Plate 2
 occlusion, 76
Retinal detachment, 175, 326; Plates 18, 30
 findings, 151

Retinal edema, 168
Retinal nerve fiber layer, 123, 124
Retinal vein thrombosis, 110
Retinal vessel(s), 65
    congenital tortuosity, Plate 6
    detail, 74
    location, 90
Retinitis pigmentosa, 75, 147, 165; Plate 16
Retinitis proliferans, 137, 164; Plate 22
Retinoblastoma, 295
Retinopathy, surface-wrinkling, 167
Retinoscopy, 357
Retrobulbar neuritis, 57
Rhegmatogenous detachment, 328
Rheumatic uveitis, 332
Rods, 7
Rotations, 297
Rubeosis iridis, 287
Rust ring, 236

S

Sarcoid, 208, 331
Schiøtz scale, 291
Schiøtz tonometer, 289
Sclera, 7, 164
Scleral crescent, Plate 2
Scleral spur, 12
Scleritis, 258
Sclerosis
    arteriolar; *see* Arteriolar sclerosis
    tuberous, 348
Scopolamine, 403
Scotoma
    Bjerrum's, 218, 225
    Seidel's, 225
Sebaceous cyst, 345
Seidel's scotoma, 225
Senile macular degeneration, 174, 178; Plates 11, 19
    findings, 152
Sensitivity, 70
Sheathing, 79
Shield, 252
Sickle cell disease, 208
Significance
    of history, 21
    statistical, 419
Size of hemorrhage, 120
Soccratic teaching, 85
Soft exudates, 139, 164; Plate 23
Specificity, 70
Square inch, 1
Star, 116
    pattern, 172
Stargardt's degeneration, 179

Statistics, 3
Stereopsis, 313
Stereoscope, 312
Strabismus
    measurement, 302, 304
    nonparalytic, 302
    paralytic, 295
Streptomycin, 390
Study objectives, 4
Sturge-Weber syndrome, 288
Sty, 39, 338
Subacute bacterial endocarditis, 209
Subconjunctival hemorrhage, 235
Subretinal exudates, 177
Subretinal hemorrhage, 162
Subretinal proliferation, 138
Sulfonamide, 390
Superior oblique, 298
Suppression, 309
Surface-wrinkling retinopathy, 167
Surgery, 421
    for strabismus, 314
Swinging flashlight test, 49
Sympathetic uveitis, 332
Symptoms, 25, 363
Syphilis, 147, 208, 331

T

Taxonomy of intellectual processes, 22
Tay-Sach's disease, 170
Tear film, 12
Temporal crescent, schematic, 92, 93
Tetracaine, 378
Tetracycline, 390
Thermal burns, 244
Therapeutic evaluation, 418
Therapy, history, 30
Thyrotrophic exophthalmos, 295
Timolol, 393, 397
Tonometer
    Goldmann applanation, 293
    Schiøtz, 289
Tonometry, 289
    contraindications, 292
Tortuosity, congenital, 77
Toxoplasmosis, 208, 213, 330; Plate 27
Triage, 16
Triflurothymidine, 391
Tropia, 307
Tropicamide, 393, 404
    dilatation, 188
Tuberculosis, 208, 331
Tuberous sclerosis, 348

U

Ultraviolet burns, 244
Uveal tract, 12
Uveitis, 330

V

Vaccinia, 344
Vancomycin, 391
Venous occlusion, 214, 287; Plate 7
    findings, 151
Vernal conjunctivitis, 262
Vessel
    caliber, 104, 105
    diameter, 103
    evaluation, 102
Viral conjunctivitis, 261
Vision, reduced, 361
Visual acuity, 35, 351
    estimation, 310
Visual field loss, 327

Visual pathways, 224
Visuoscope, 80
Vitamin A intoxication, chronic, 208
Vitelliform degeneration, 179
Vitreous hemorrhage, 127, 239
Vitreous traction, 327
Von Hippel-Lindau disease, 75, 177
Von Recklinghausen's neurofibromatosis, 206, 348

W

Warm compresses, 372
Water, toxicity, 410
White diagnostic sequence, 163

X

Xanthelasma, 346
Xylocaine, 379

Y

Yoke muscles, 299